AF838119

Creating Beauty
Cosmetic Surgery & The Beauty Industry

Creating Beauty - Cosmetic Surgery & The Beauty Industry

Published by:
The Foundation for Cosmetic Surgery
400 Newport Center Drive, Suite 800
Newport Beach, California 92660
ffps2007@yahoo.com

Printed in the United States of America

ISBN: 978-0-9799438-05

The Foundation for Cosmetic Surgery is a non-profit organization # 23-7076052

Table of Contents

Acknowledgments

The Foundation for Cosmetic Surgery is a non-profit organization whose primary goal is education. This book is designed to educate.

The philosophy of the Foundation is non-political, promoting a multi-disciplinary approach to the field of cosmetic surgery.

The Foundation of Cosmetic Surgery is indebted to all the doctors who have served on the Board of Advisors;

William Beeson, MD
Robert Cattani, MD
Donn Chatham, MD
Edwin Cortez, MD
Sheldon Kabaker, MD
R. James Koch, MD
Corey Maas, MD
Harry Mittelman, MD
Louie Patseavouras, MD
Steven Pearlman, MD
Daniel Rousso, MD
Norman Shorr, MD
Edward Terino, MD
S. Randolph Waldman, MD

It is grateful to the numerous doctors who have contributed to the scientific meetings over the past 20 years.

The Foundation for Cosmetic Surgery would also like to acknowledge the tireless work and contributions of the editorial staff and its contributing authors;

Editorial Staff:

Debbie Antoniono
Marissa Chery
Diane Riddell
Maggie Zieback

Contributing Authors:

H. George Brennan, MD
Patrick Ryan Brennan
Aram Bonni, MD
Robert Cattani, MD
Candace Chatham
Nikolas V. Chugay, DO
Cherie Lundquist-Grochow
Arthur J. Helliwell, DDS
Sheldon S. Kabaker, MD
David Lee, DPM
Lisa McGill
Joyce Scherer
E. Douglas Whitehead, MD

The work of the Foundation would be impossible without the help and support of the following companies;

Anthony Products
BioForm Medical
British Custom Tailors & Shirtmakers
Canaday Group
Canfield Imaging Systems
Coapt Systems
Cosmedix
Derma Sweep
Design Veronique
Dispensing Solutions
Einstein Medical
Ellman International
Elsevier Journals
Elsevier Saunders and Mosby
EMed
Gaylee Spa
Hanson Medical
Implantech Associates
Is Clinical by Innovative Skincare
Jan Marini Skin Research
Lumenis
Maloney Development Associates
Marina Medical Instruments
Medical Justice Services
Medicis Aesthetics, Inc.
Microsurgery Instruments
Nextech Systems
Obagi Medical Products
Ocean Breeze Surgical
PlasticSurgery.com
Reliant Technologies
Shippert Medical Technologies Corp
Snowden Pencer
Surgical Specialties Corporation
Thermage
TransMotion Medical
Tulip Medical Products

Forward

This is a lighthearted, *show & tell* effort to educate the lay sector. It puts cosmetic surgery in perspective and it depicts realistically the magic of cosmetic surgery and as importantly it dispels myths and misconceptions. It is the ultimate guide and resource in cosmetic surgery, as we know it today. As the reader, you will be informed, entertained and guided to further information to expand your horizons based on your individual preference and interest.

You will also learn the history of beauty and cosmetic surgery with a potpourri of fascinating photographs.

The chapter, Consultation with a Cosmetic Surgeon, includes the evaluation, the surgical experience and post surgical experience. You will learn a self-analysis system to answer the basic question "am I ready?"

A chapter on actual patients before and after photographs of examples of the miracles of cosmetic surgery from head to toe will follow.

The next chapter will deal with public patients who have had cosmetic surgery showing you before and after photographs. This is followed by a chapter on "what if?" public faces had cosmetic surgery. The results will be simulated using computer-morphing techniques.

You will be educated as to all current accepted procedures and modalities both surgical and non-surgical in the quest for ultimate enhancement of appearance.

Finally, there will be a chapter on all the legitimate specialties in organized healthcare and the beauty industry that deliver the state-of-the-art possibilities.

Introduction

Cosmetic surgery is the epitome of the marriage between art and science. Cosmetic (aesthetic) surgery is a subspecialty of plastic surgery. Plastic surgery derives its name from the Greek root ***plastikos*** – (meaning to mold or give form). Commercial plastics have the same derivation.

In cosmetic surgery synthetic materials are rarely used but commercial plastic is never used.

Plastic surgery has two broad categories: reconstructive and cosmetic. Reconstructive surgery corrects defects whether they are birth defects, burn defects and defects secondary to accidents or surgery, attempting to achieve normal appearance and function.

Virtually every surgical specialty whether it is neurosurgery, thoracic surgery, gynecological surgery, or orthopedic surgery involves reconstructive surgery.

The psychodynamics in reconstructive surgery are vastly different than cosmetic surgery. In reconstructive surgery the patient's greatest hope is to be normal once again.

In cosmetic surgery the patient is happy, healthy, well adjusted and normal; void of injury, defect or disease.

This patient simply wants to look better.

The cosmetic surgery patient is basically saying "Doctor, this is what God gave me and I want you to do better."

The happy reality is that they look better. Cosmetic surgery is the only happy area of organized medicine.

History

By: Patrick Ryan Brennan

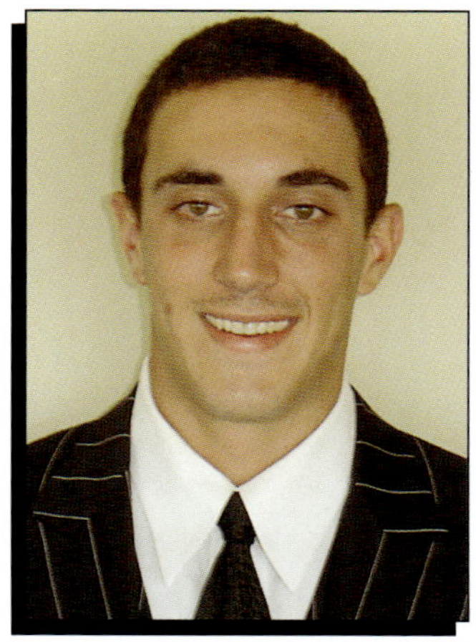

The field of cosmetic surgery began when Narcissus saw his reflection in nature's mirror.

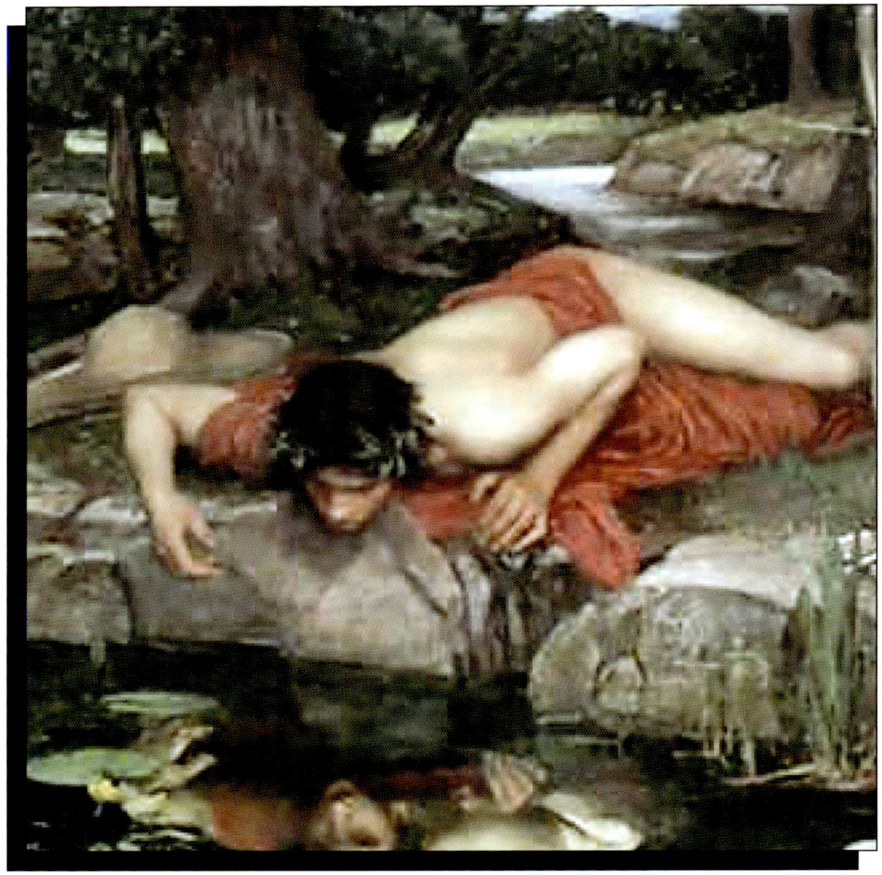

Since then man has been obsessed with changing his appearance either by adornment.

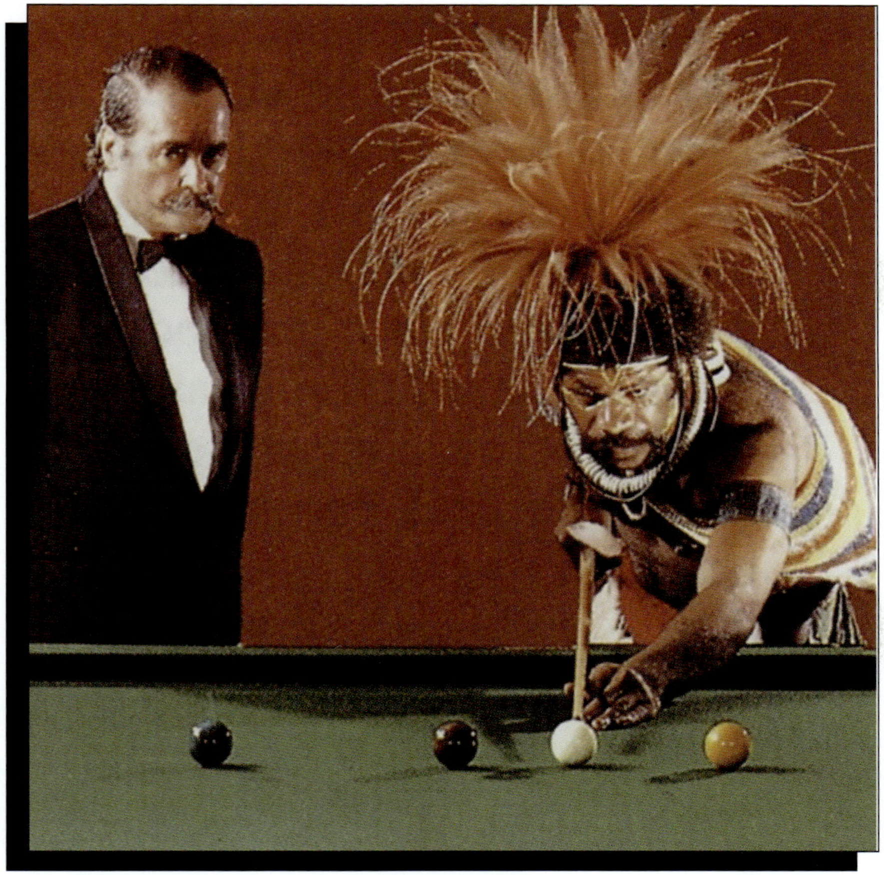

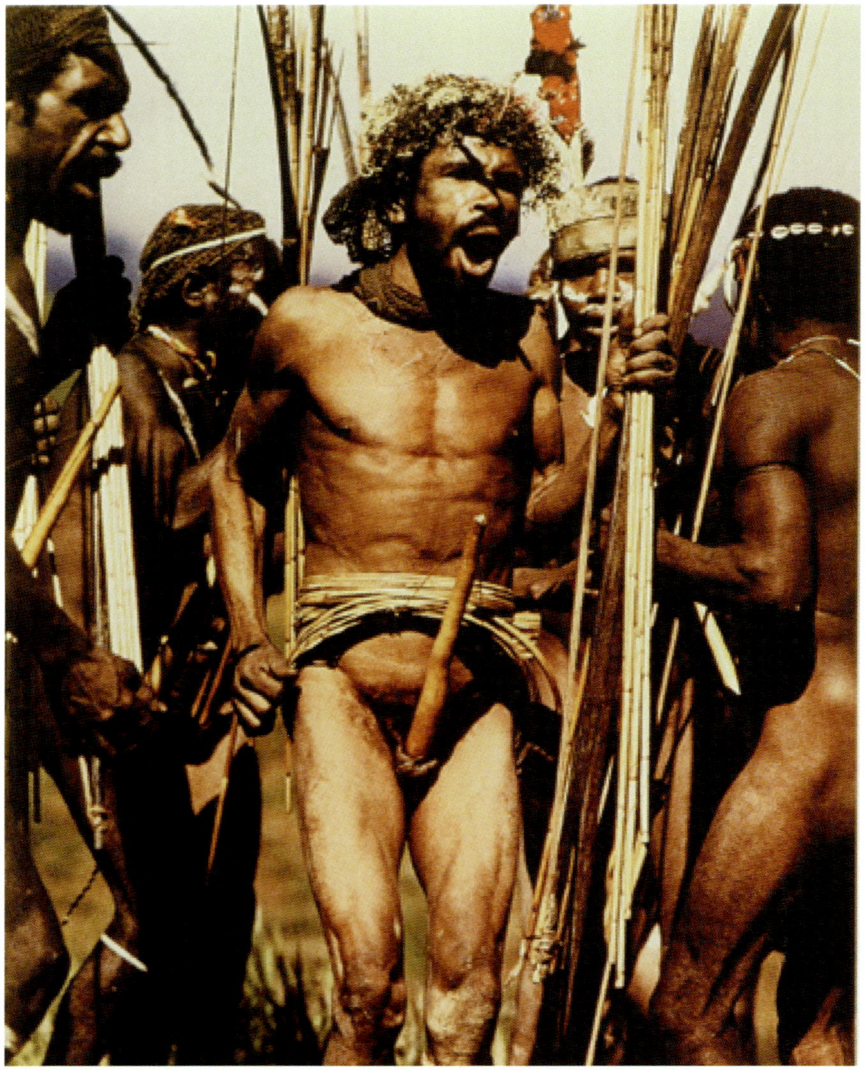

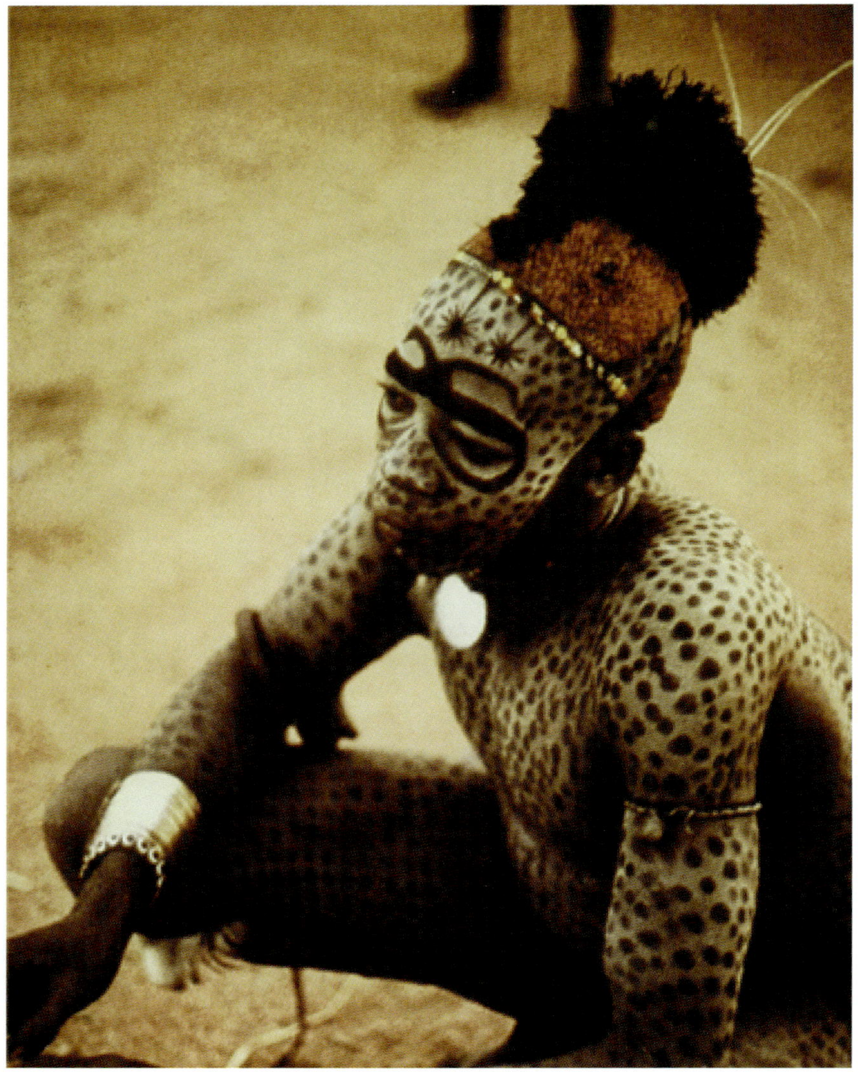

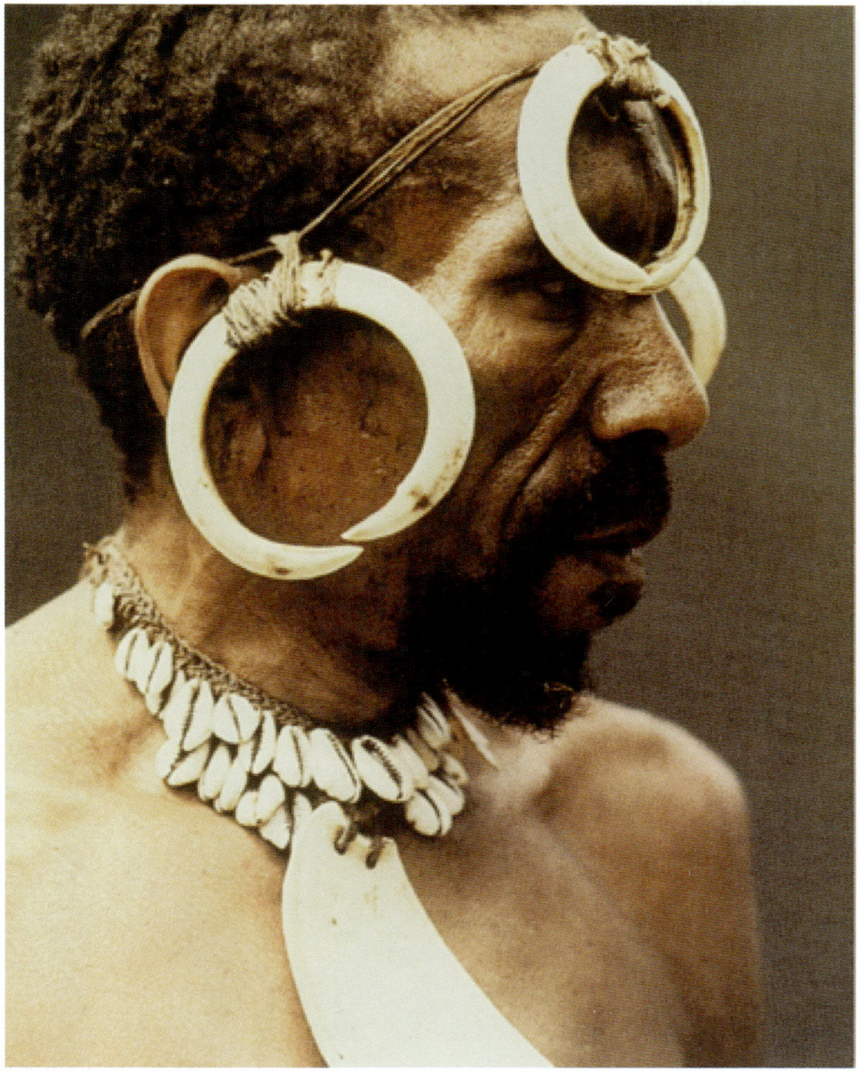

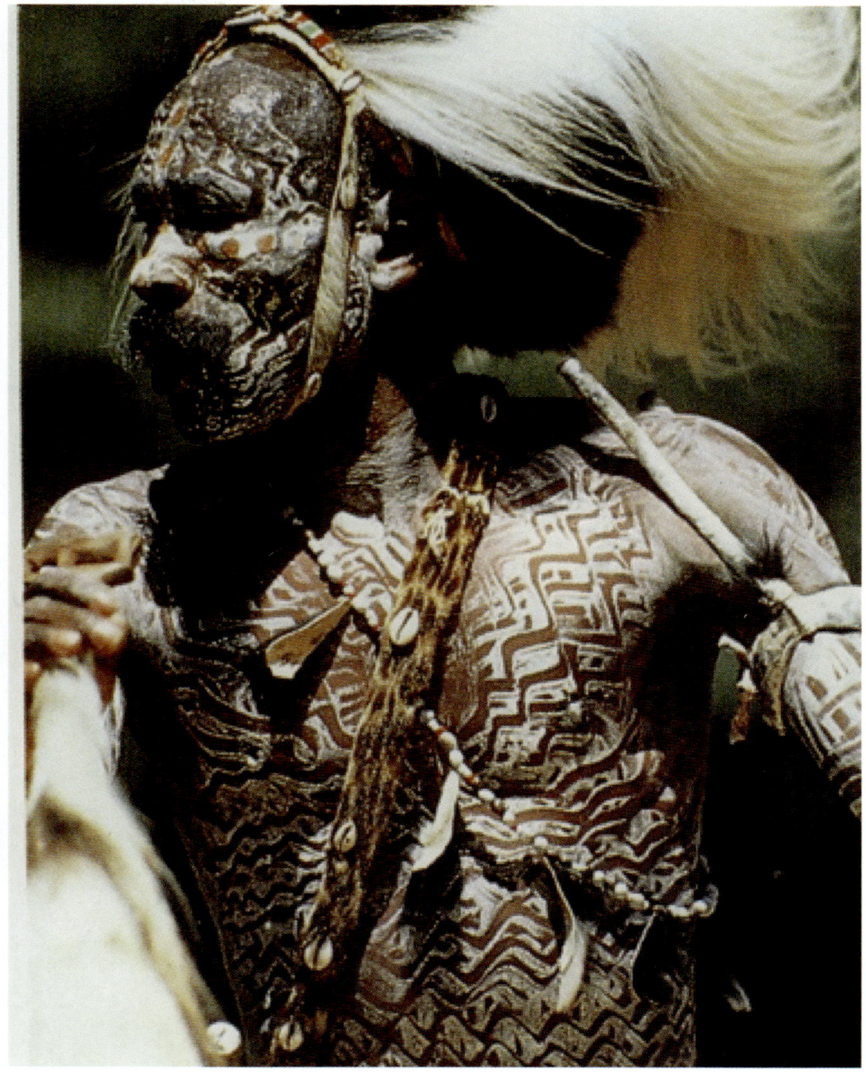

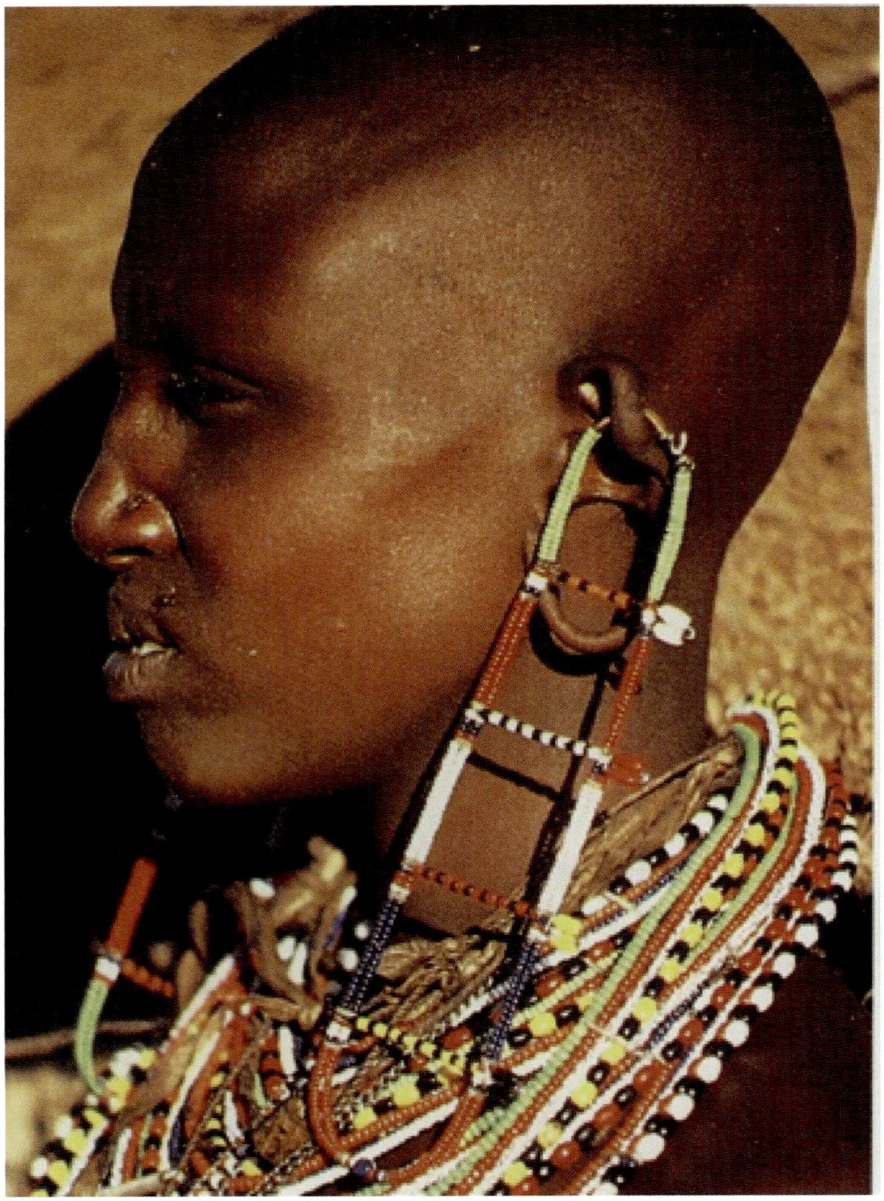

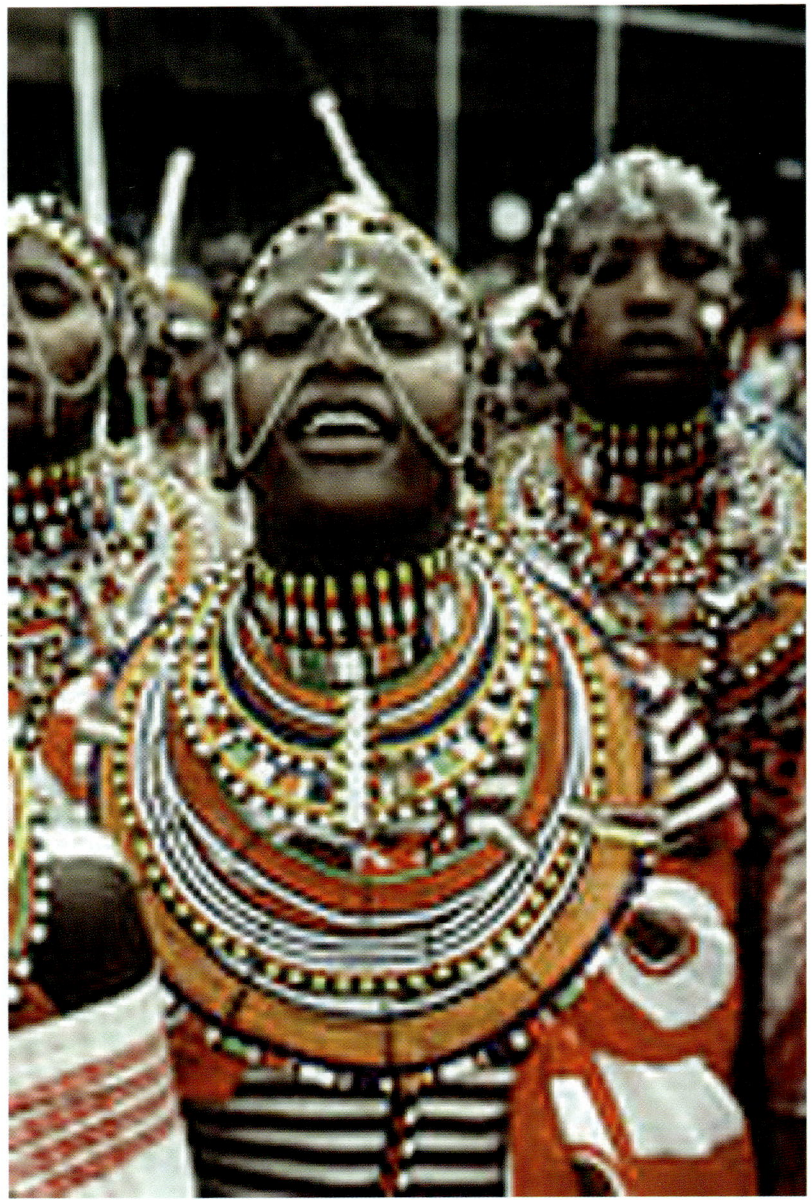

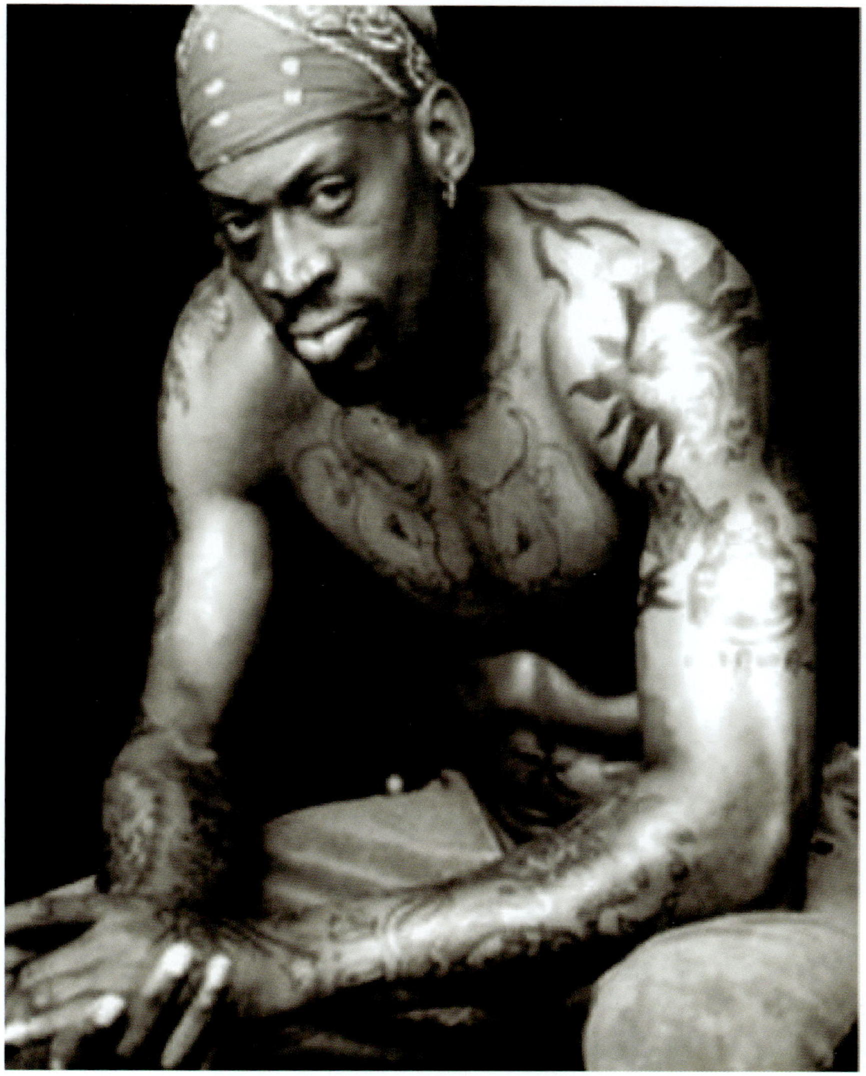

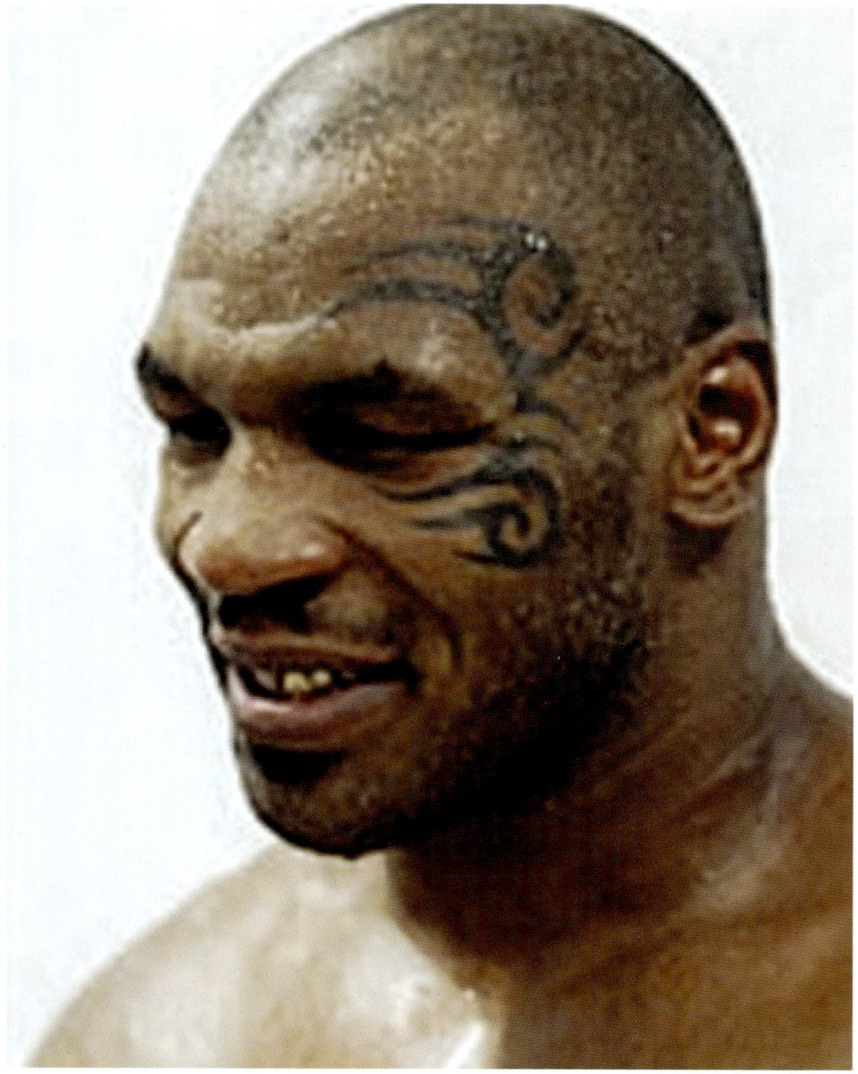

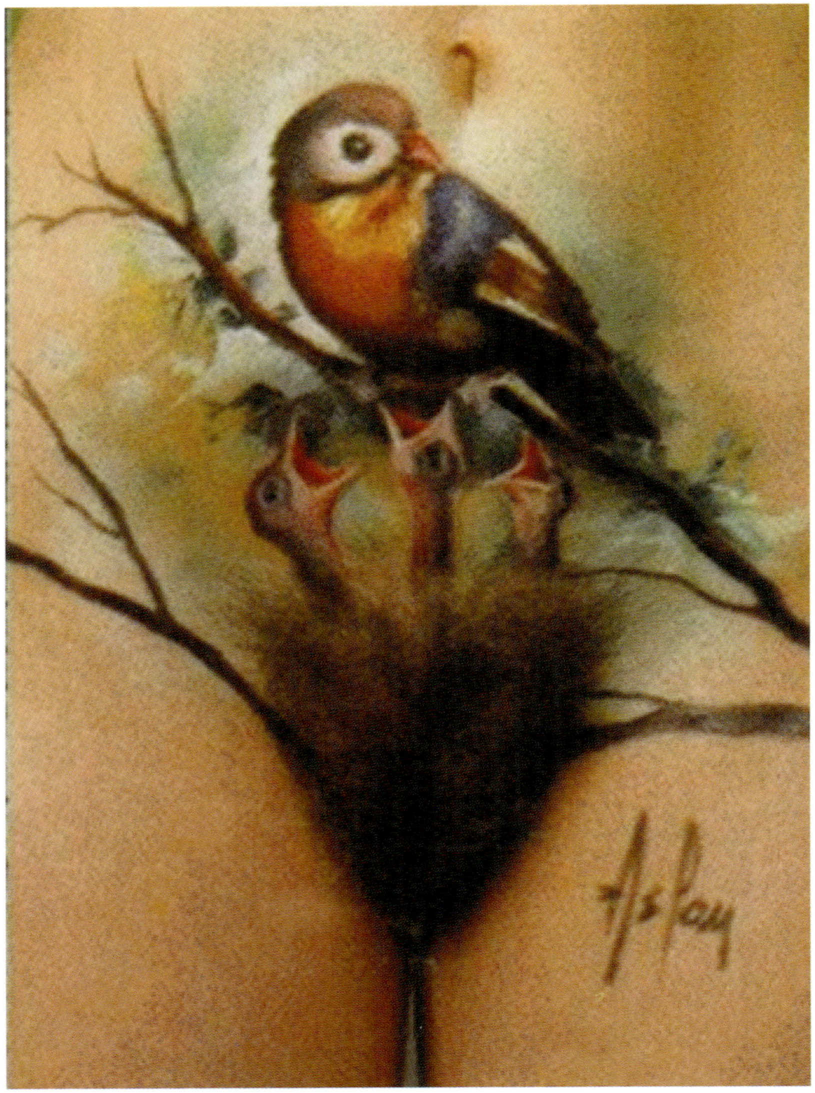

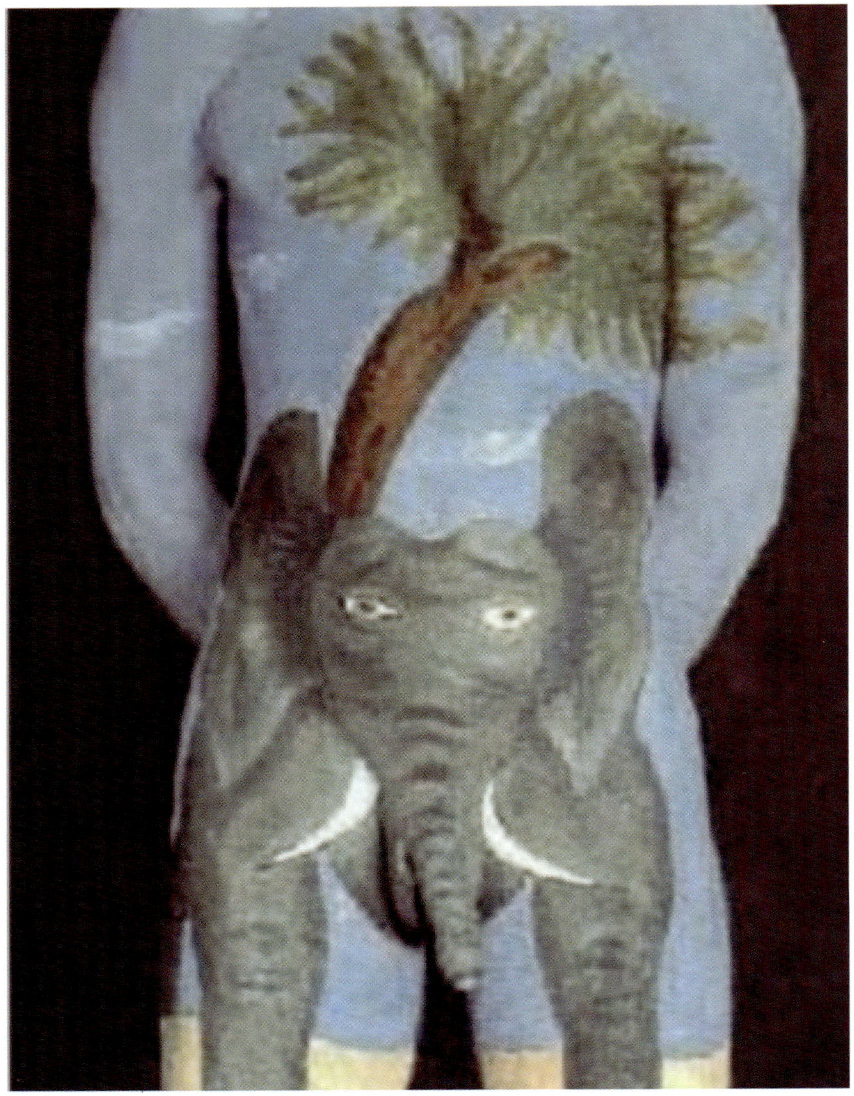

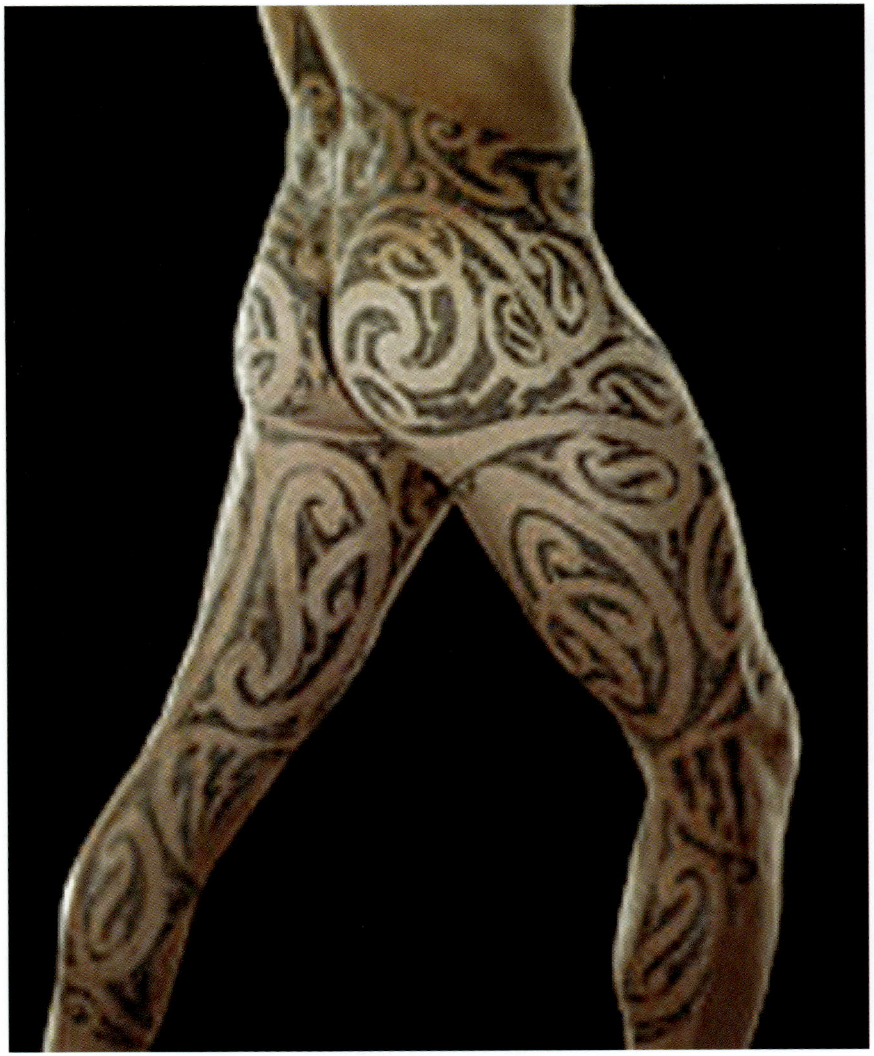

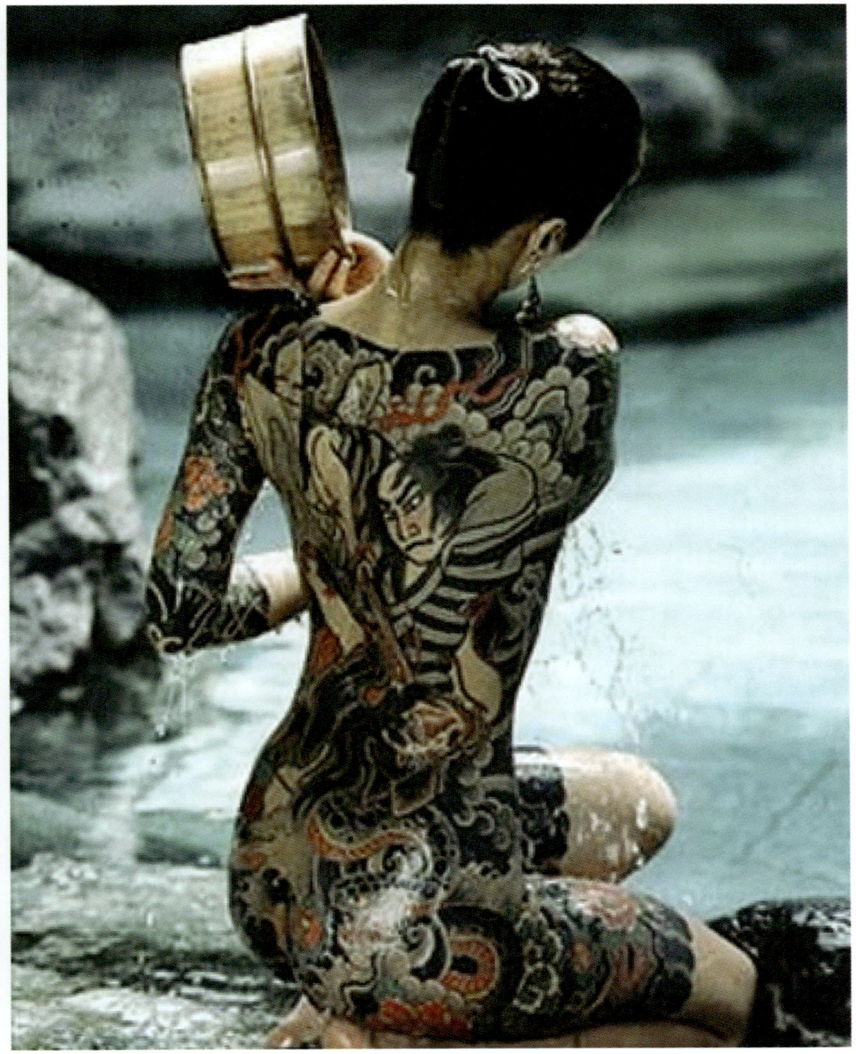

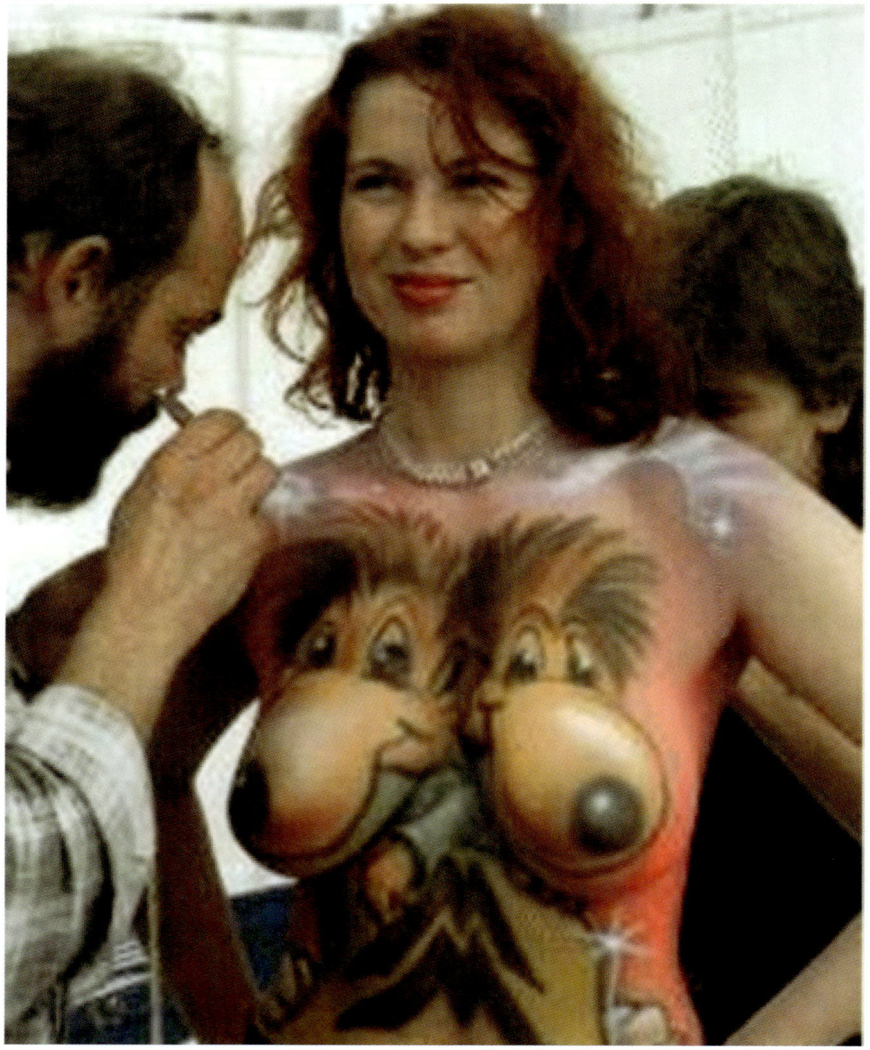

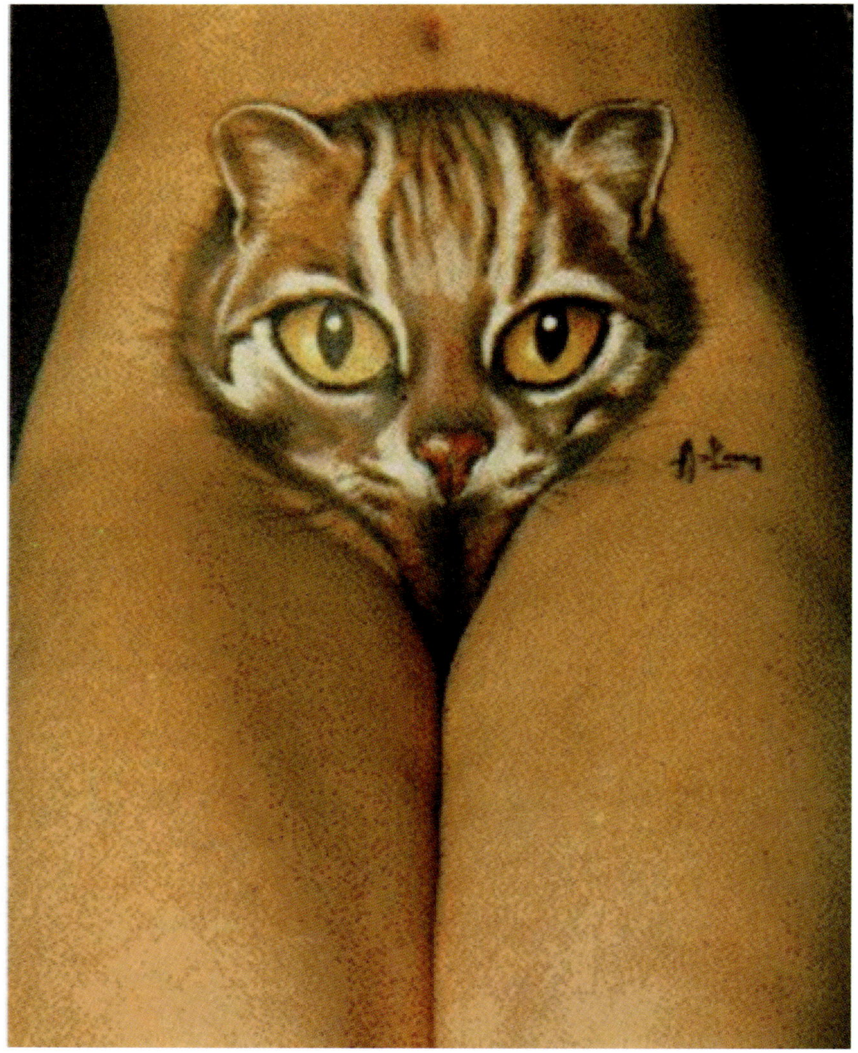

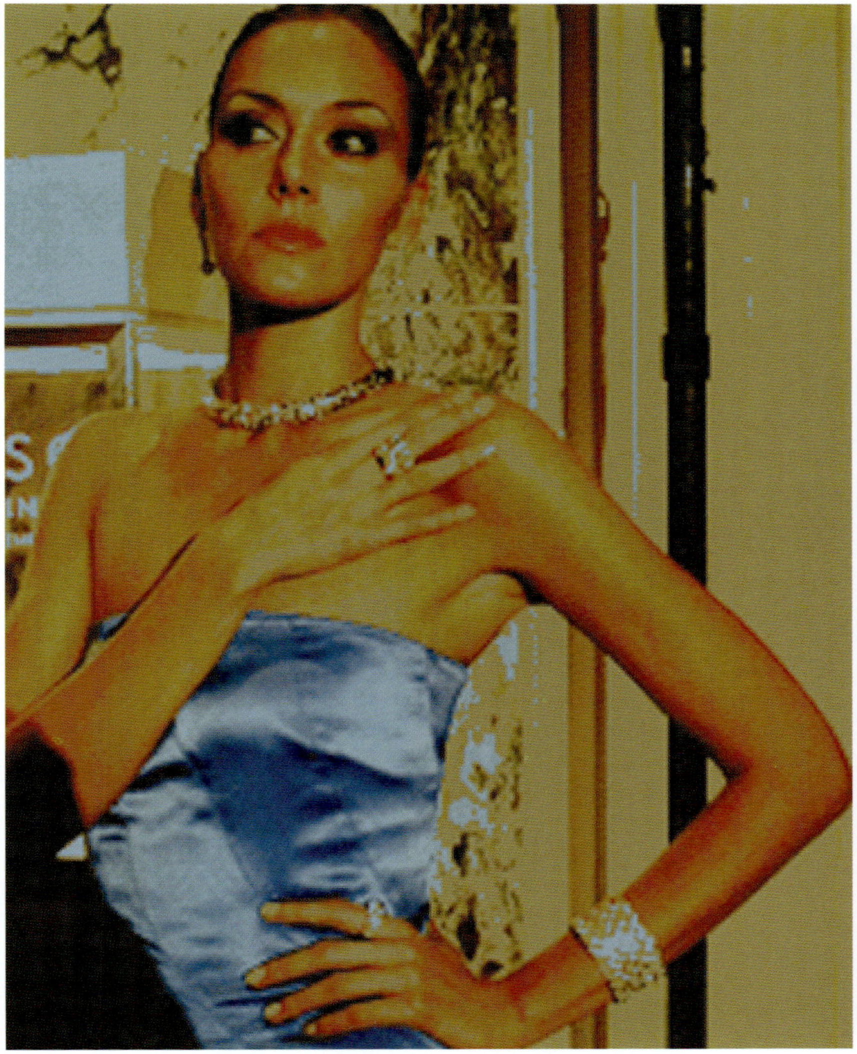

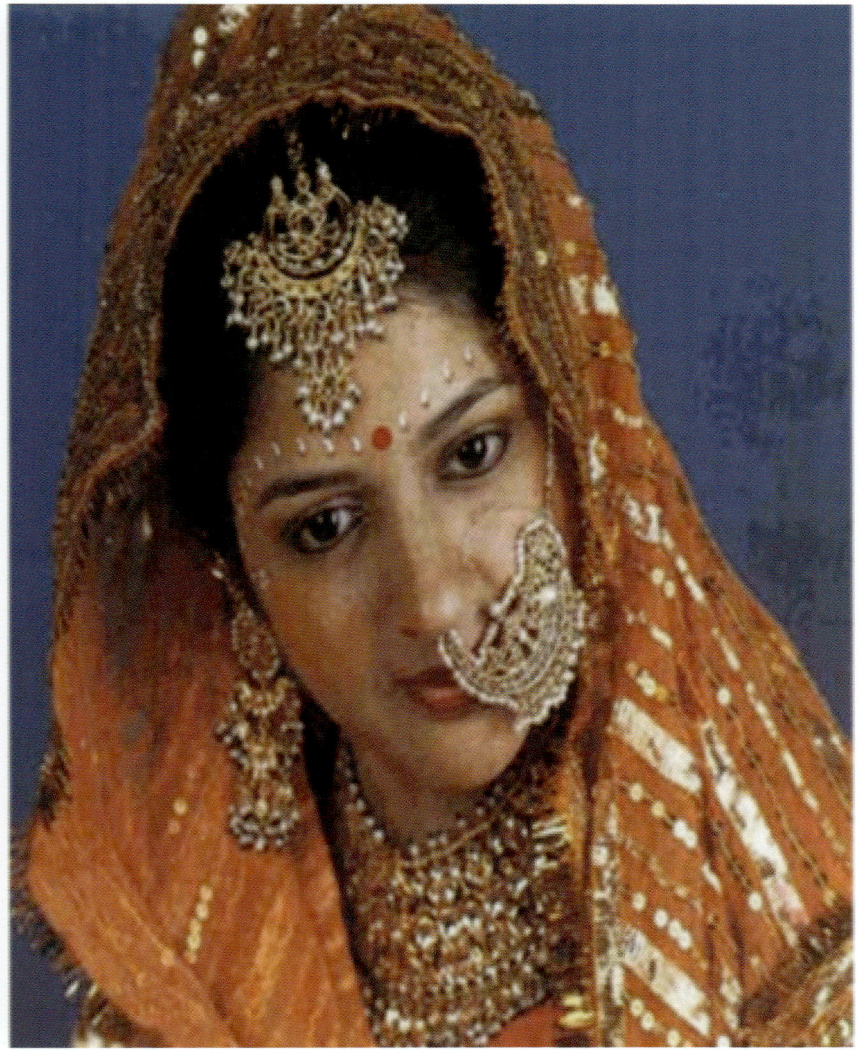

or by physical alteration.

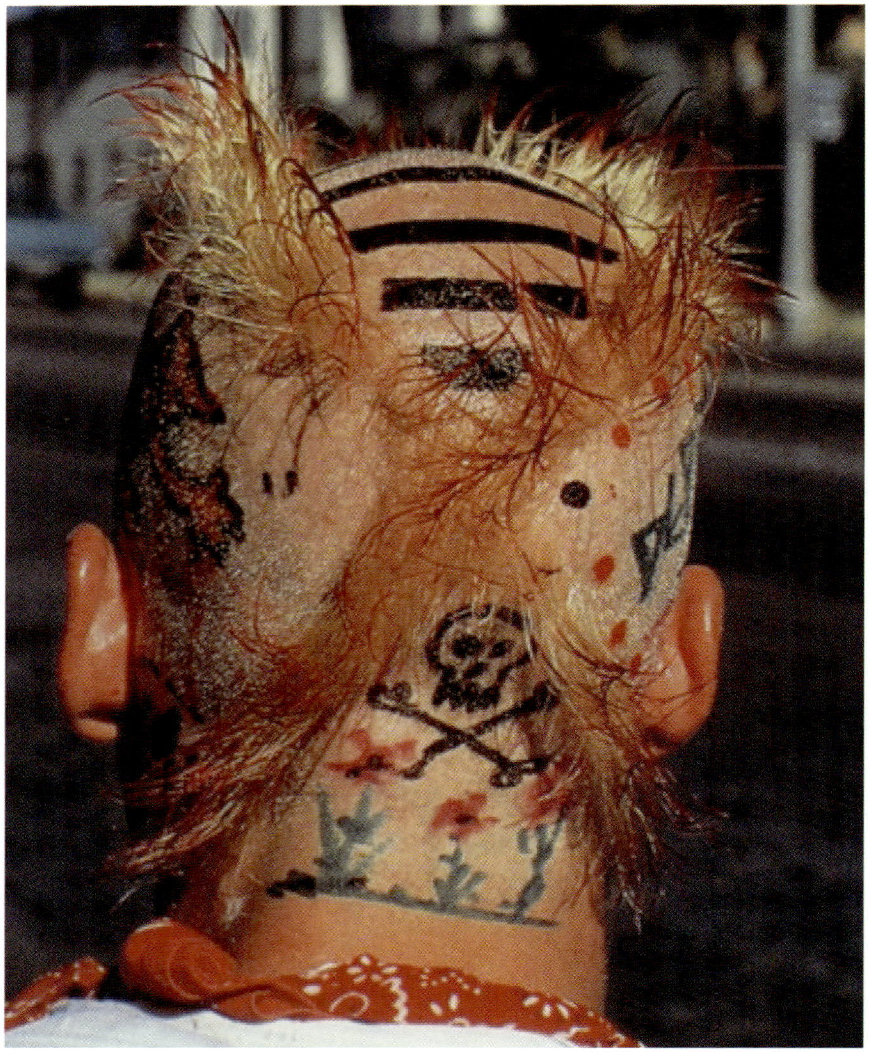

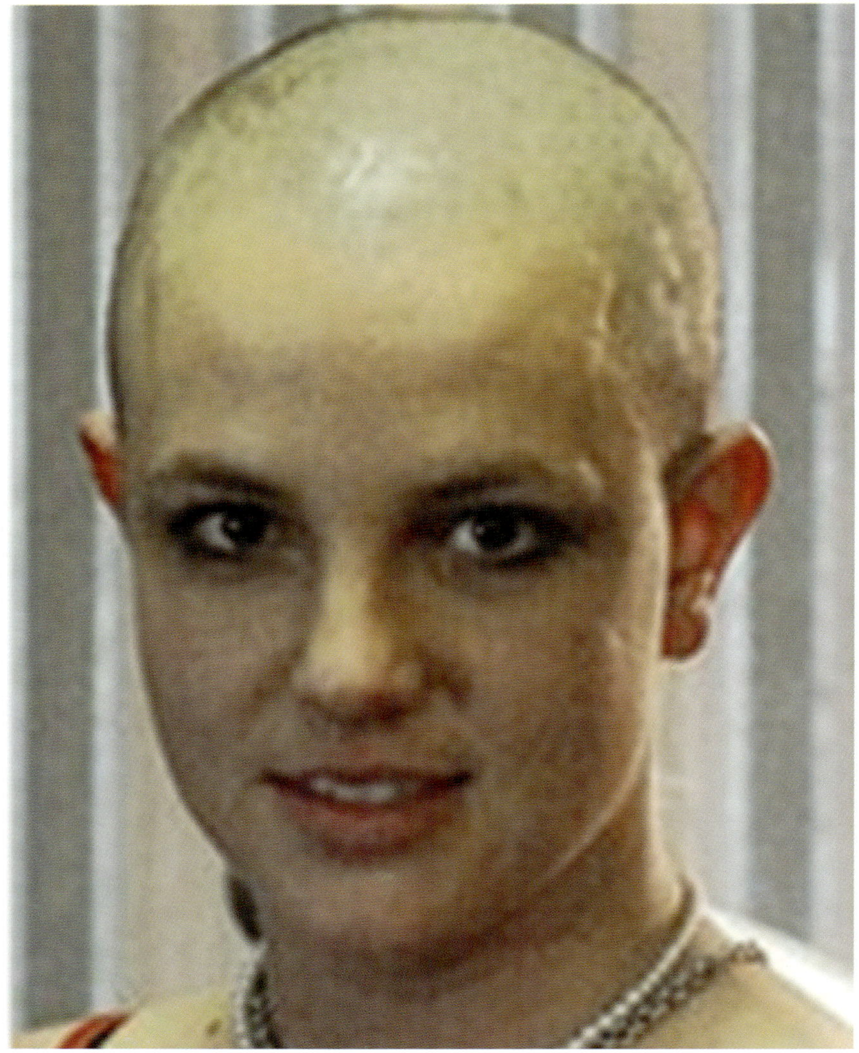

Britney Spears 2007

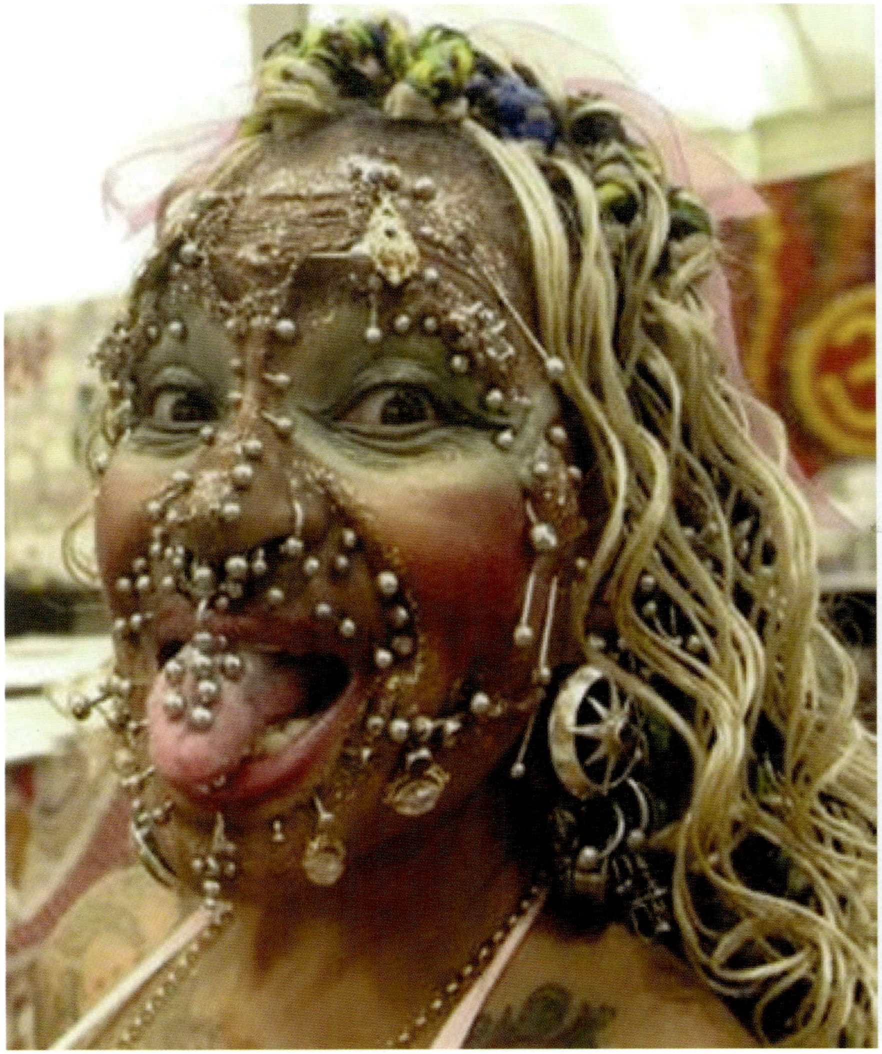

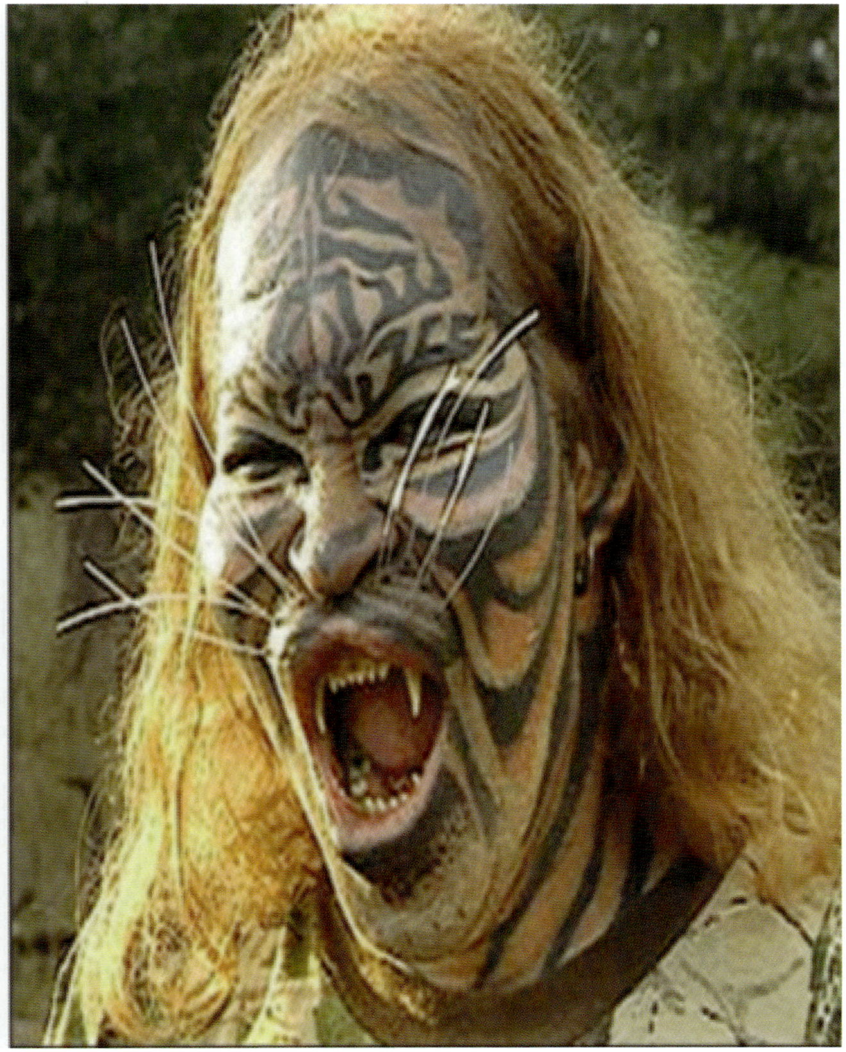

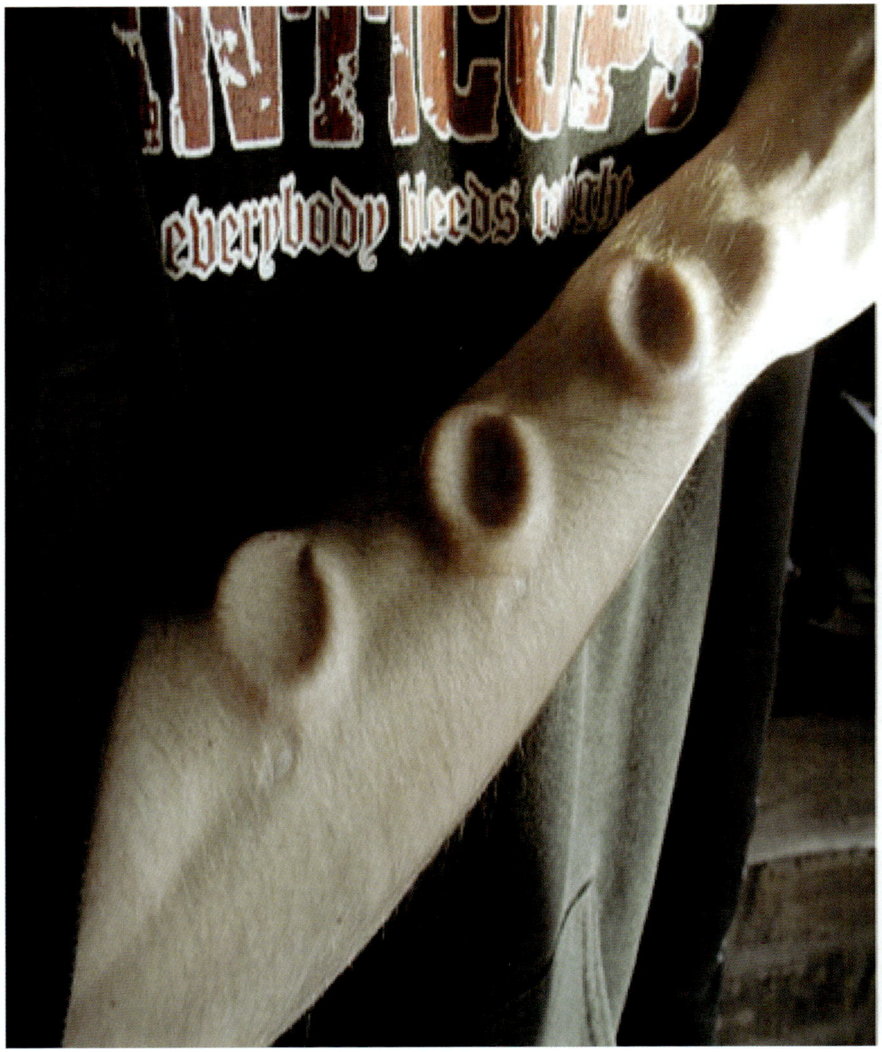
everybody bleeds

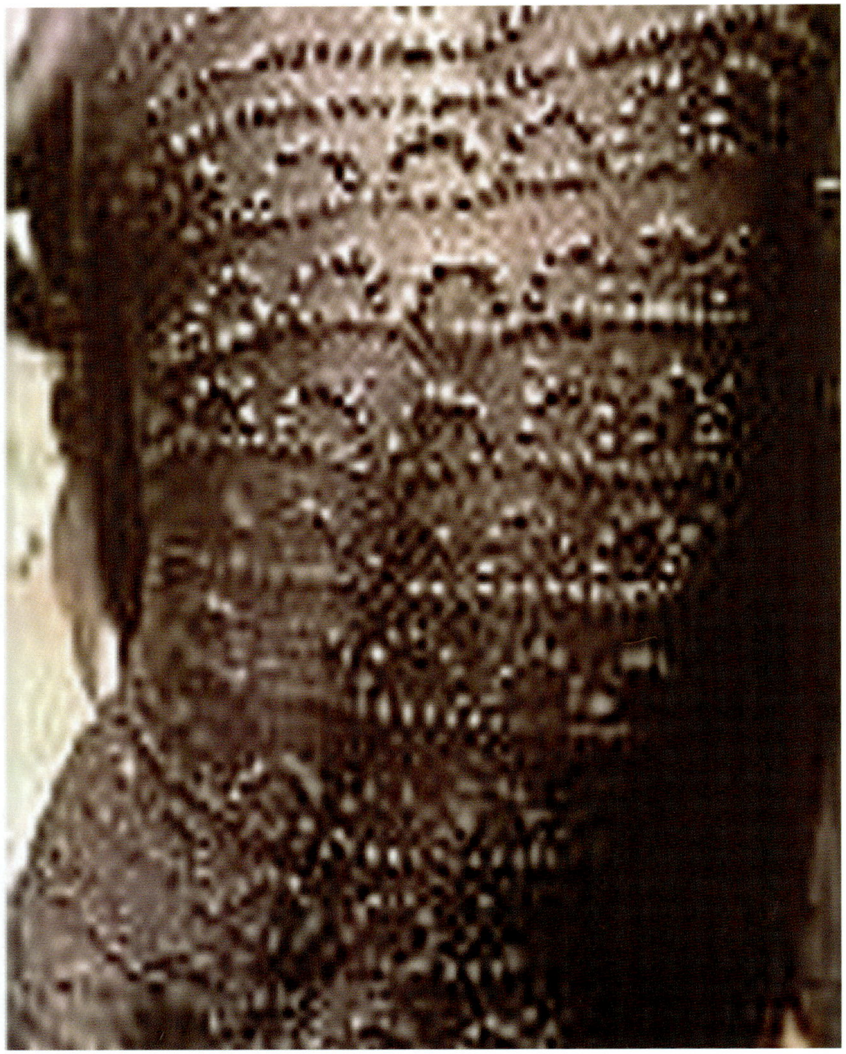

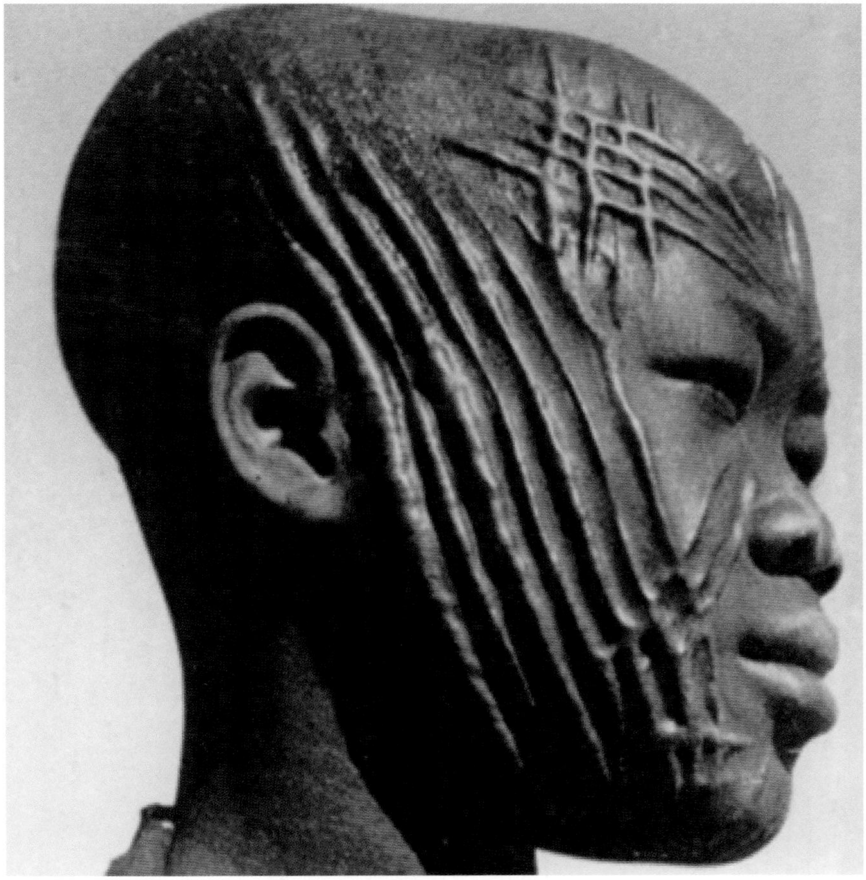

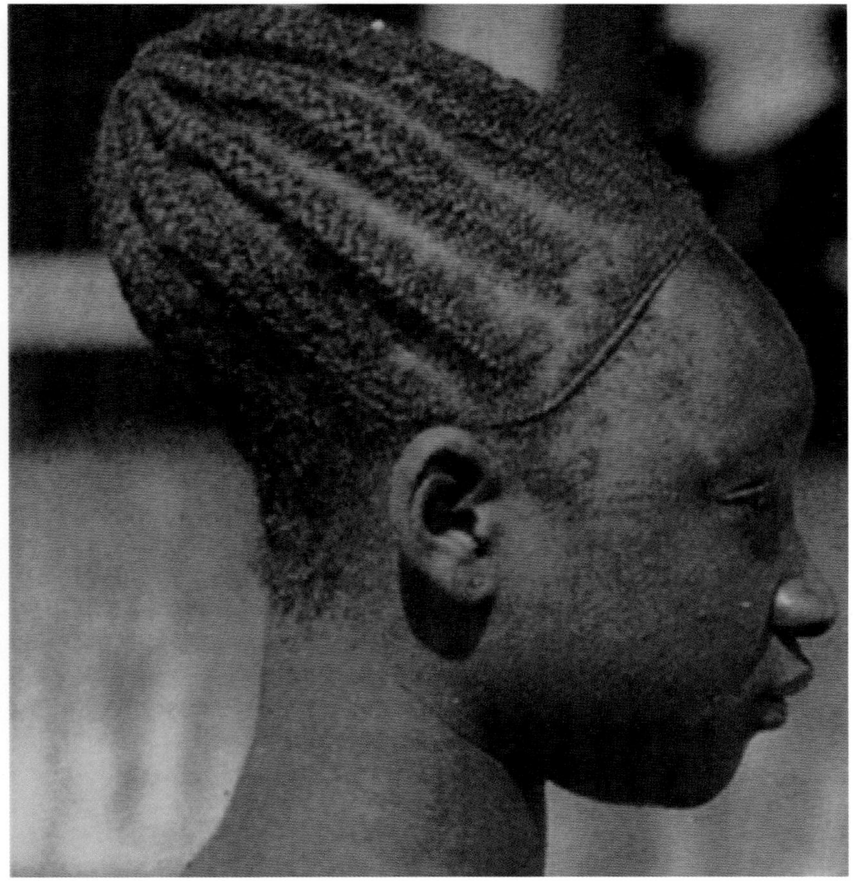

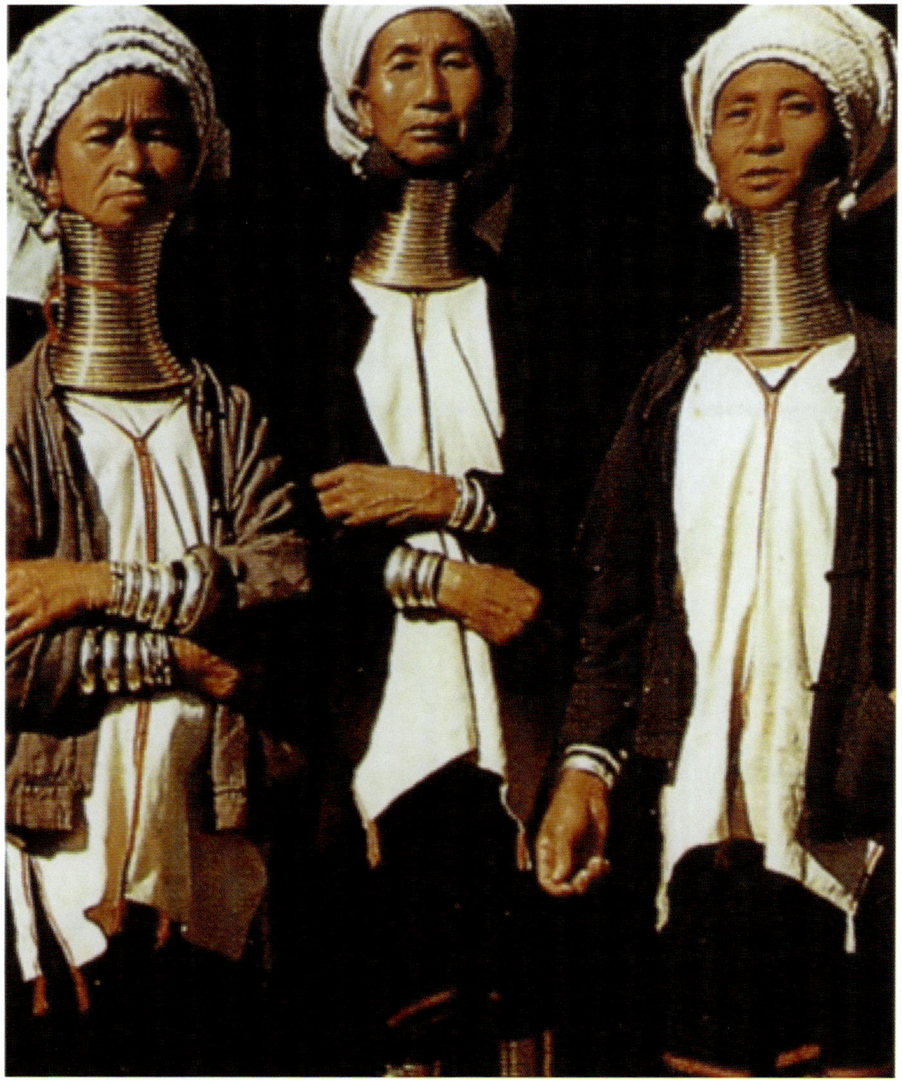 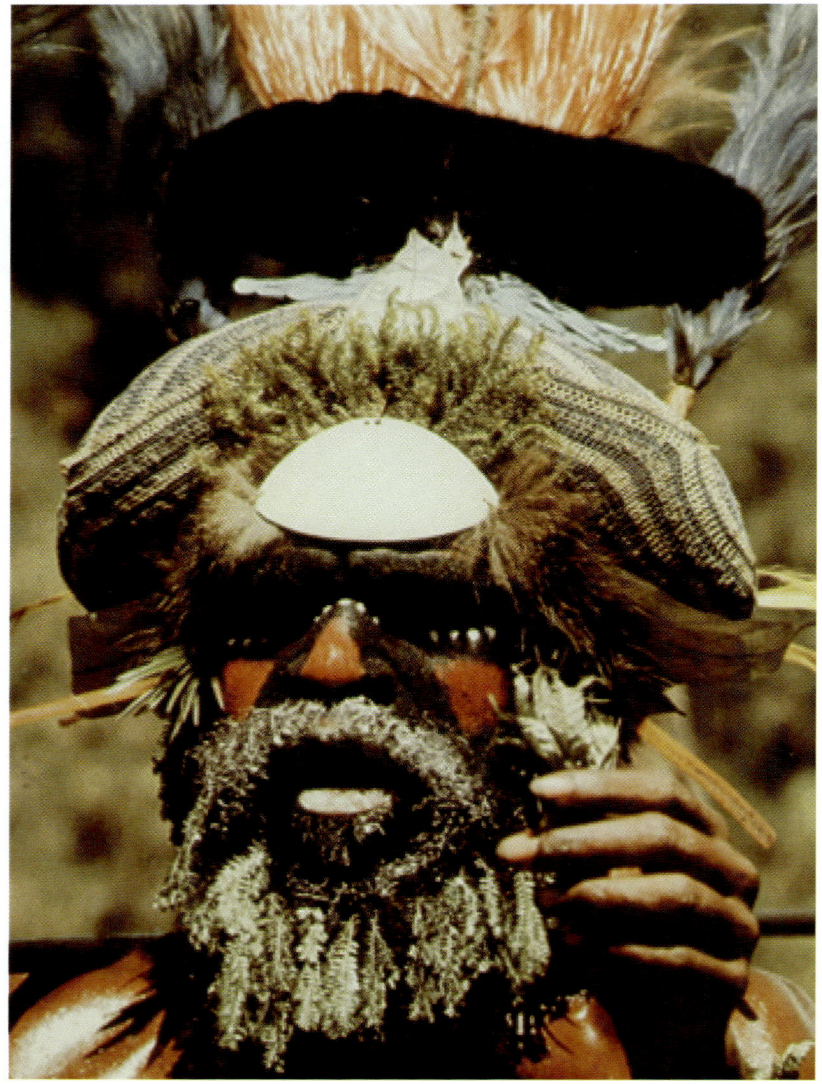

In modern western culture the civilized method of physical alteration is cosmetic surgery.

Since childhood, all of us have been programmed by the mirror. The mirror has had a tremendous impact on man. All of us have daily interactions with mirrors. Can any of us in civilized society function even one day without a mirror?.... try it!!

In Snow White the witch is tormented when she constantly asks the mirror "who is the fairest of them all?"

This sends us an early message about the perception of beauty.

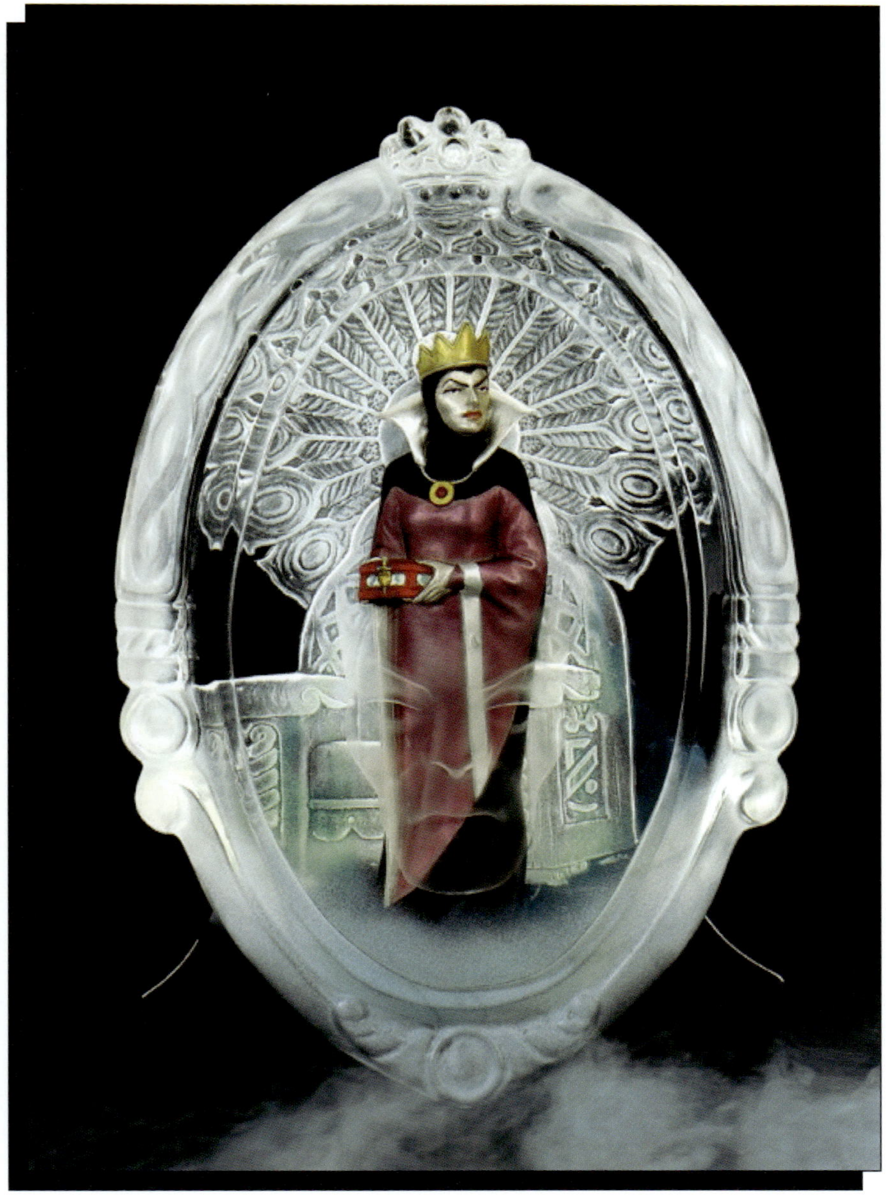

Art is replete with the introspection of the mirror. Rockwell's famous painting, "A girl at the mirror", shows the adolescent in transition pondering her future appearance.

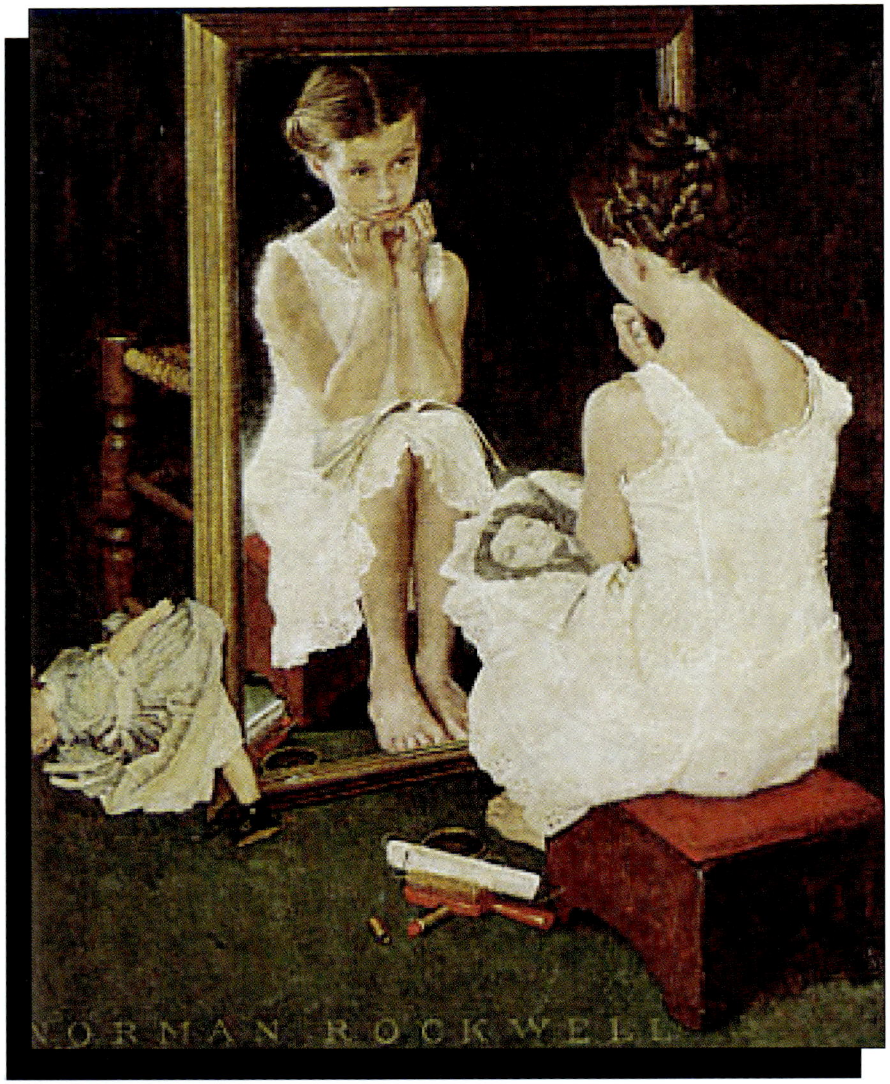

Even classic artists who seemingly should be preoccupied with their creations on canvas historically have produced self-portraits; an impossible feat but for the mirror.

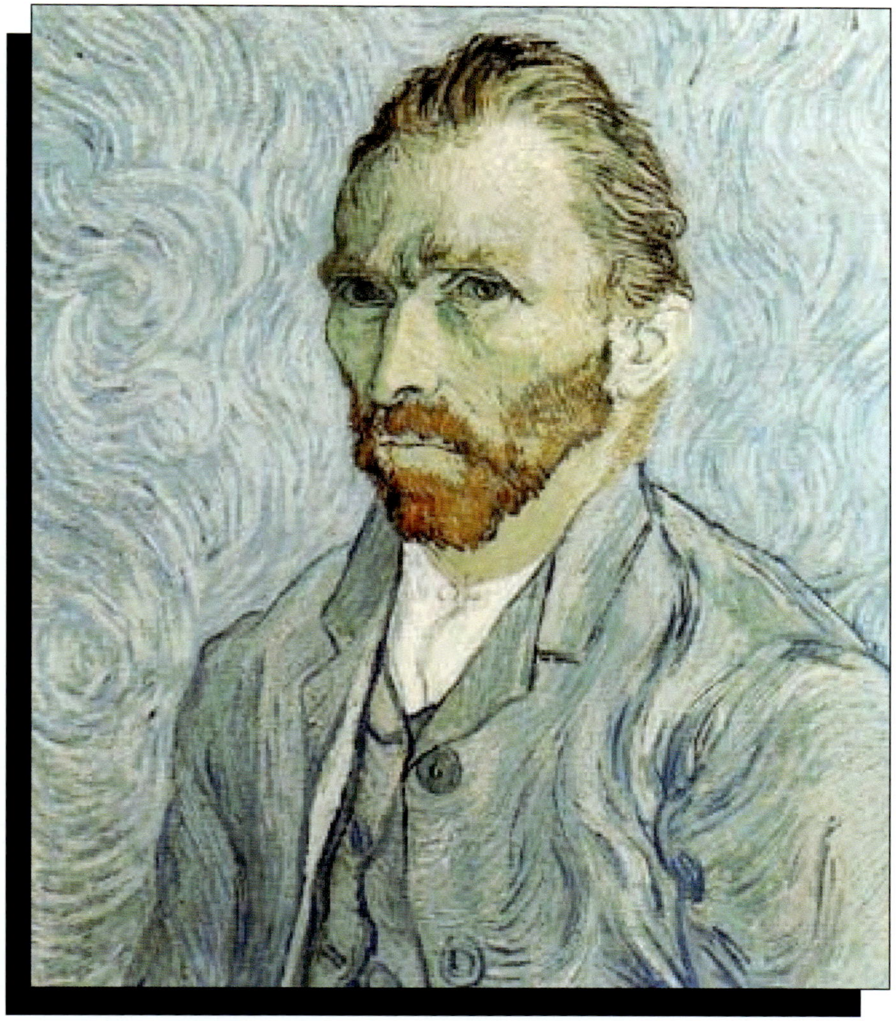

Perception is reality and the perception of beauty varies from person to person, culture to culture and with time. Perceived beauty creates comfort, self-confidence and self-esteem. The emphasis on appearance in our culture has created a multi billion-dollar industry. This is driven by the media, performing arts and the fashion industry including; clothing, jewelry, cosmetics and a variety of solutions for eternal youth. The historic quest for the Fountain of Youth is universal.

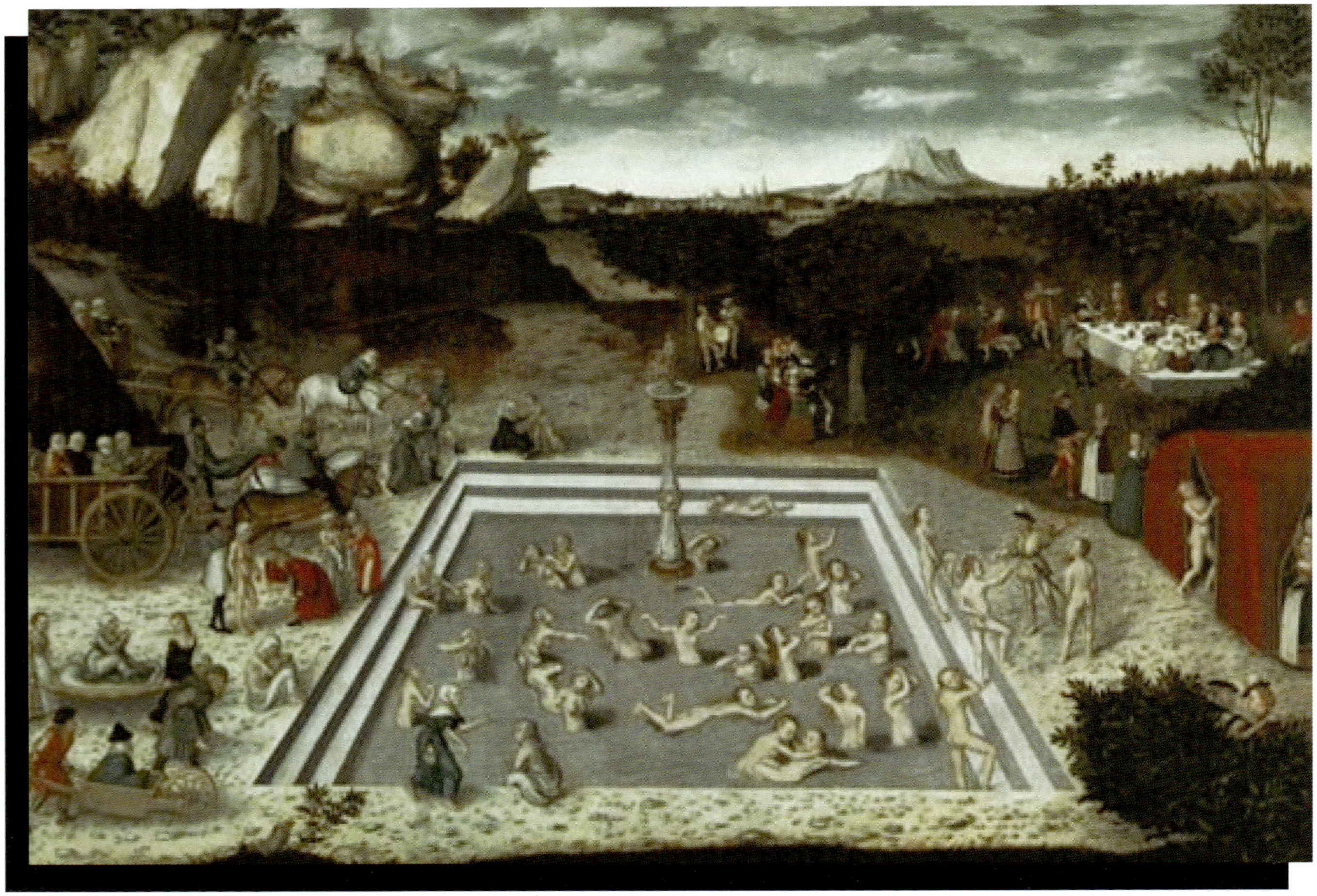

Beauty can be defined by a series of lines, angles, curves, contours and proportions which are referred to as "tenets of beauty." We study model faces, faces that do not require an education, faces that "earn a living" by merely standing in front of a camera. This is true of the male or female model.

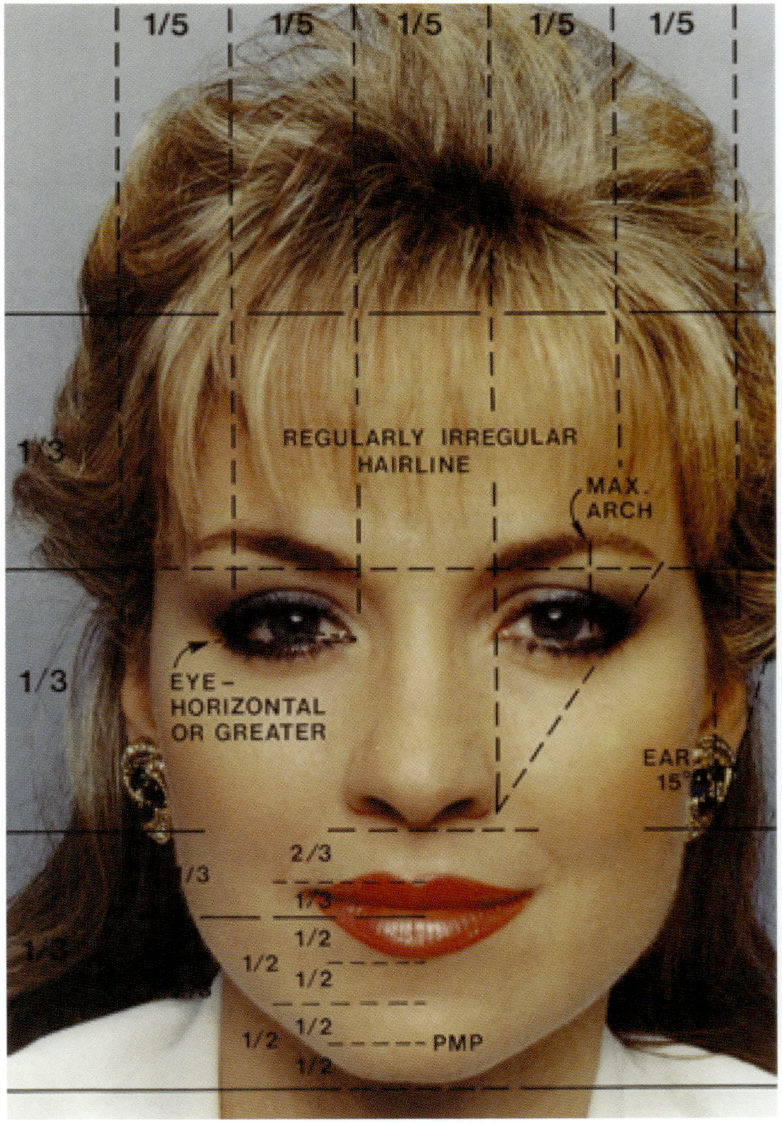

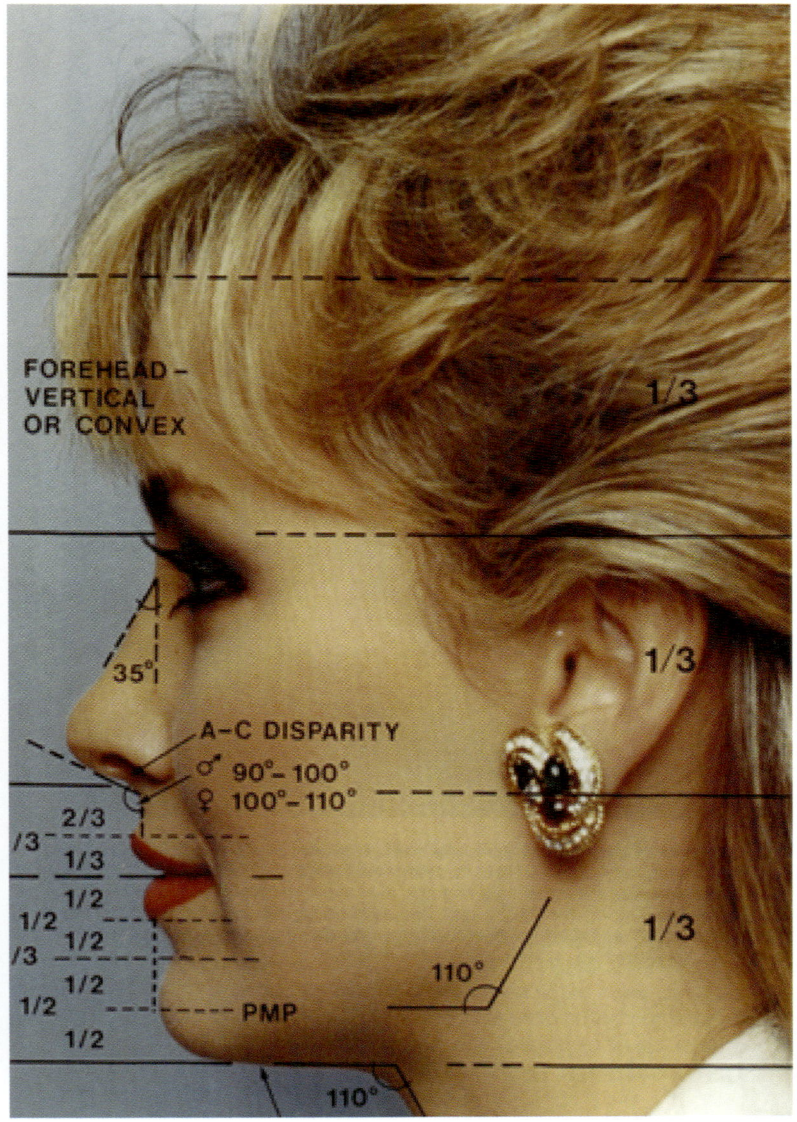

Invariably, the beautiful female model face or the handsome male model face will conform to the tenets of beauty.

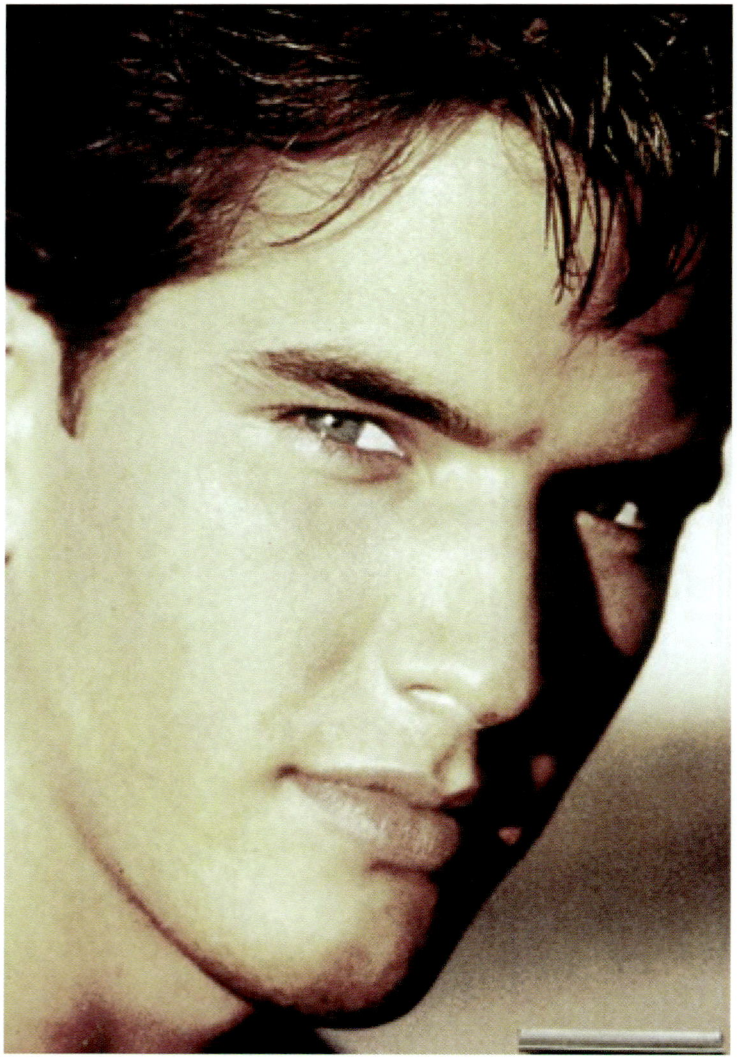

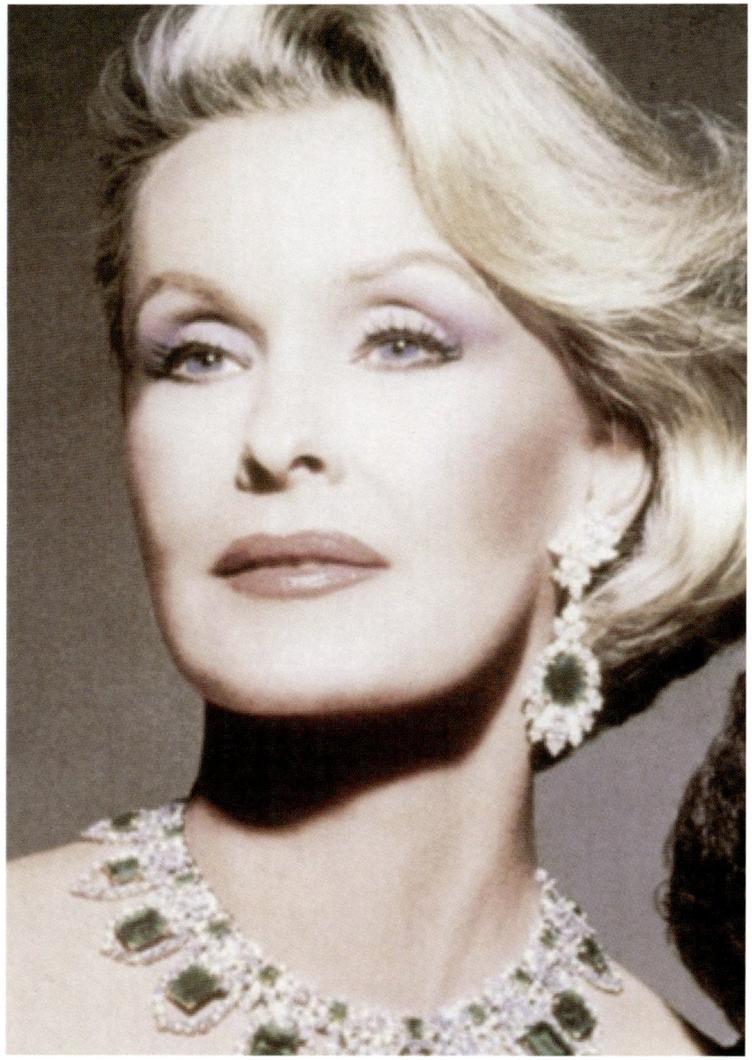

If, we are not endowed with natural beauty, the mirror and social encounters may undermine our self-confidence. Even if, one is endowed with youthful beauty, time often erodes and is not kind.

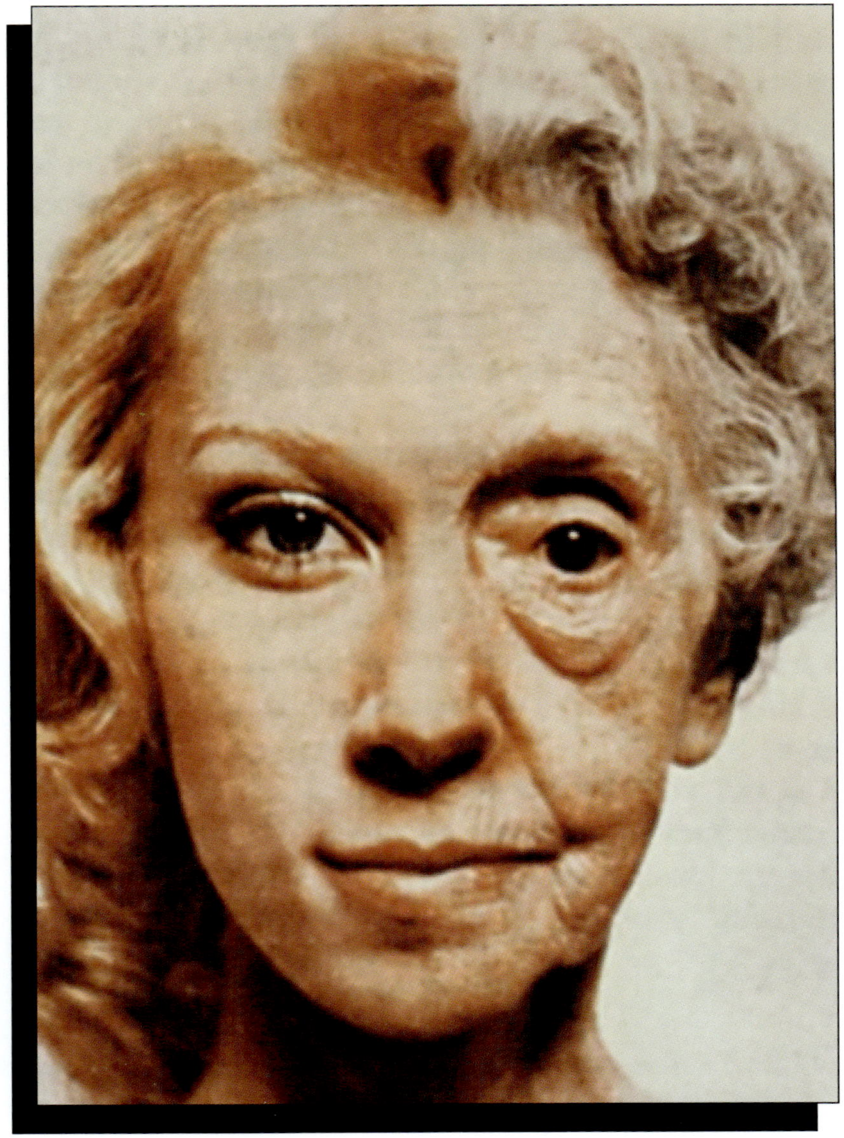

Classic beauties are not immune to the devastation of time based on heredity, lifestyle and environmental factors.

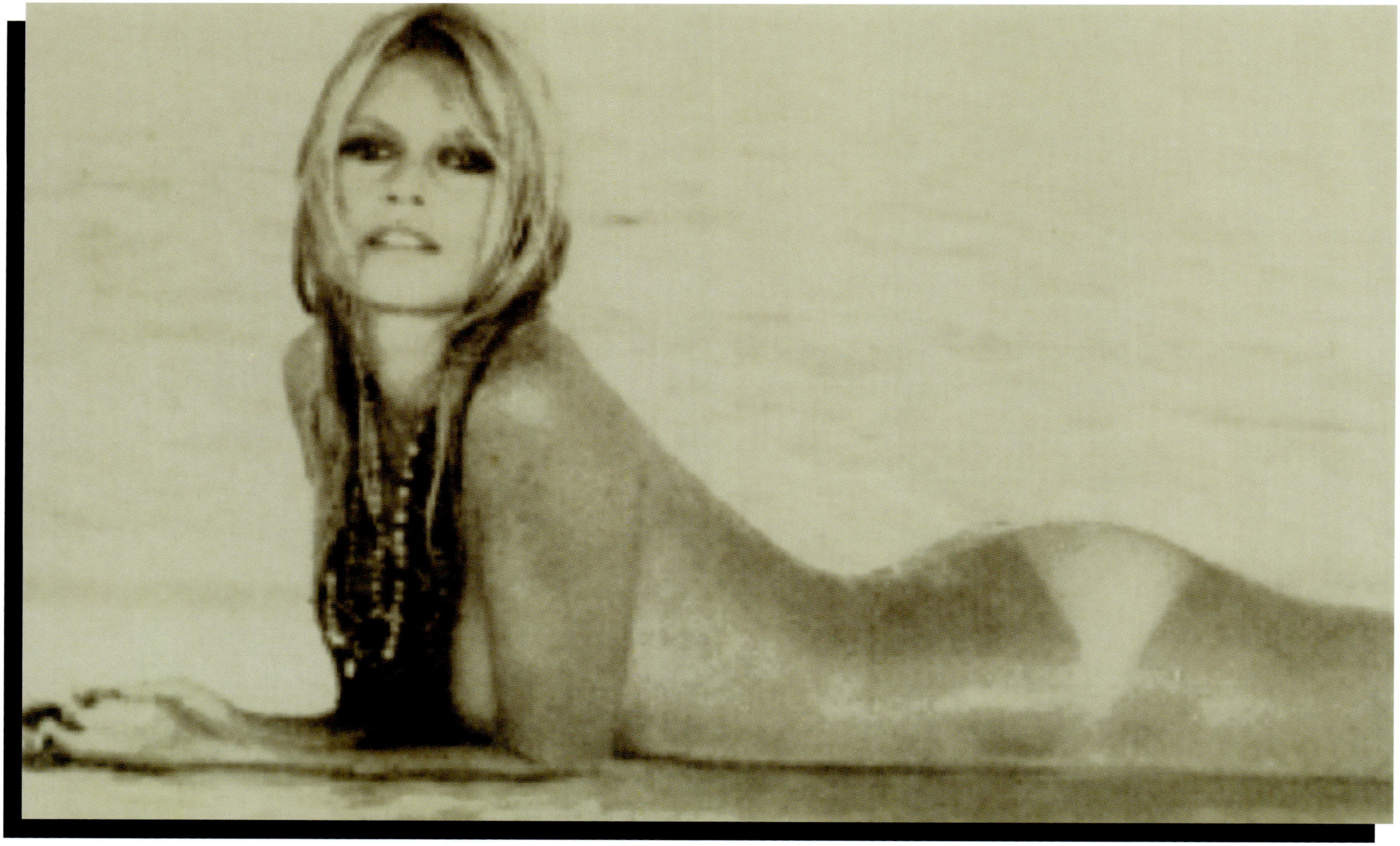

Brigitte Bardot as a young classic beauty.

Brigitte Bardot showing the painful deterioration of her natural God given beauty.

"It's better that I live like an ostrich, with my head in the sand," Bardot once said. "When I pull my head out, I am so blue I cannot stand it."

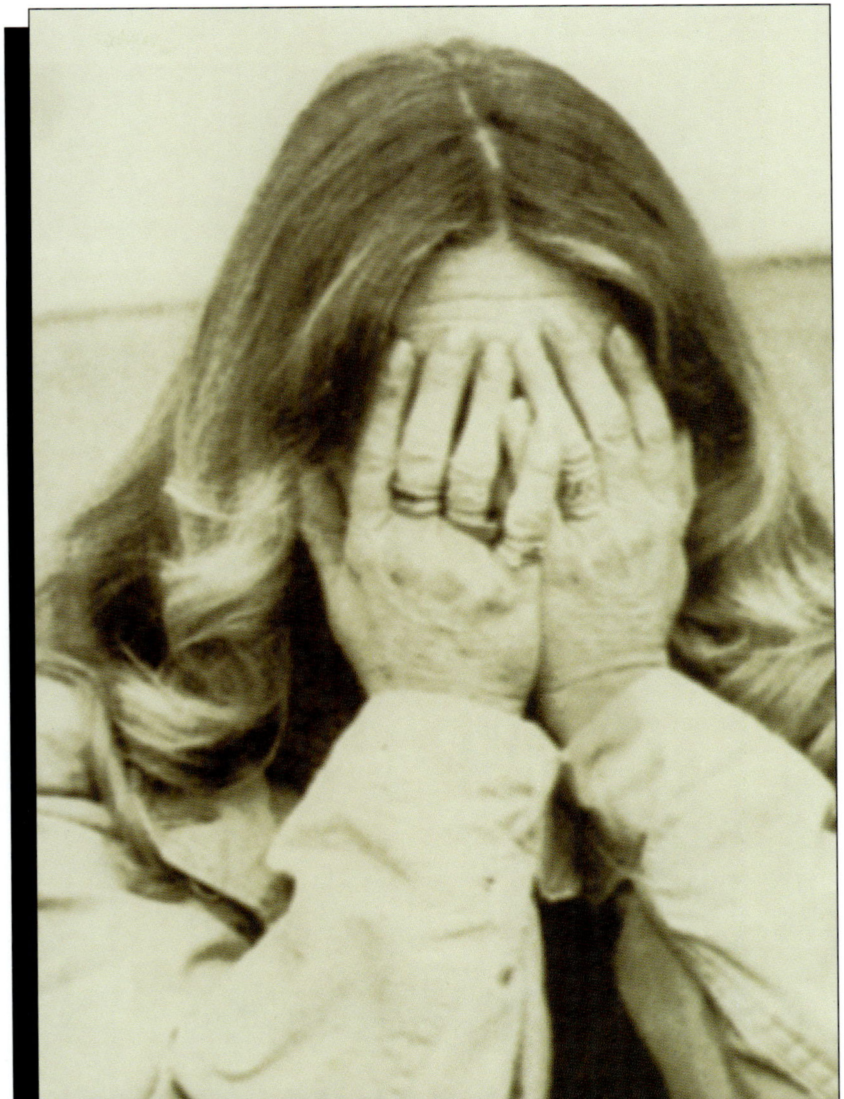

Studying youthful and mature male and female faces is a sobering reality check. Cosmetic surgery can often be a simple solution.

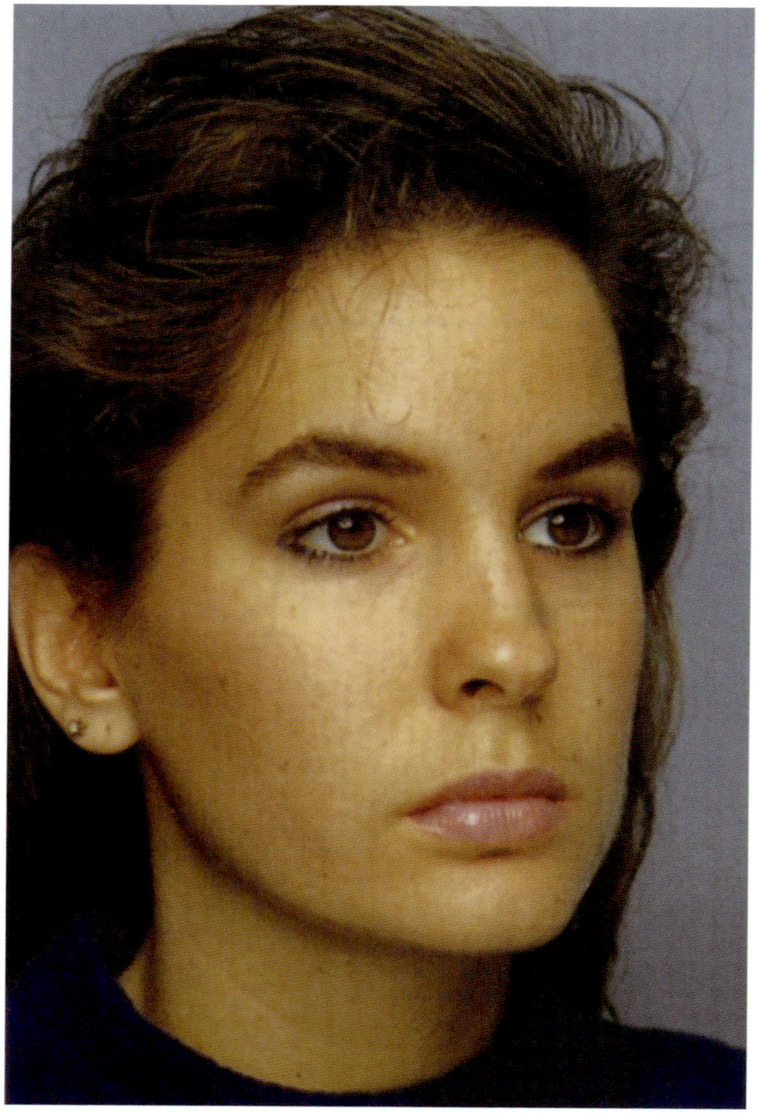

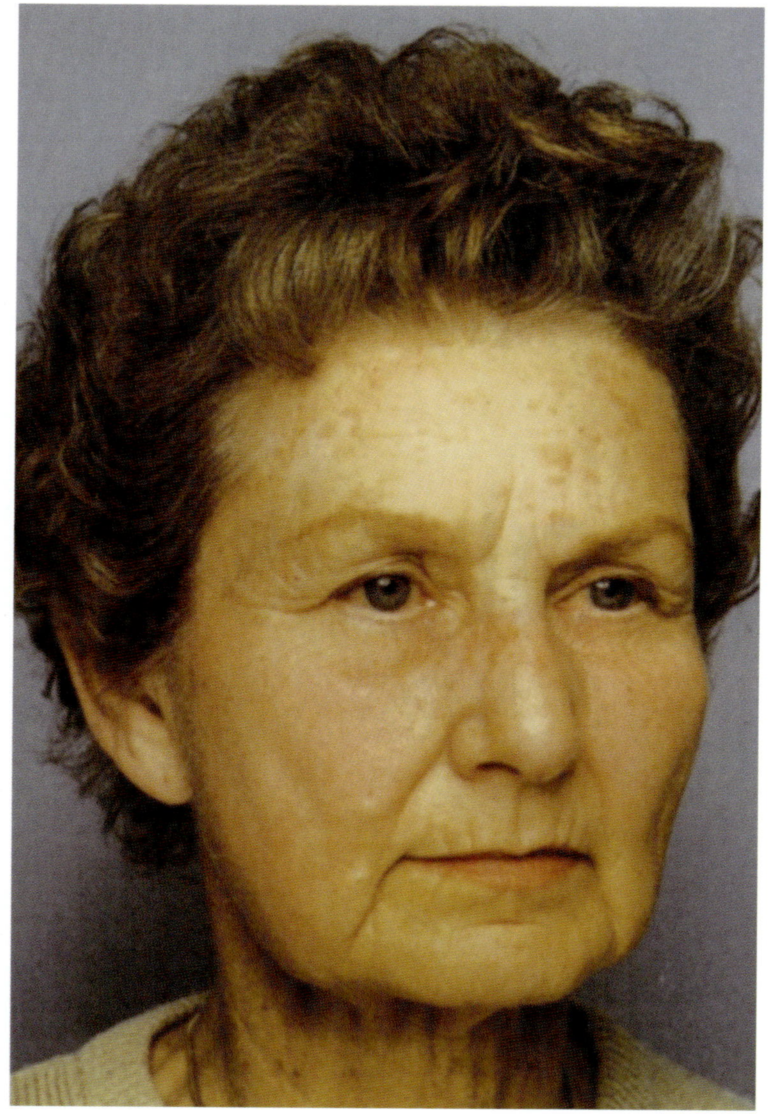

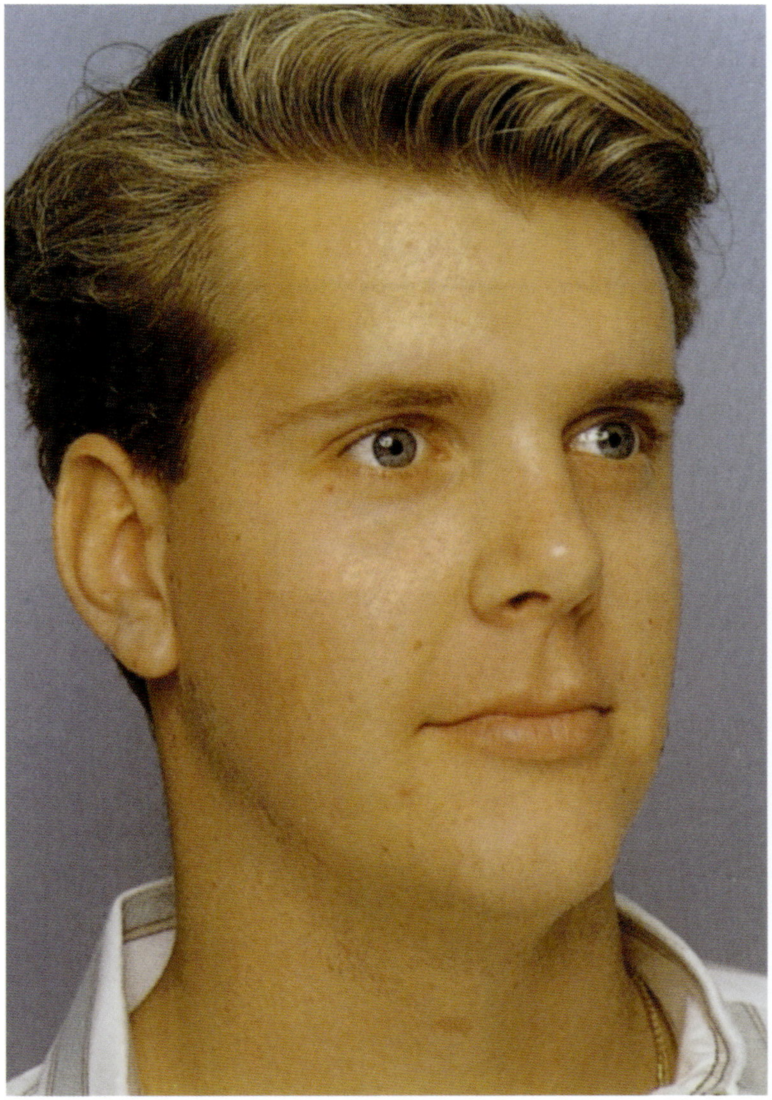

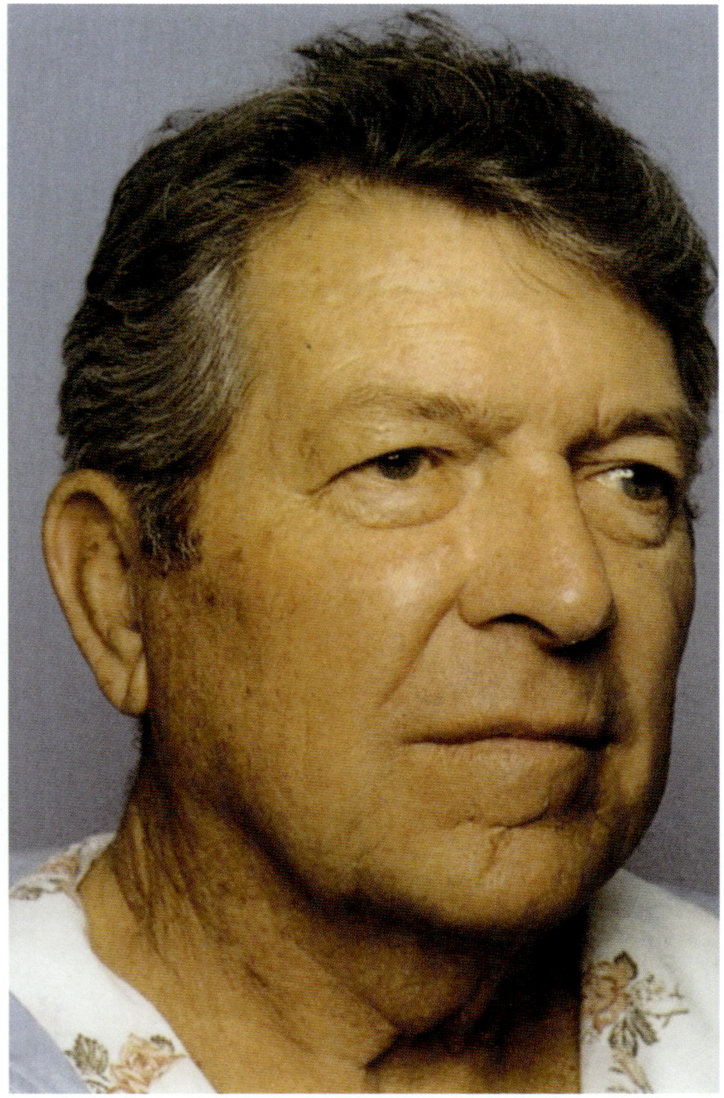

Whether it is designed to create beauty in the younger patient

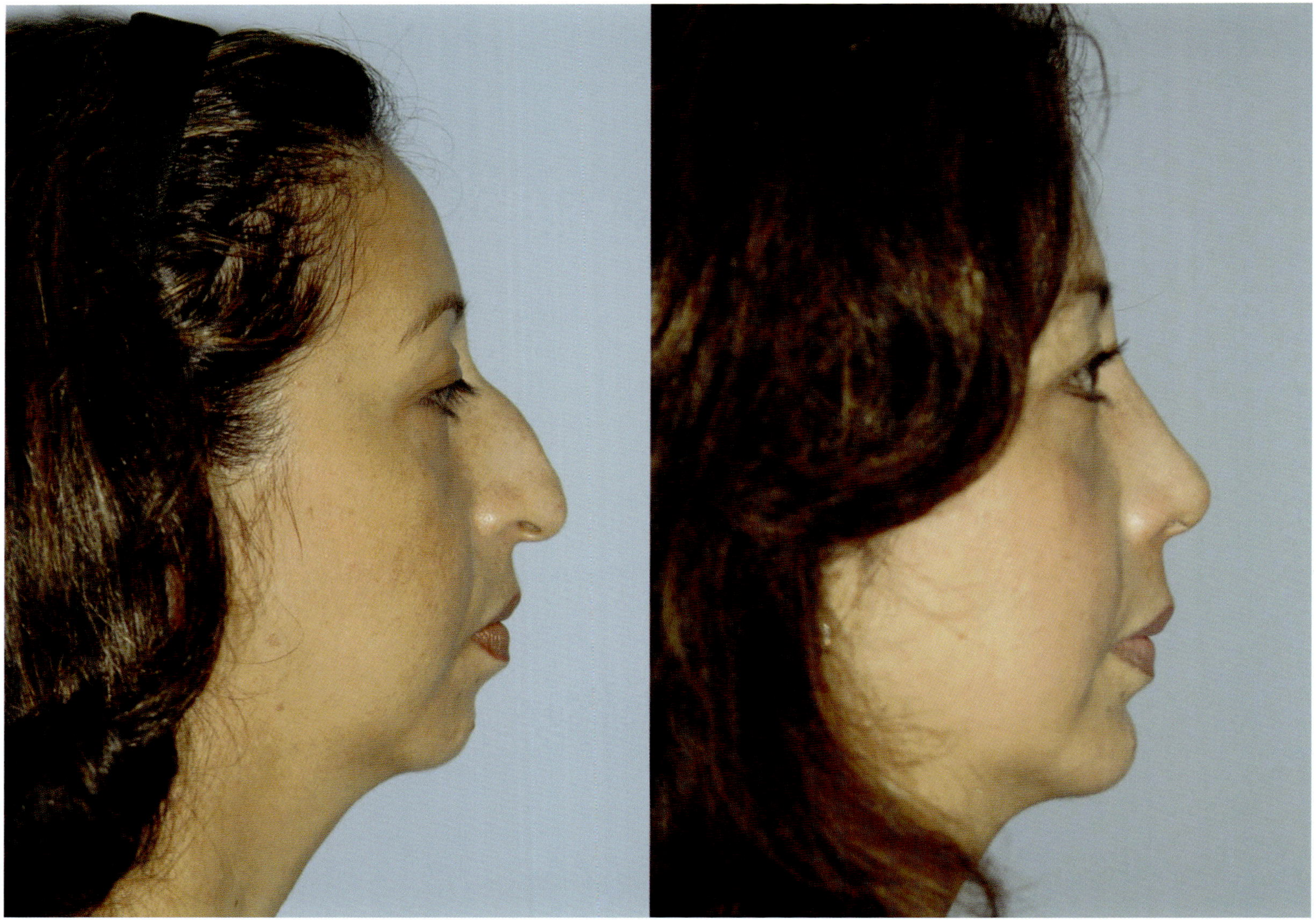

or to reverse the ravages of time in the mature patient.

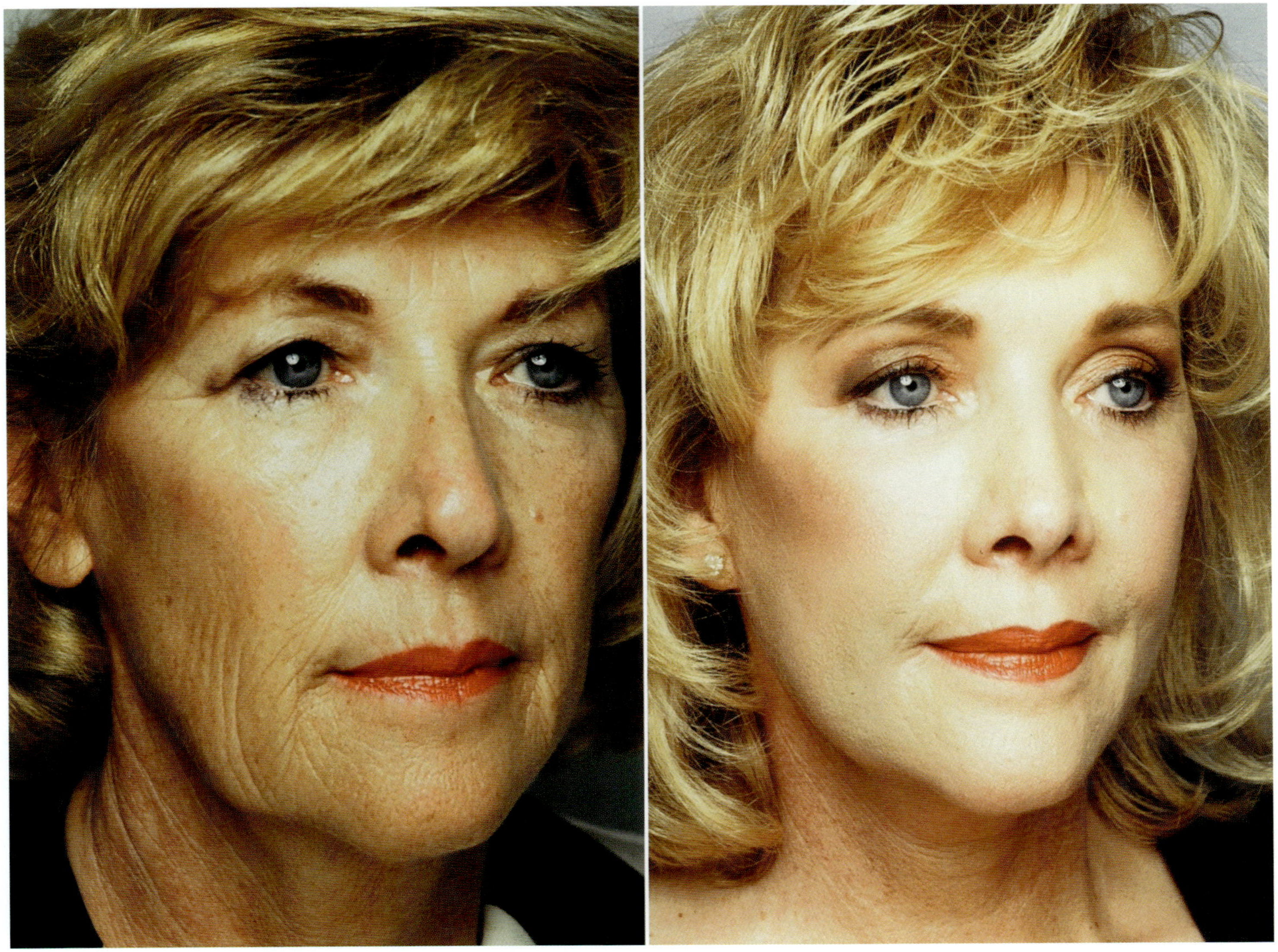

The Beauty Industry

By: Lisa McGill

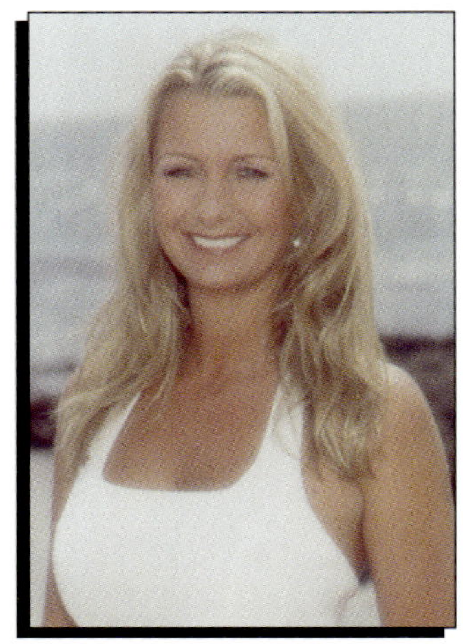

Beauty does better. It's a fact. In our society it is true that every culture has standards for physical attractiveness that can have a tremendous influence in many areas of our lives. Although we know that it is who we are in the inside that really counts, we can not ignore the fact that physical characteristics play a huge role in society. For example, forming personal relationships, being accepted into social groups and opening doors to careers and other opportunities are all predicated on our beauty. It is unrefuted that all things being equal.... Beauty breeds success.

The beauty industry knows this and that is why it is a multi-billion dollar industry, which starts influencing us as newborns. We are bombarded with images of beautiful babies, children and young adults starting with the Gerber baby.

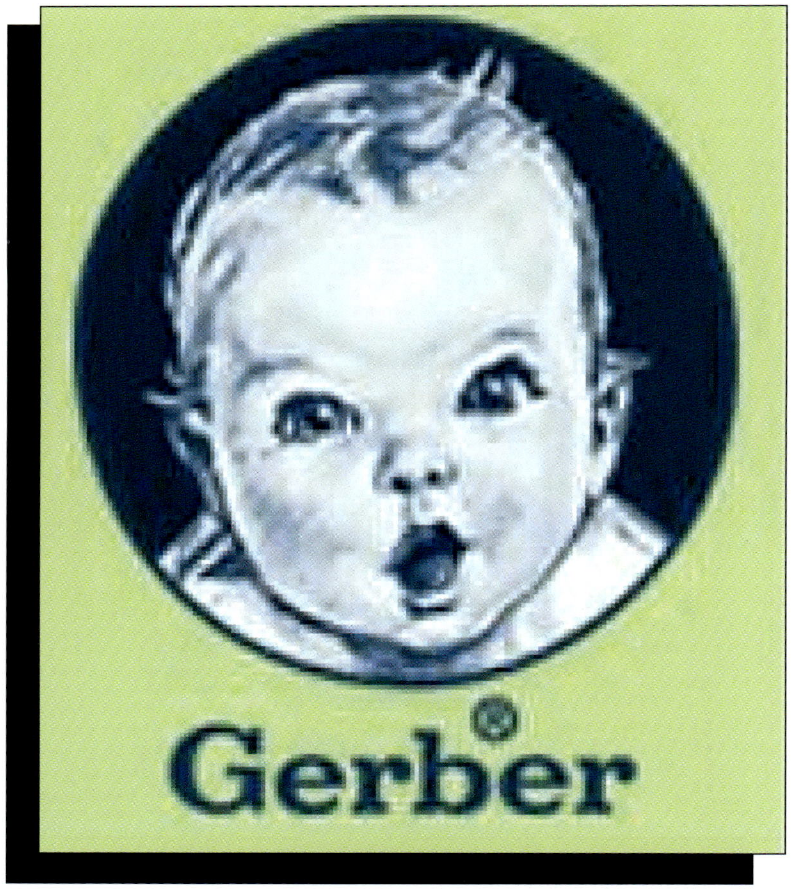

Beauty is especially relevant when we consider our children's future. Whether we like it or not, beauty can often mean the difference between acceptance and rejection in many situations. Have you ever seen an unattractive Prom Queen? Some parents have taken this to the extreme and the controversy over young girls in beauty pageants has grown. Many feel that these girls are being dressed up to look and act like adults and being made to be "Sexy too Soon."

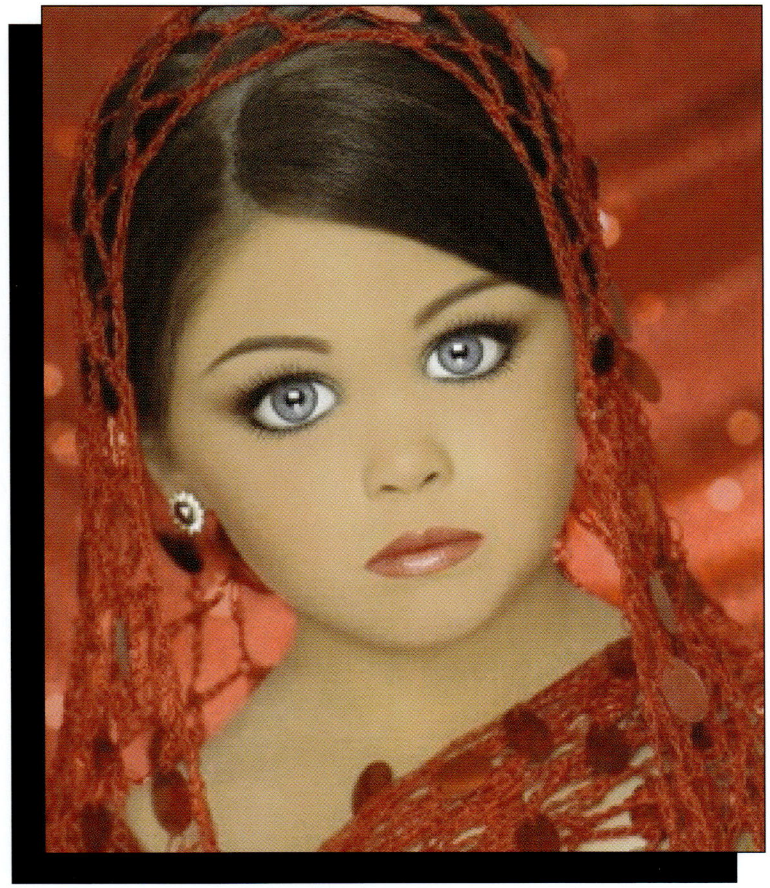

Have you ever stopped to think just how much money weekly/monthly/yearly you spend on beauty products? Whether it's getting your hair done, getting your nails manicured, buying clothing and make up……it adds up. On a daily basis we create beauty. Very few of us are blessed with natural beauty. Therefore, we must either create it daily or permanently with Cosmetic Surgery. We are consistently reminded of the many cosmetic procedures and options available to us, whether it's Britney Spears breast augmentation or your best friend having her nose done. People of all ages are recognizing that cosmetic surgery is increasingly more accepted among women and men. You can find study after study that focus on which waist-to-hip ratios or facial features people find most attractive, and these studies have captured society's attention. Many of us today are not content to "grow old gracefully" and that is why we have written this book; to help society become better educated.

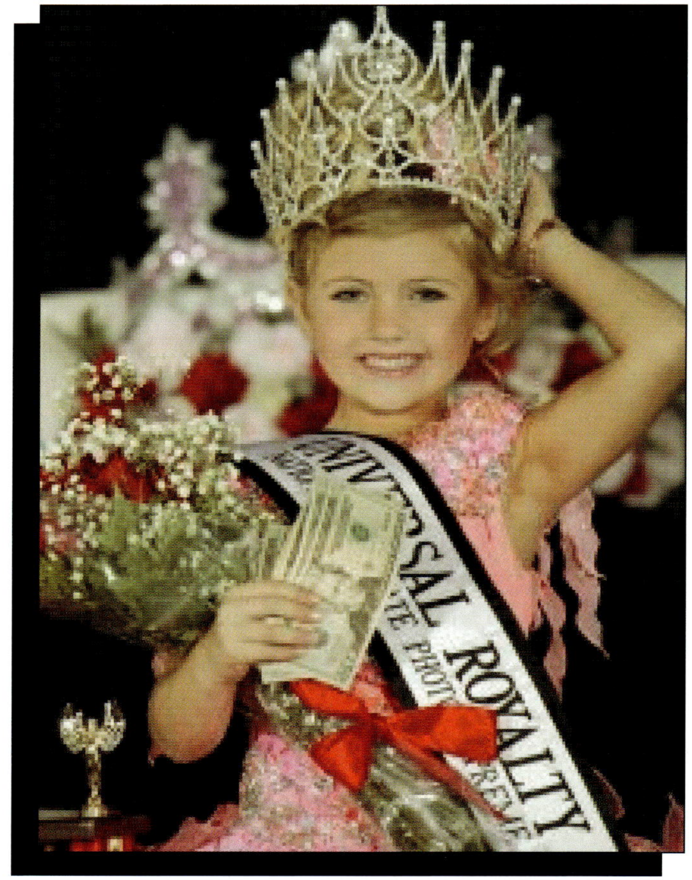

Modern Society's answer to growing old gracefully is to have cosmetic surgery.

The Universal Royalty, Miss Teen USA , Miss USA, Miss Universe, Mrs. America and Mrs. World are some of the most popular beauty pageants that have us intrigued by the world of beauty and glamour.

Dr. Brennan,

Thank you for everything! You have opened a lot of doors for me! Thanks for the #1 care!

-Nadia Moeller

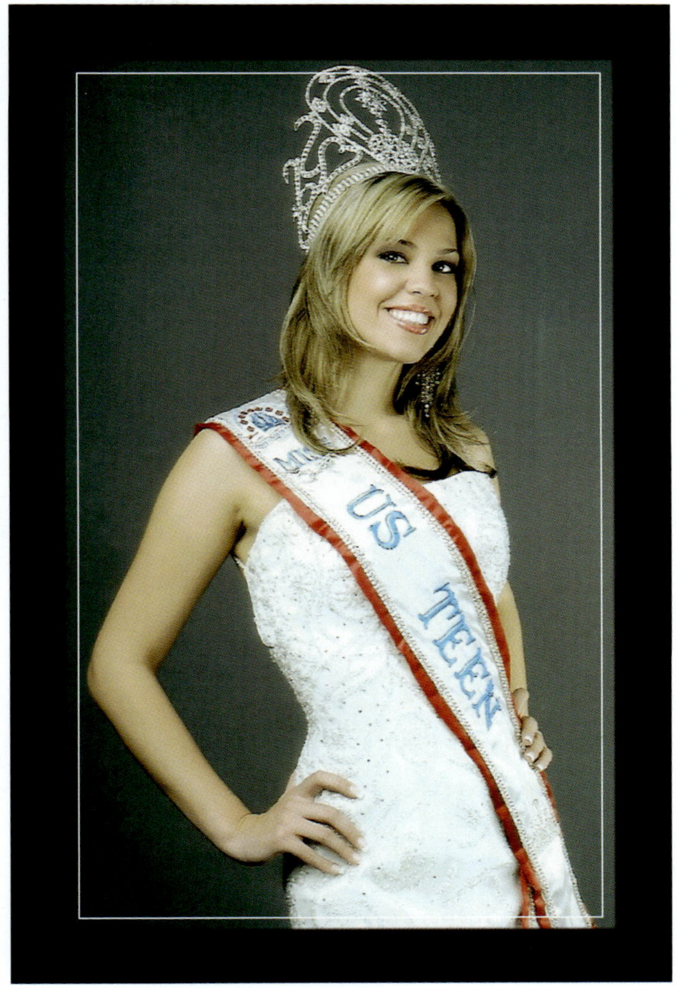

Miss US Teen 06-07 - Nadia Moeller

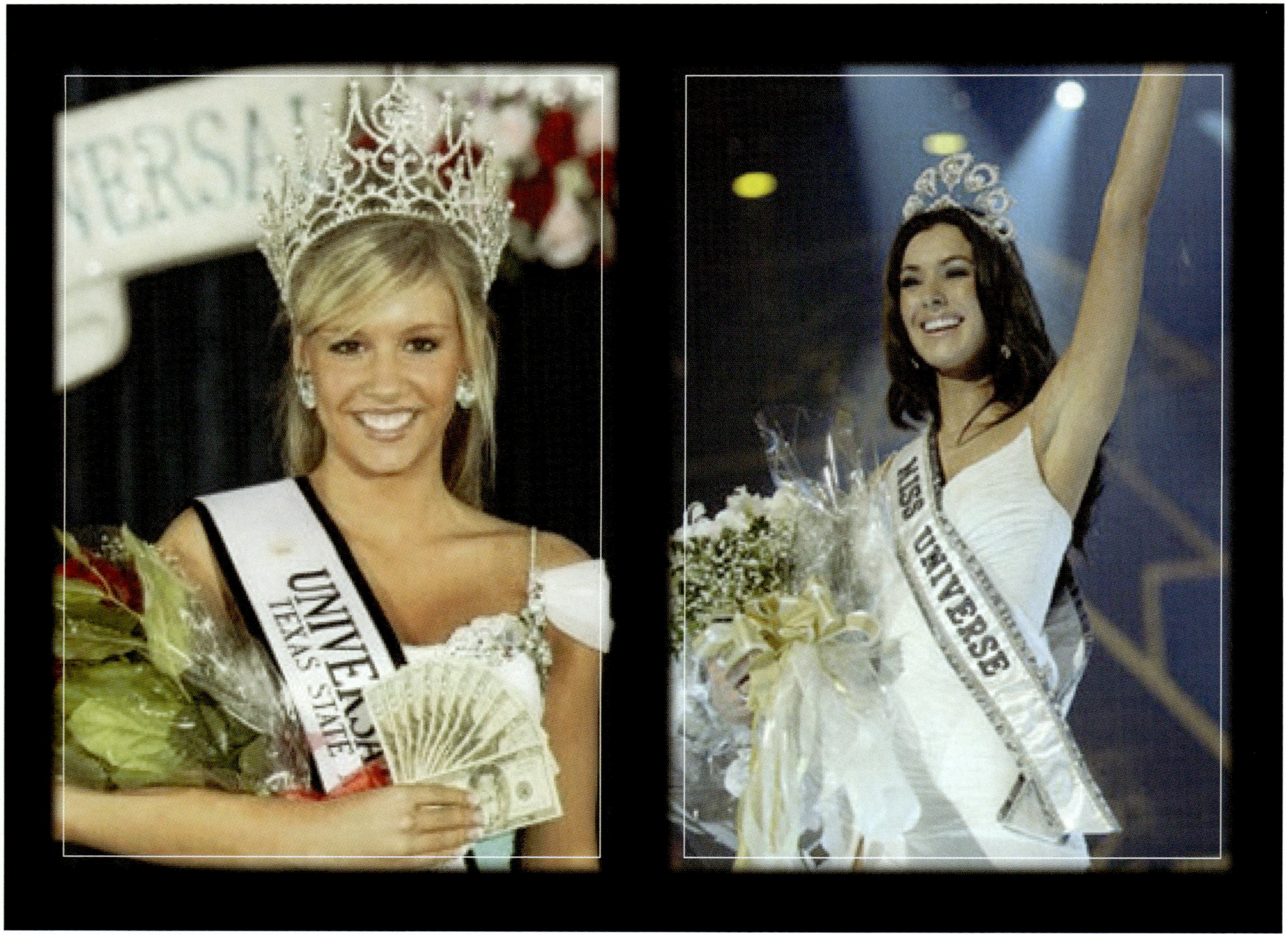

Miss Universe

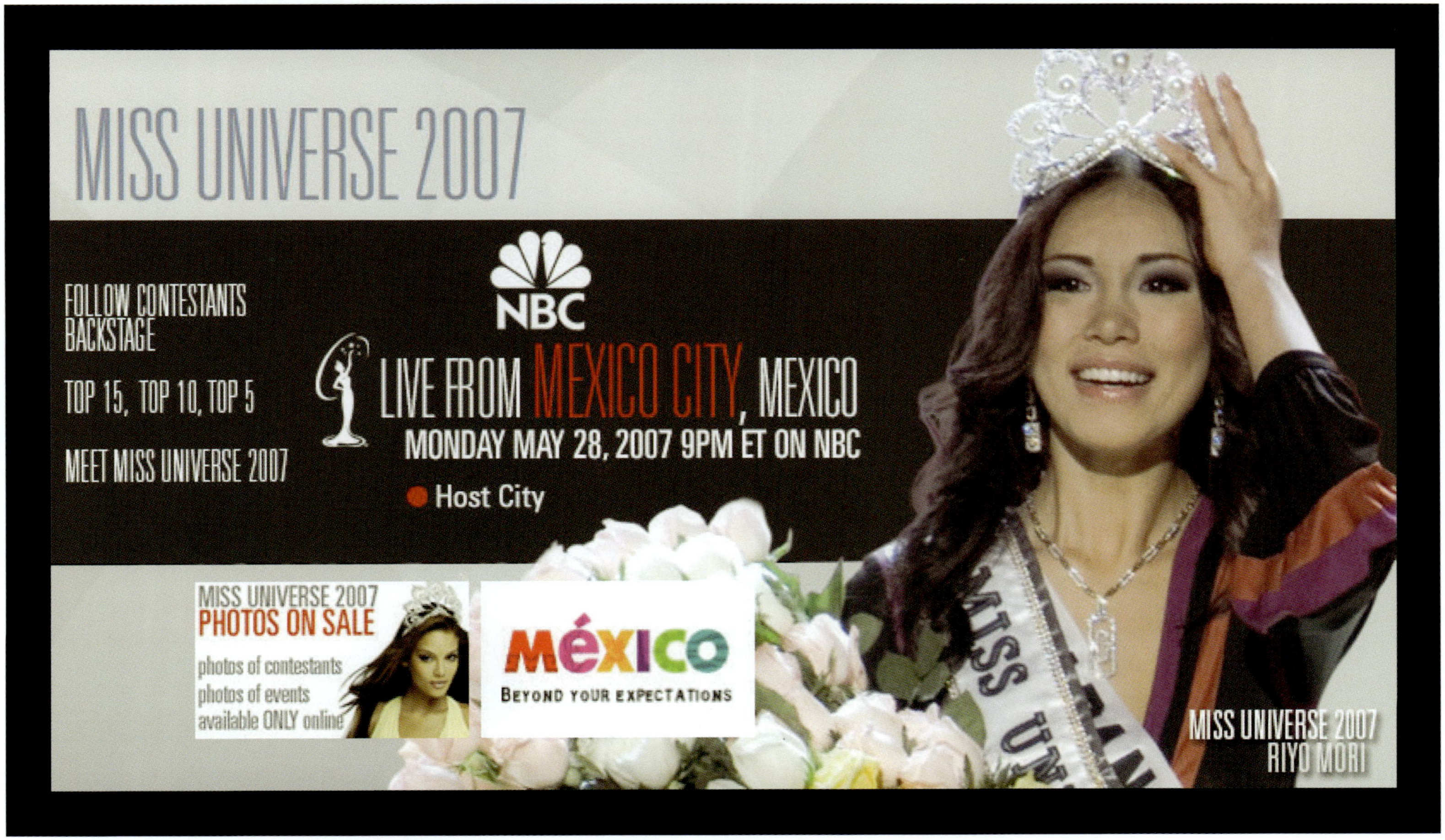

Miss Universe 2007 - Ryo Mori

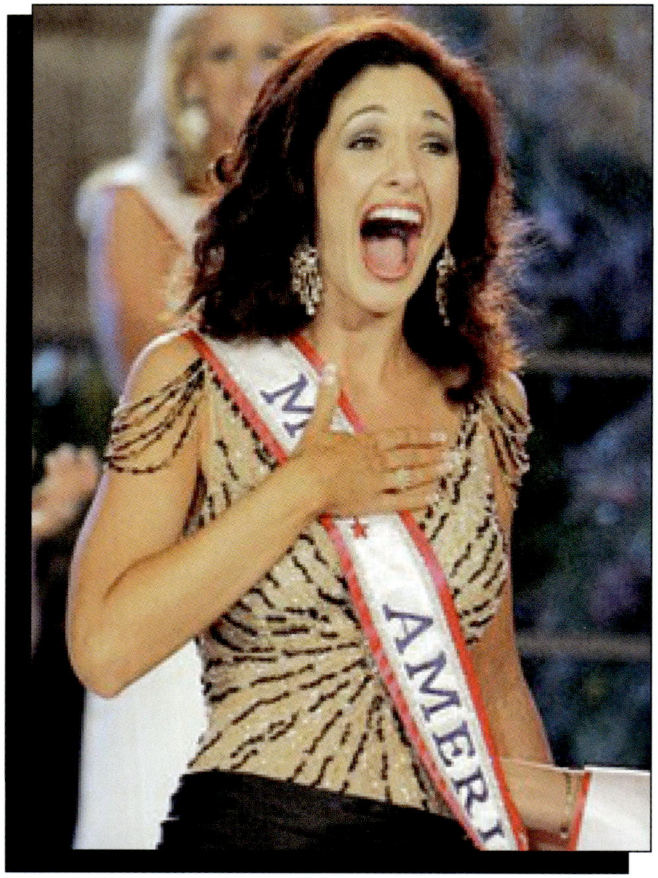

Mrs. America

Consultation with the Cosmetic Surgeon "Am I ready?"

By: H. George Brennan, MD, FACS

Consultation with the Cosmetic Surgeon "Am I ready?"

The patient should take the consultation with the cosmetic surgeon very seriously. They have to realize that cosmetic surgery is unlike common medicine.

Cosmetic surgery is simply a desire based on a psychological need to look better. The patient is void of illness, injury, or disease.

Cosmetic surgery is strictly elective.

Cosmetic surgeons can explore various possibilities with the prospective patient using either the mirror, photographic examples or by simulating results on the computer.

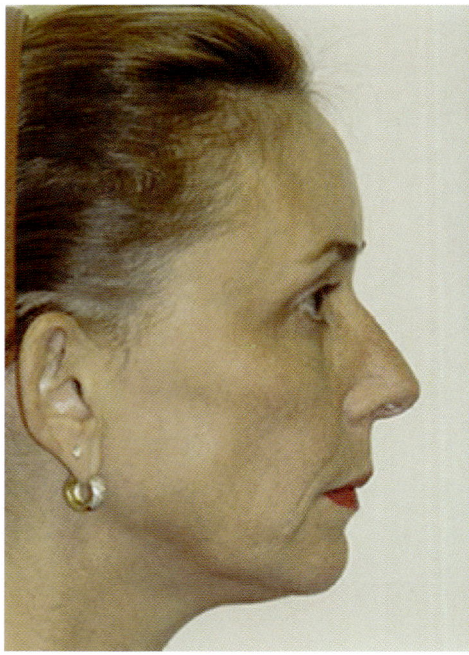

Before

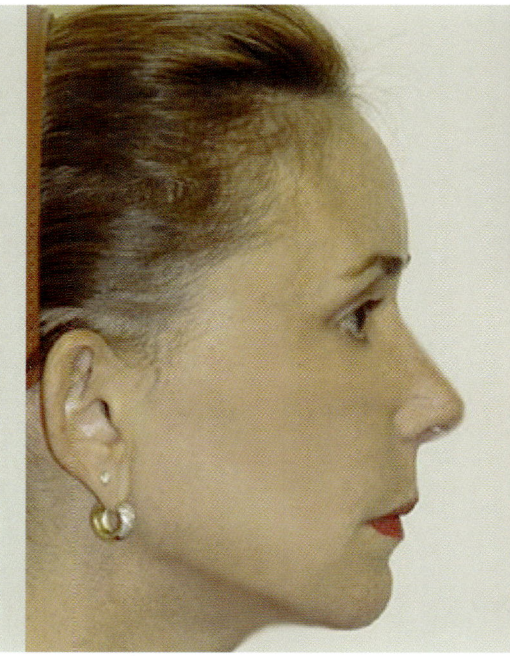

Simulated Results

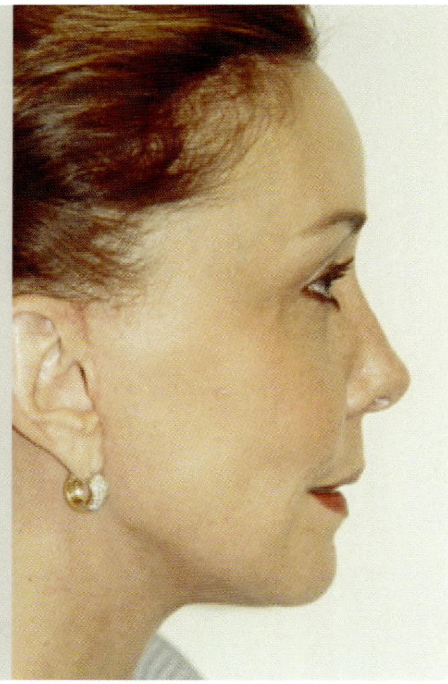

Actual Results

The patient must then understand their own body and appearance. They have to know realistically what can, and more importantly, what cannot be achieved. They must know what to expect before, during and after surgery. They must know the upside and potential downside including potential complications.

They must study all aspects, obtain advice from their core support group, consult their mirror and make their individual decision. In the final analysis this is simply an elective decision made between the patient and the mirror. The mirror guides and dictates the patient's decision. Once that decision is made, the cosmetic surgery is performed in an attempt to achieve the best possible results.

The cosmetic surgeon has often been referred to as the psychiatrist with a scalpel.

Consultation with the Cosmetic Surgeon "Am I ready?"

In facial cosmetic surgery, patients must understand that there are basically three realms. They present with conditions that will respond to;

1. *Surgery*
2. *Relaxing over active muscles of facial expression*
3. *Reversing sun damaged skin*

Even though the three are inter-related the patient needs to separate their conditions and the treatments.

The patient must also realize that the surgeon is, from a technical standpoint, dealing with four anatomical elements.

1. *The skeletal framework*
2. *The muscle*
3. *The fat layer between the skin and the muscle*
4. *The skin*

In facial cosmetic surgery any given patient may require any or all of these procedures
(see example on page 46)

Preparing for Surgery

On the initial consultation the patients medical history including any previous illnesses, adverse social habits, allergies, medications and previous surgeries must be revealed.

The general physical examination and the examination of the specific areas in question will be performed.

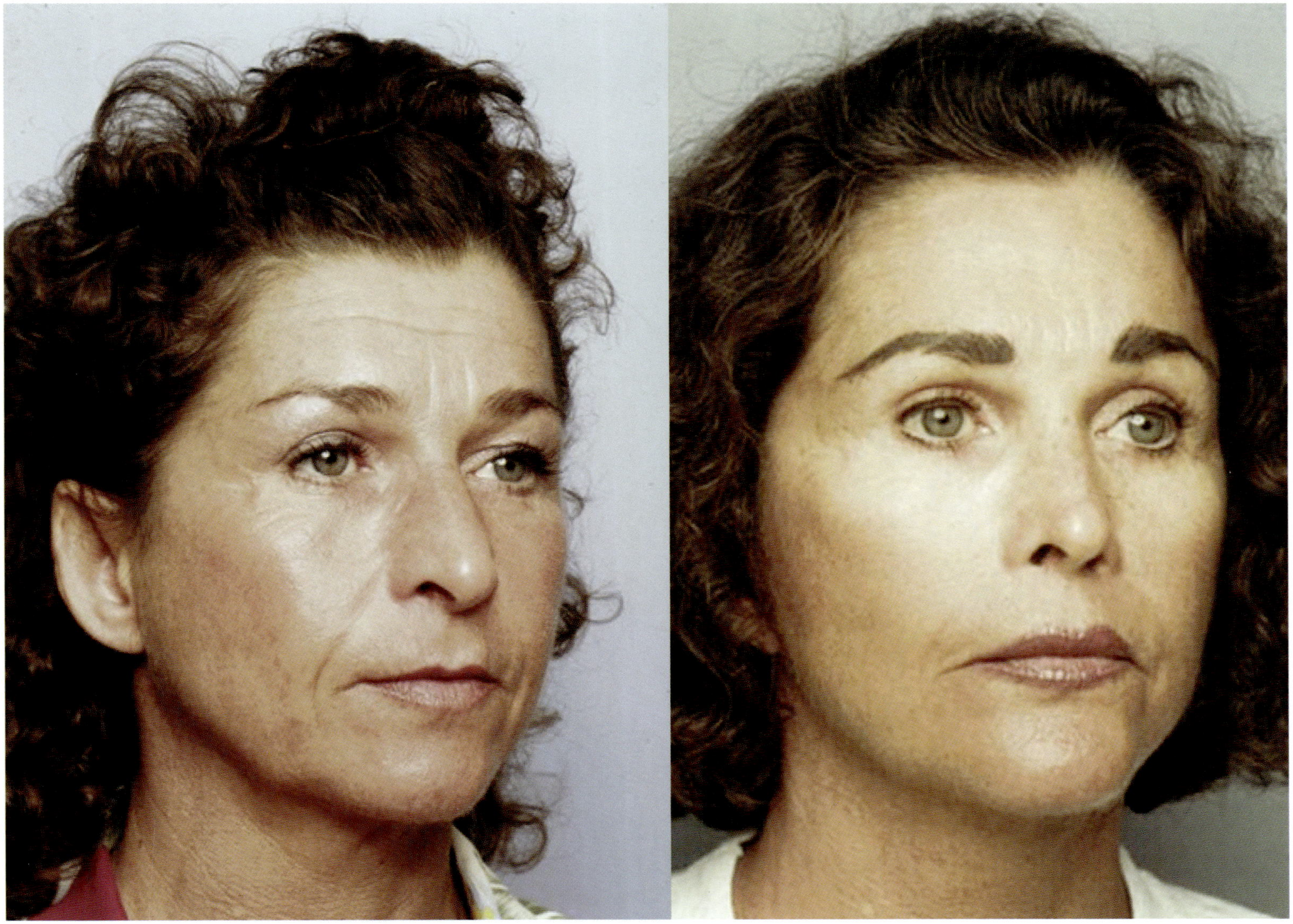

Example of a patient improved by treating all four anatomical elements including

1. The skeletal framework 2. The muscle 3. The fat layer between the skin and the muscle 4. The skin

Consultation with the Cosmetic Surgeon "Am I ready?"

Any appropriate diagnostic studies will be recommended including blood, EKG's and urine tests, possible x-rays and on occasion, more sophisticated diagnostic studies. It is sometimes necessary to consult with the patient's current treating physicians. Consultations with other doctors may also be necessary.

You will be given extensive consents that will inform you of all the likely as well as the unlikely possible results from cosmetic surgery.

The good news is that in cosmetic surgery the four most common conditions that occur are;

1. *Temporary Bruising*
2. *Temporary Swelling*
3. *Delayed Healing*
4. *Scar*

While other conditions and complications can occur they are unusual.

Day of Surgery

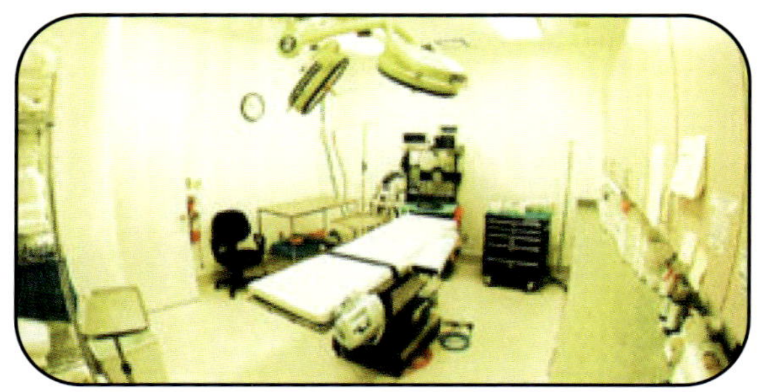

Most commonly cosmetic surgery is performed in an outpatient-accredited facility. It is very important to refrain for eating and drinking after midnight the day prior to surgery. Normal hygiene and no cosmetics are recommended the morning of surgery. The patient is to wear comfortable casual clothing, and preferably bring no valuable possessions. On admission, a review of the procedures is performed and intravenous established and various monitors are placed on the patient.

Consultation with the Cosmetic Surgeon "Am I ready?"

Anesthesia varies depending on the complexity of the procedure. In any case, the anesthesia is extremely safe. The patients are safer, statistically, in the accredited facility under anesthesia than they are in their vehicles driving to the facility.

There are four levels of anesthesia:

1. *Local*
2. *Conscious sedation*
3. *Unconscious sedation*
4. *General*

Methods of anesthesia are a decision that is made between the anesthesiologist and the patient. All aspects of anesthesia are discussed thoroughly with the patient. All of this is with the concurrence of the operating surgeon.

On completion of the surgical procedure the appropriate dressings are applied and the patient is transferred to the recovery room for close monitoring.

Once the patient has recovered from the anesthesia, which is usually less than an hour in duration, a decision is made either to discharge the patient to a care giver of their own choice or the patient has the option to stay overnight in the facility under nurse observation.

The following morning - the dressings are removed, appropriate sutures are removed, the hair is shampooed and the patient is then discharged with the appropriate instructions and advice.

Patients are allowed to resume their personal hygiene, non-strenuous activities and normal diet, even the day after surgery.

Consultation with the Cosmetic Surgeon "Am I ready?"

During the first week the patients follow their normal daily hygiene routine and are to engage in their normal daily activities.

The expectation is that within a week the patient can be out in public without a stranger recognizing their surgery. In a week, the patient will likely be presentable but not perfect. They themselves will recognize that they are still healing but it is uncommon for a stranger to recognize that the patient has recently had surgery performed.

The patient continues to improve as times goes on. However, patients must understand while they and the surgeon have common goals it is possible for them to have;

1. *Temporary bruising*
2. *Temporary swelling*
3. *Delayed healing*
4. *Unusual scar formation*

All of these conditions are possible but not probable. With time all of these conditions improve.
It is important to monitor the incisional healing in case that scar tissue develops. While problematic scars may occur, they are unusual and usually treatable.

The ultimate desire of the patient and doctor alike is to have satisfactory results, minimal inconvenience and a happy and healthy patient who has achieved their goal in looking better and feeling much better about themselves.

Patients must understand the pros and cons and if in their mind the anticipated improvement out weighs the negatives, (time, expense, risks, inconvenience, etc) then and only then and with the concurrence of their mirror should they choose elective surgery.

Private Patients - Head to Toe

HAIR RESTORATION

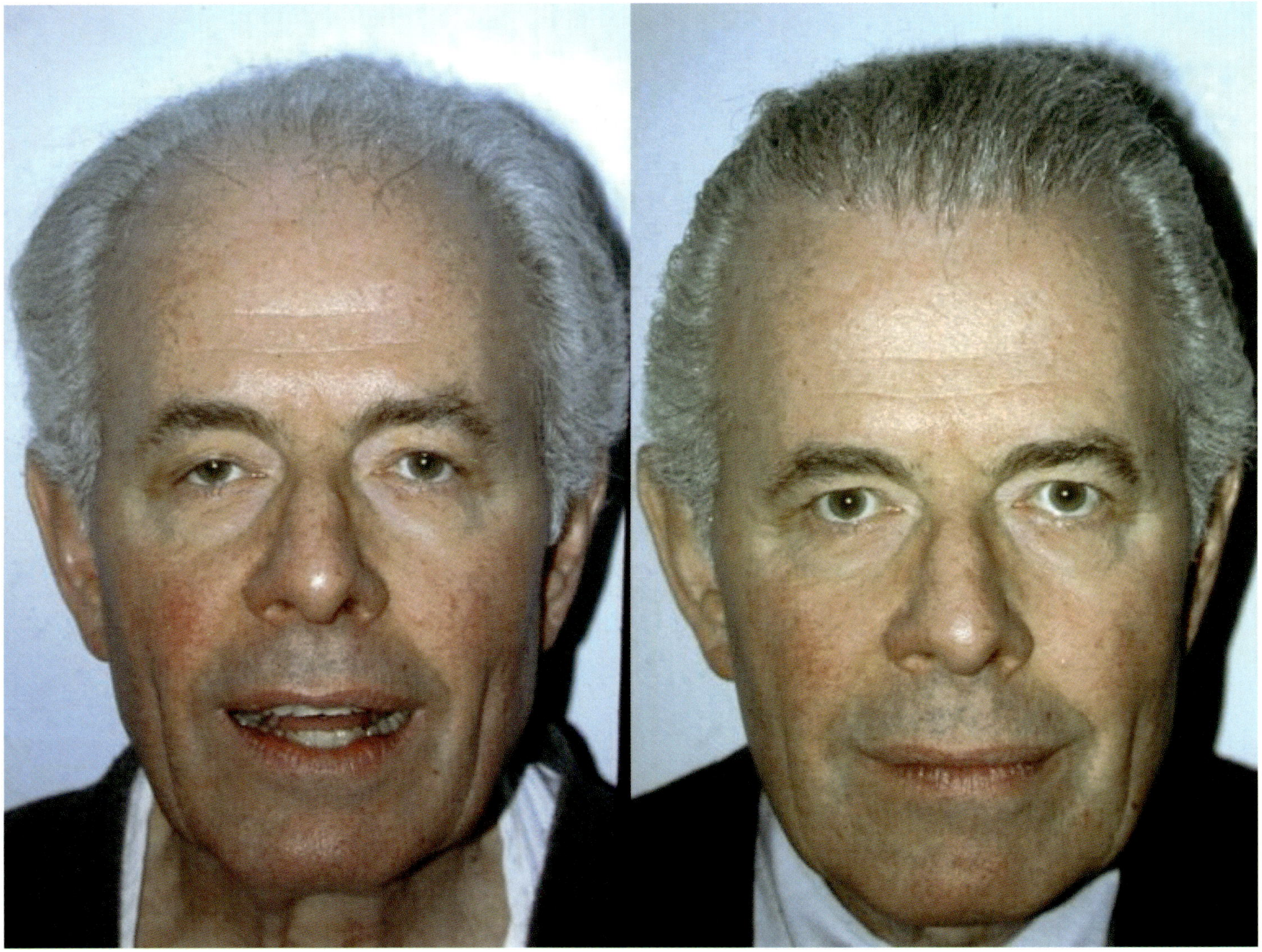

Courtesy of Dr. Sheldon Kabaker, MD
www.kabaker.com

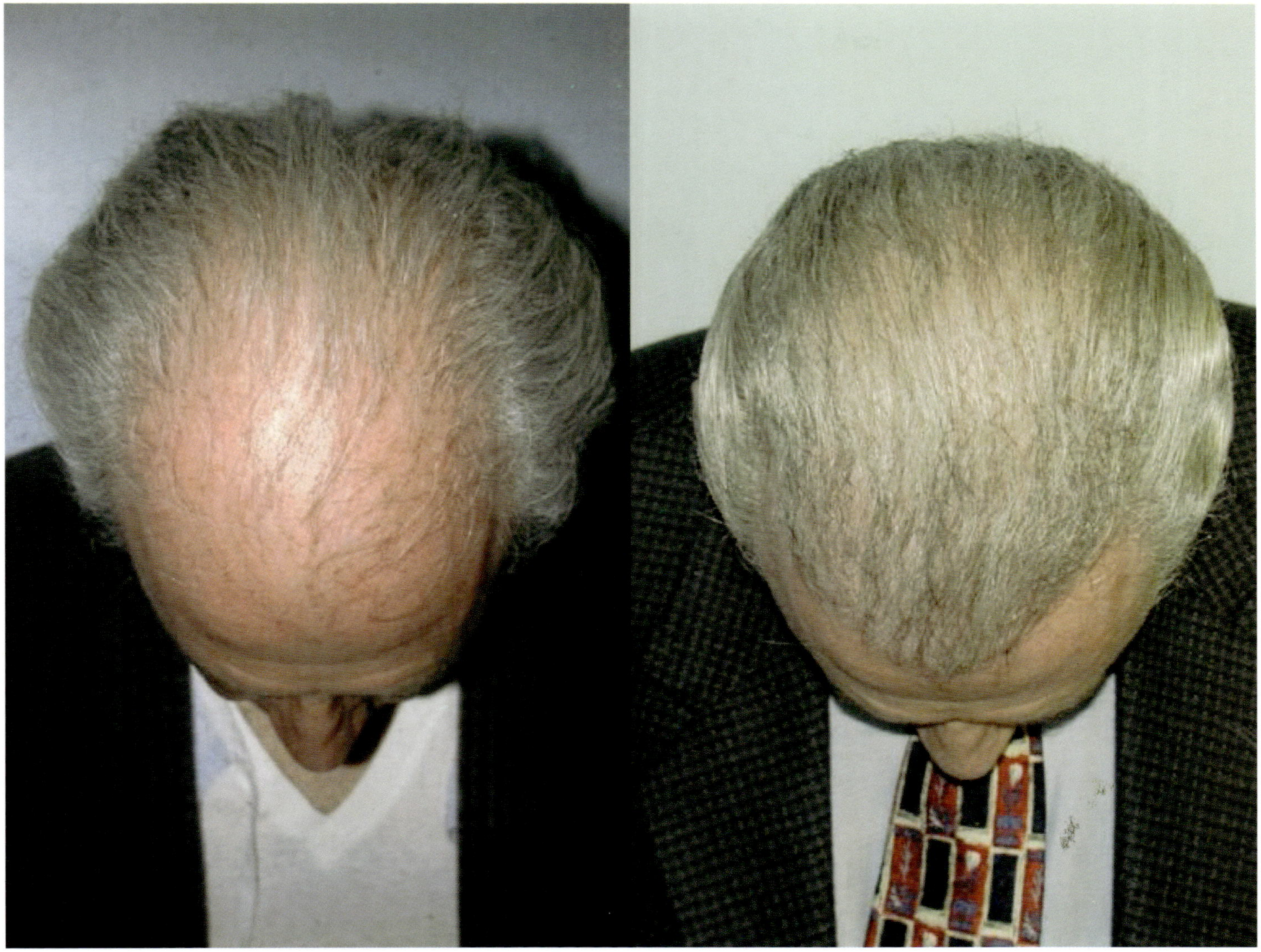

Courtesy of Dr. Sheldon Kabaker, MD
www.kabaker.com

For patients concerned with a high or tall forehead (usually women) a hairline lowering procedure works quickly and efficiently.

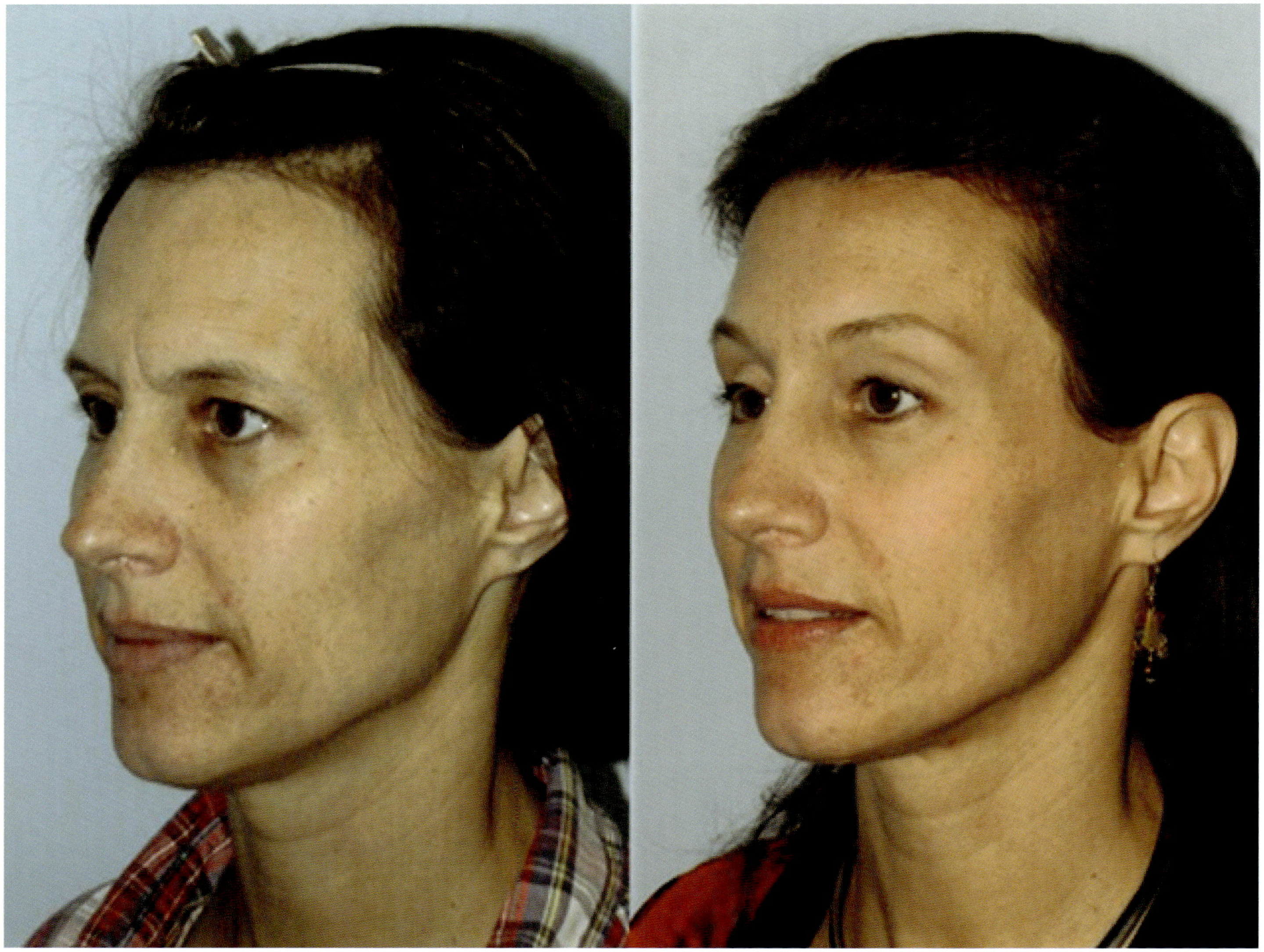

Courtesy of Dr. Sheldon Kabaker, MD
www.kabaker.com

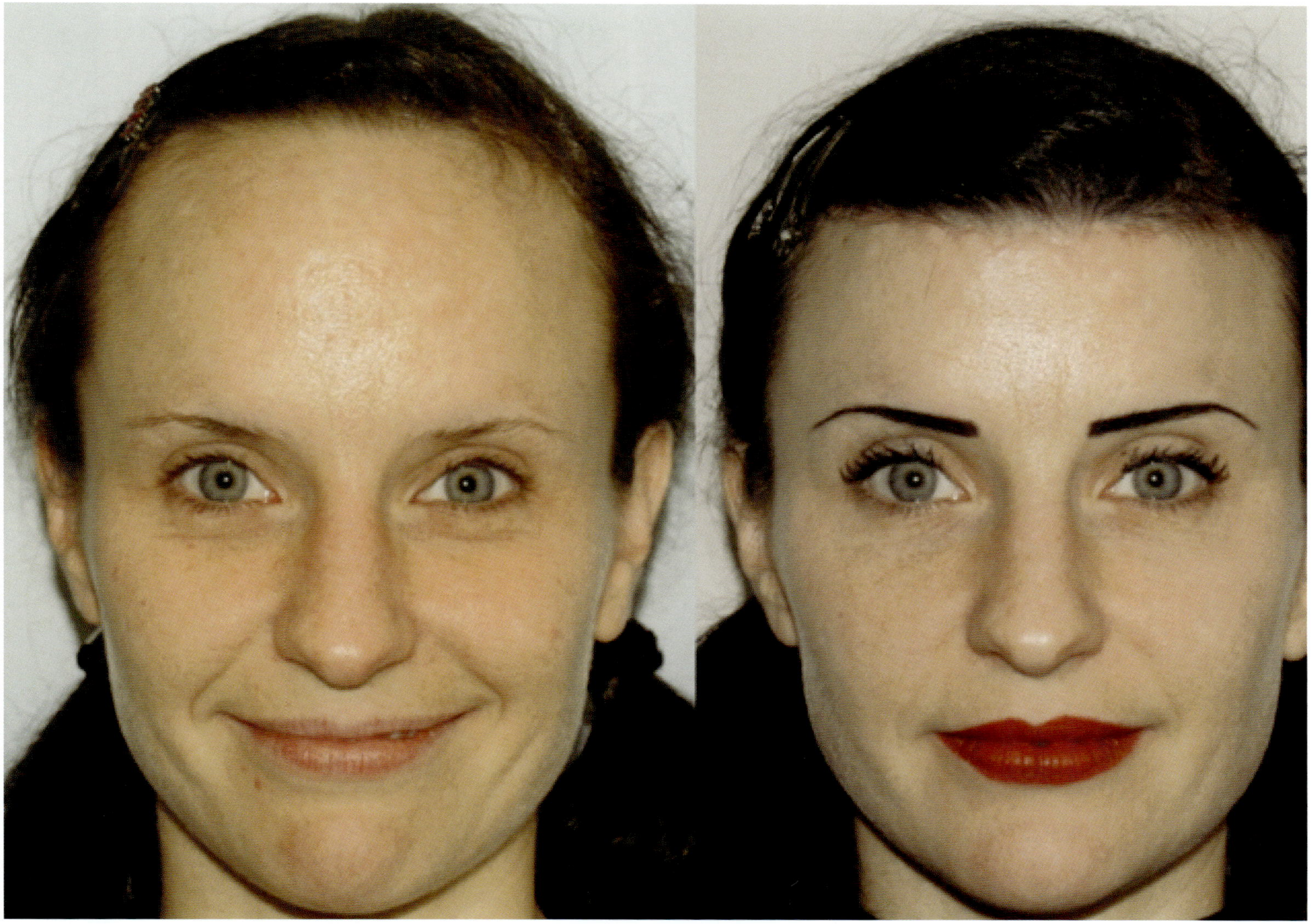

Courtesy of Dr. Sheldon Kabaker, MD
www.kabaker.com

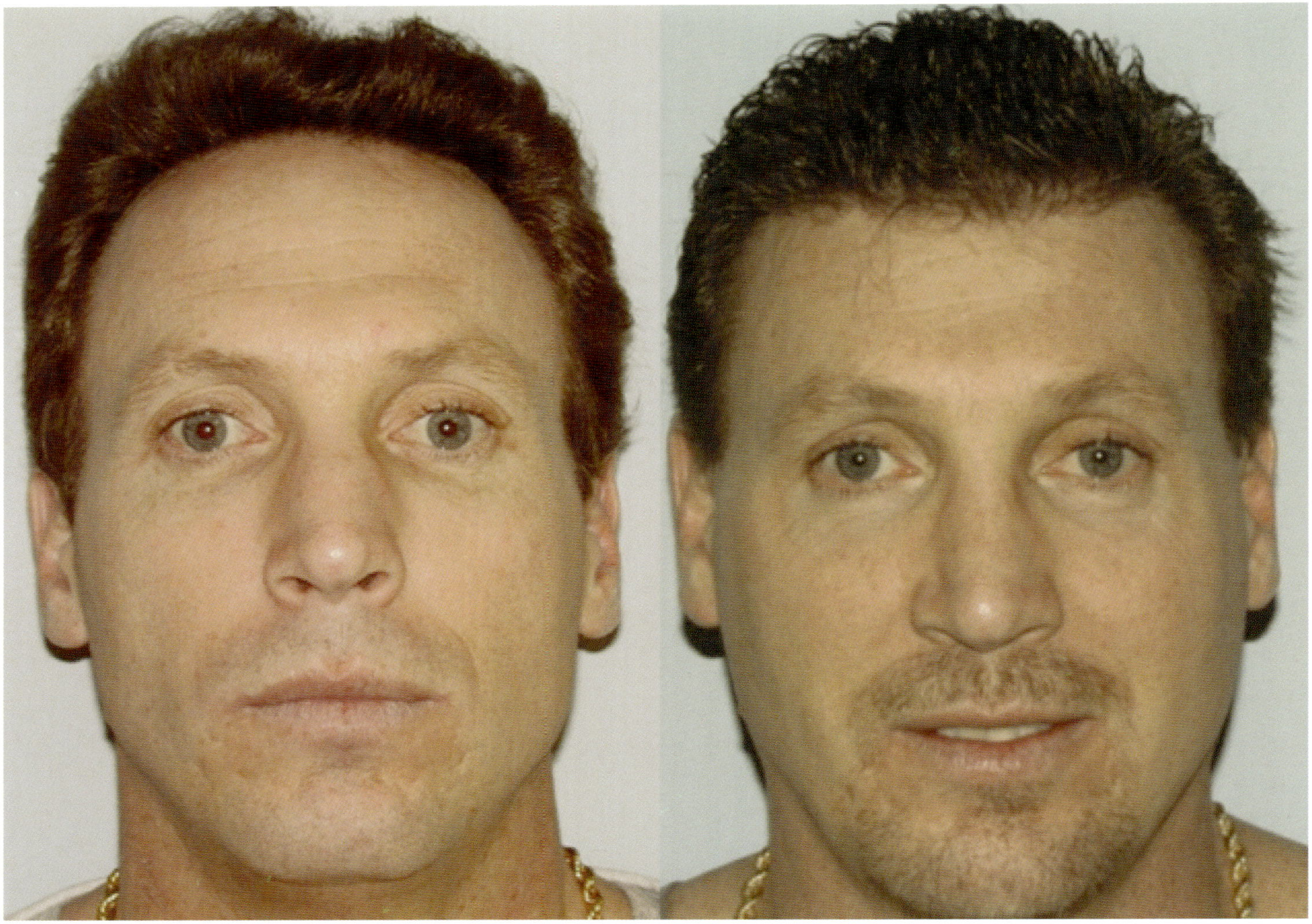

Courtesy of Dr. Sheldon Kabaker, MD
www.kabaker.com

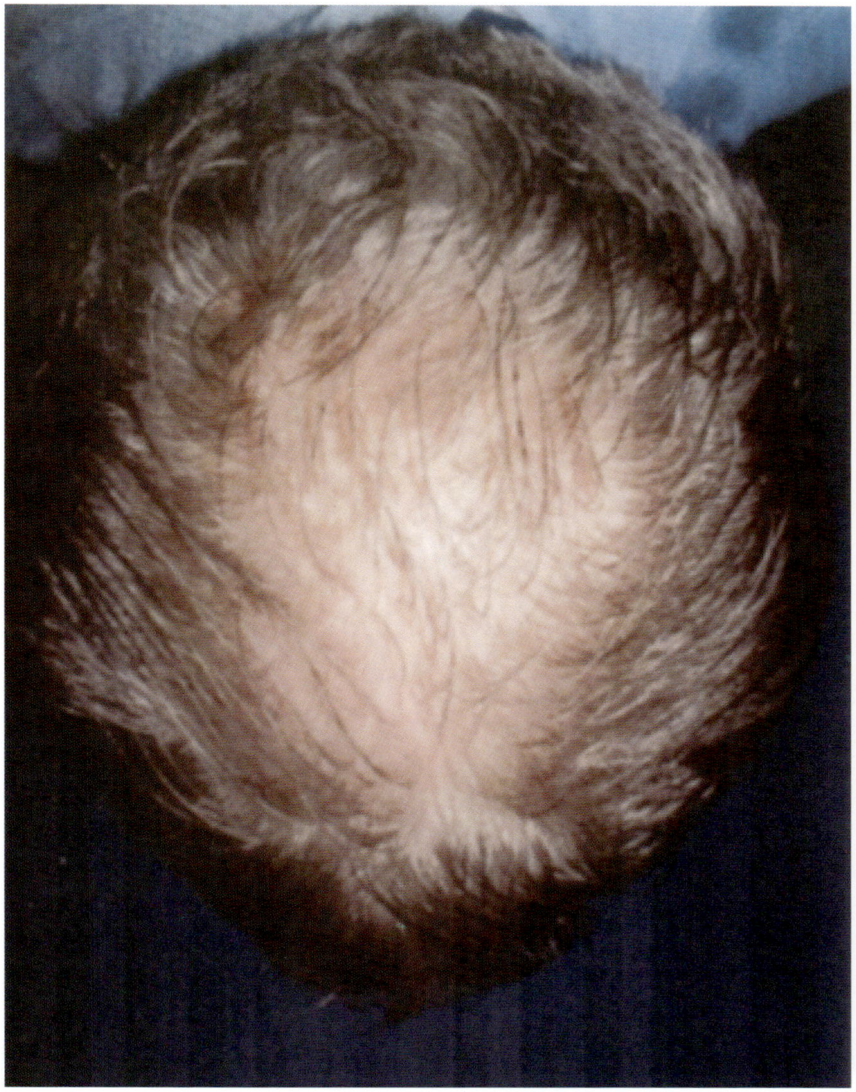

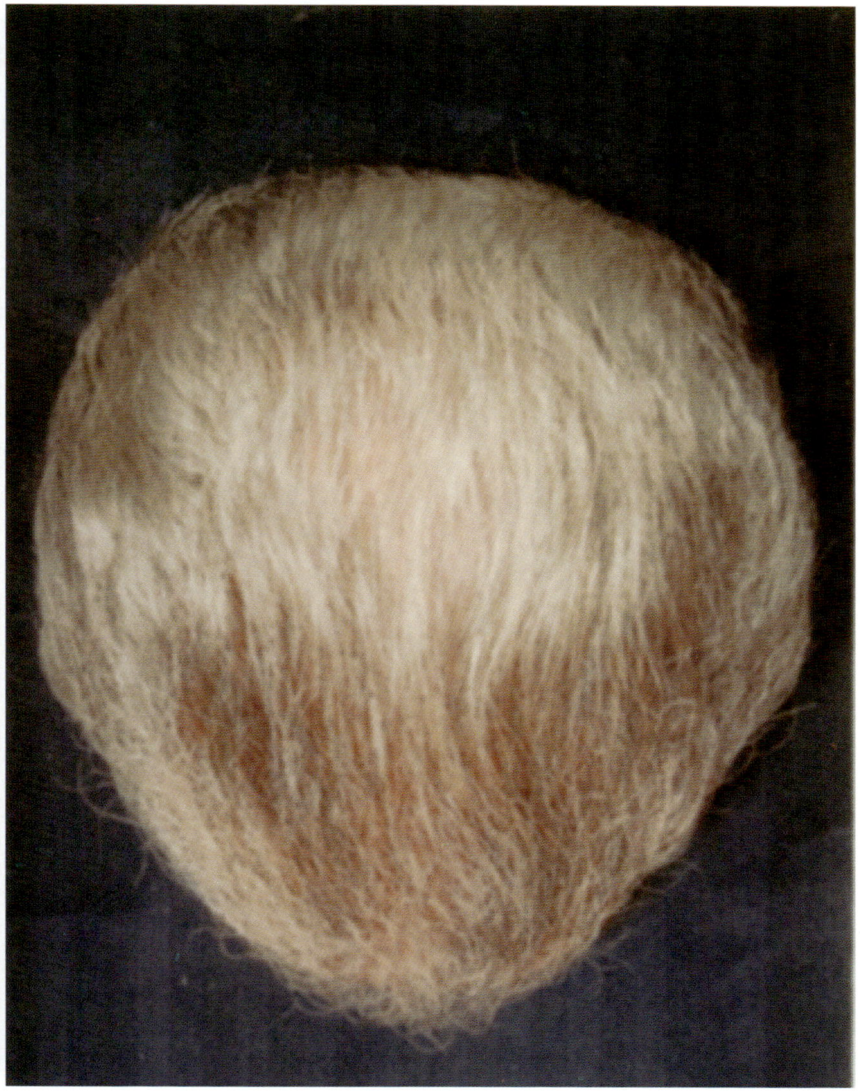

Courtesy of Dr. Robert Cattani, MD
www.drcattani.com

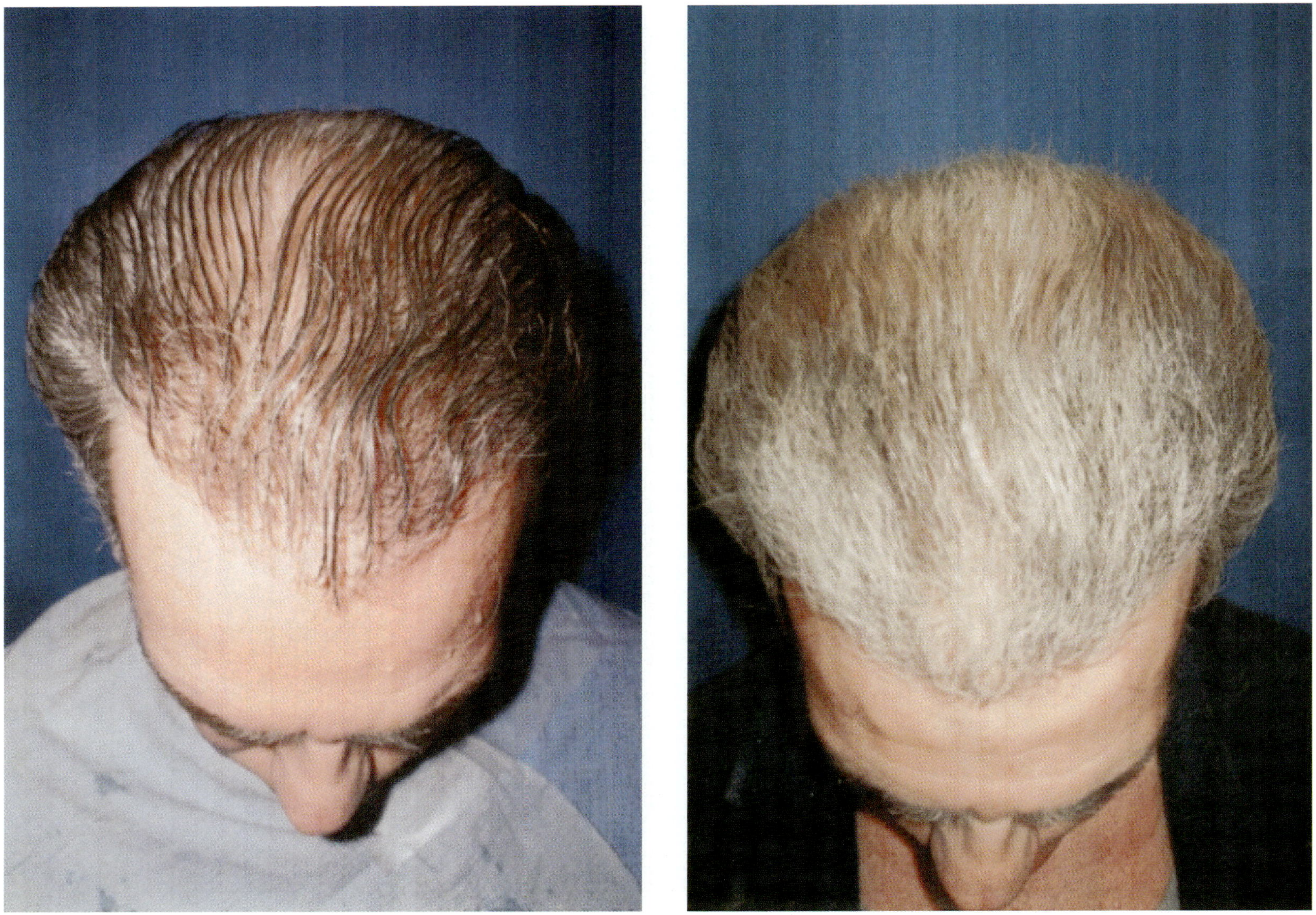

Courtesy of Dr. Robert Cattani, MD
www.drcattani.com

POSITIONING PROTRUDING EARS

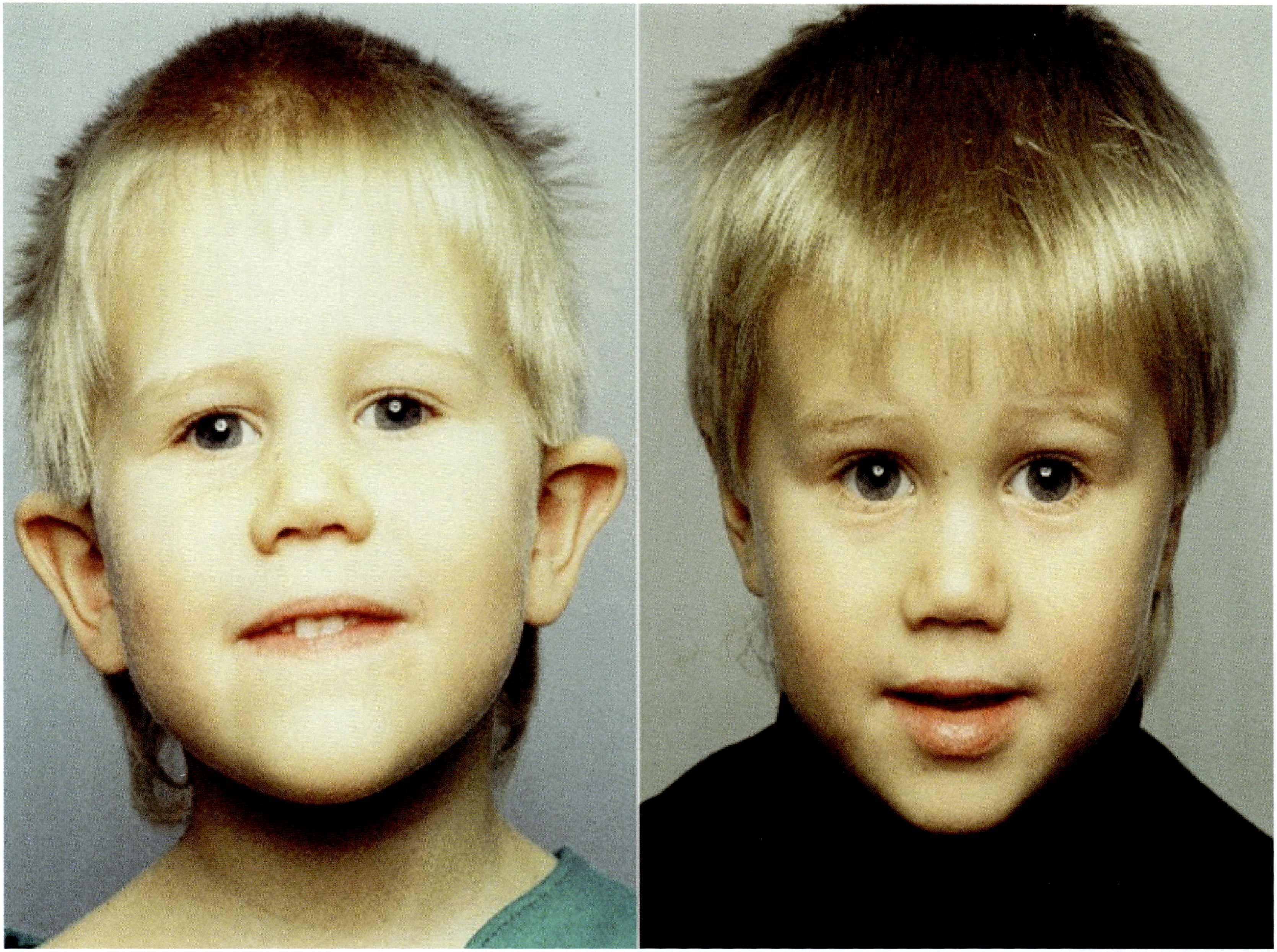

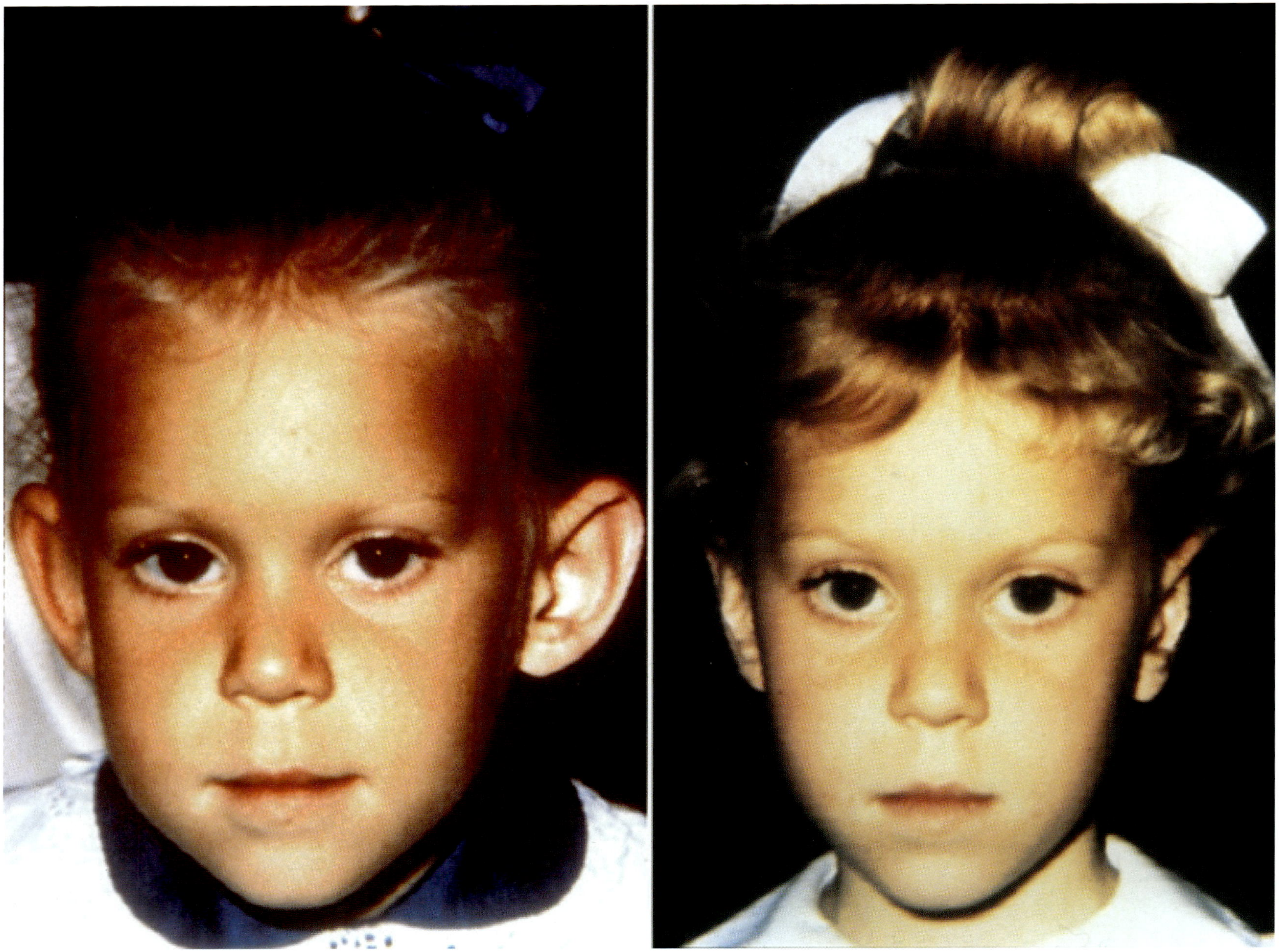

59

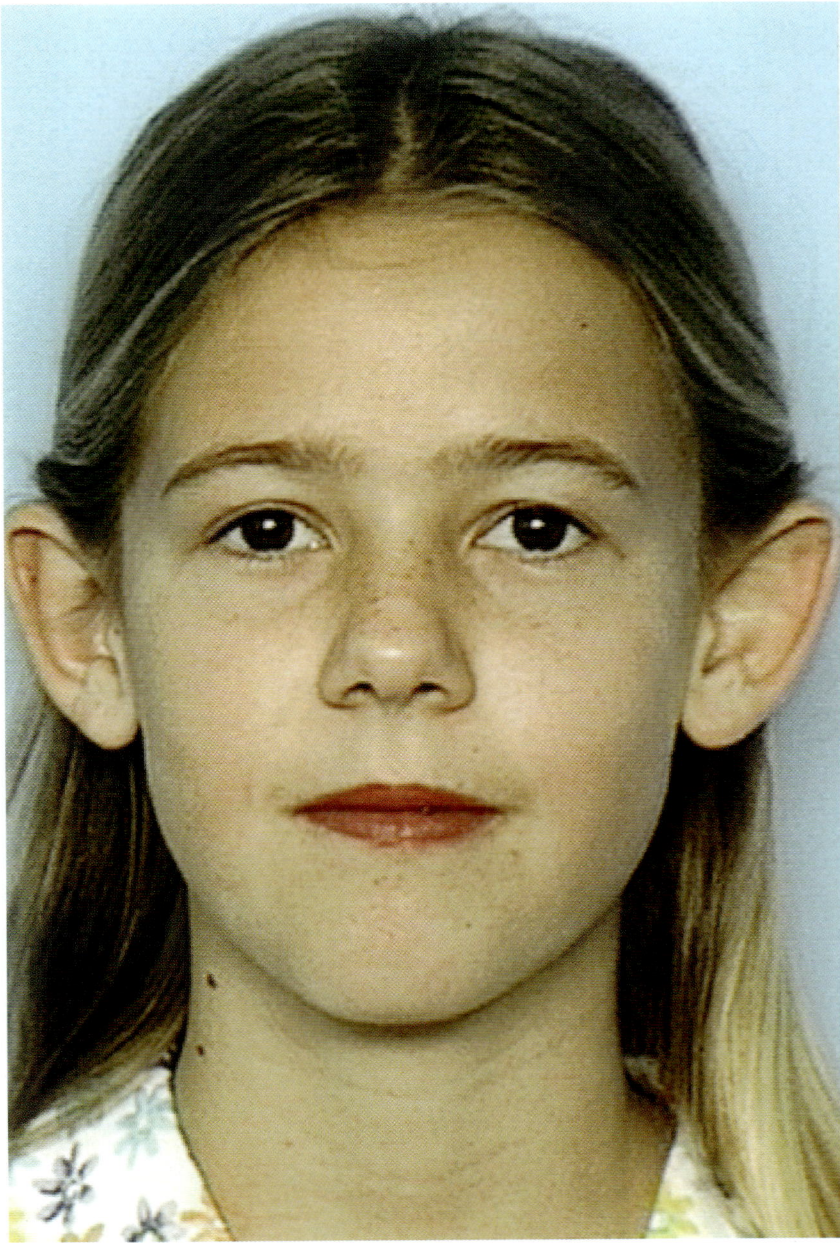

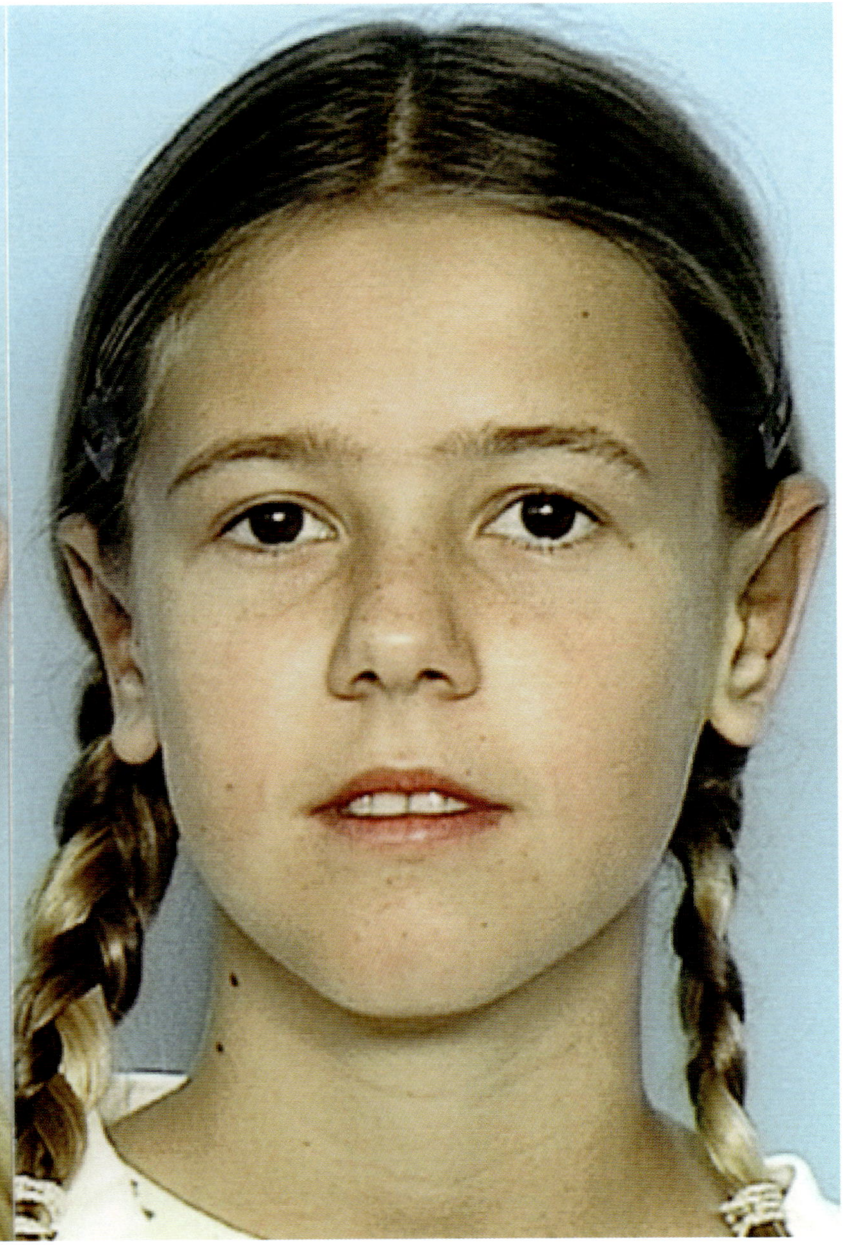

FACIAL REJUVENATION

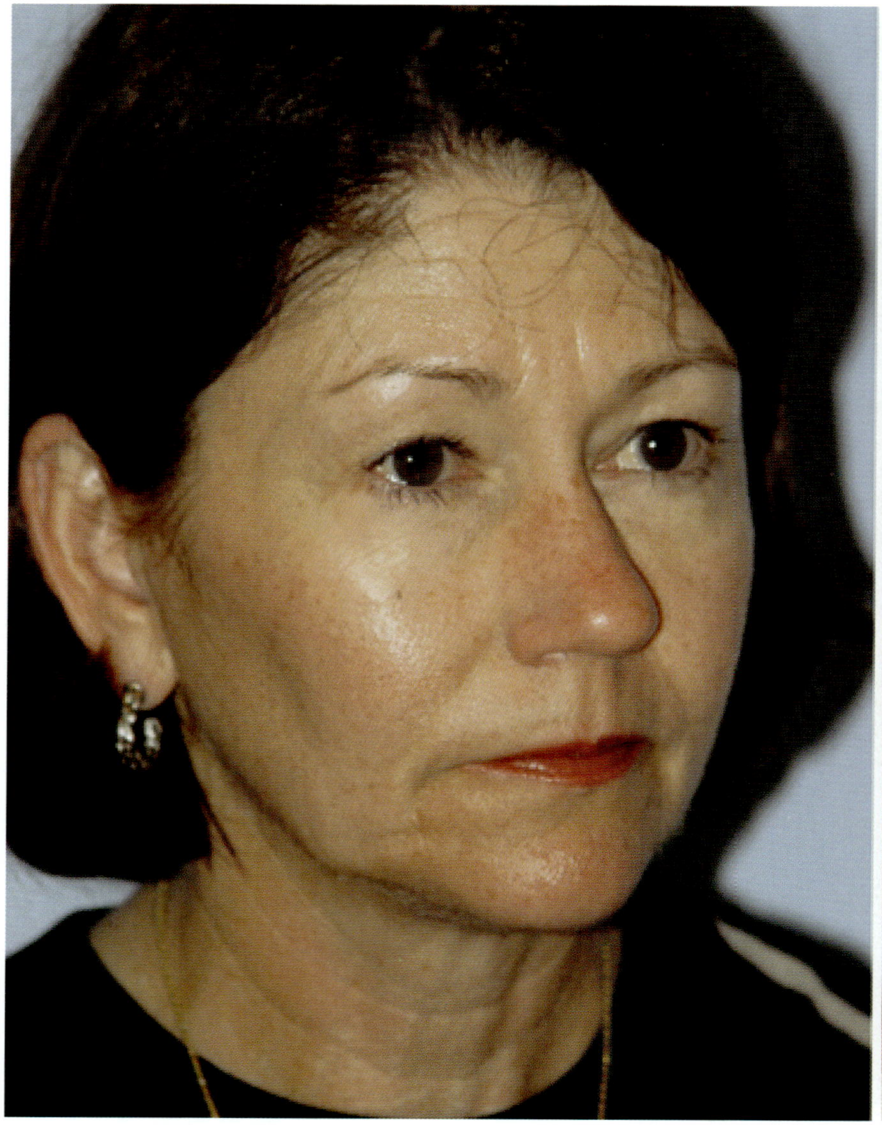

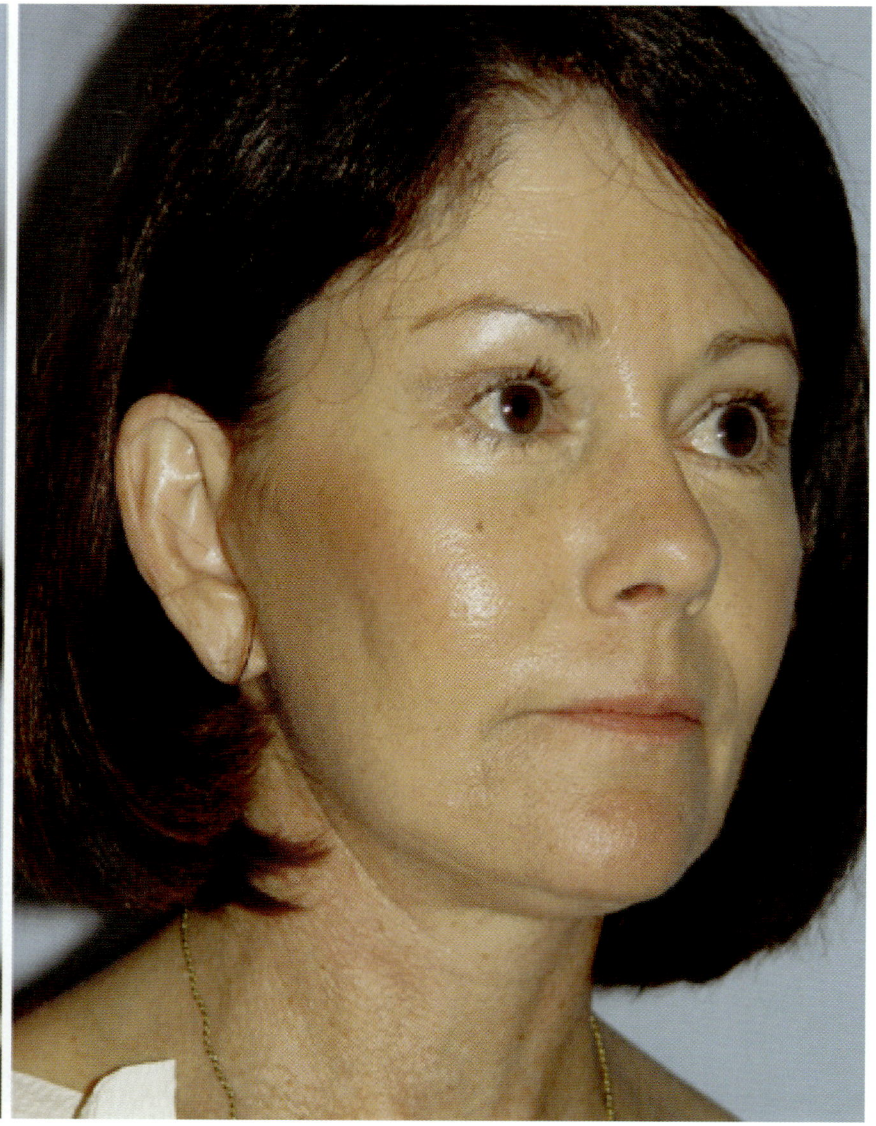

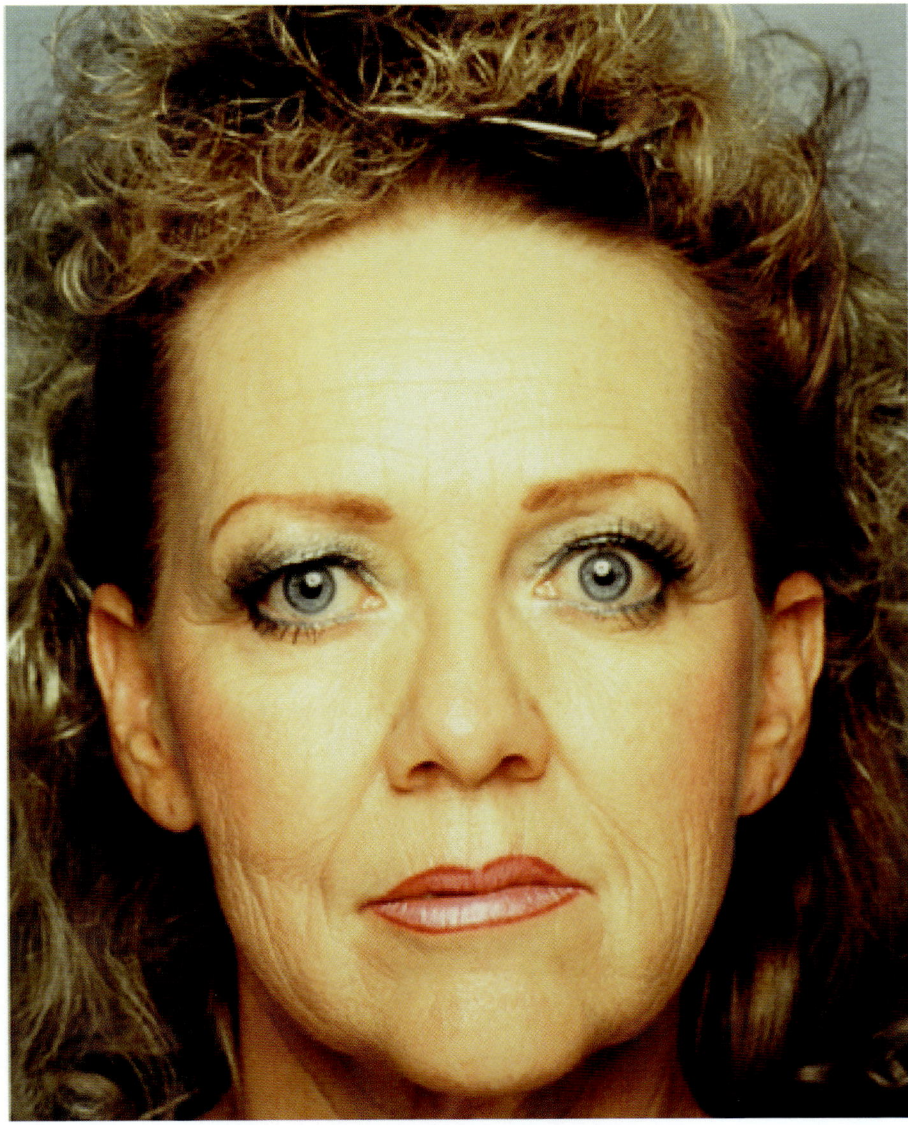
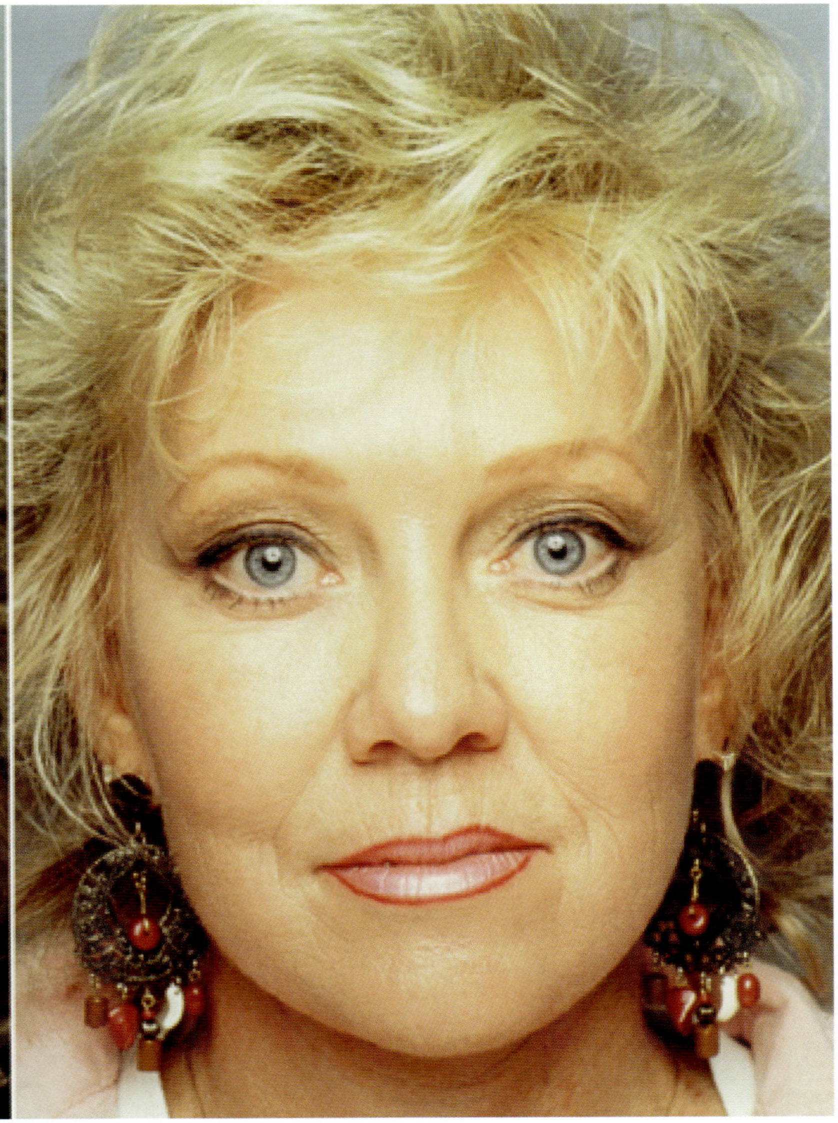

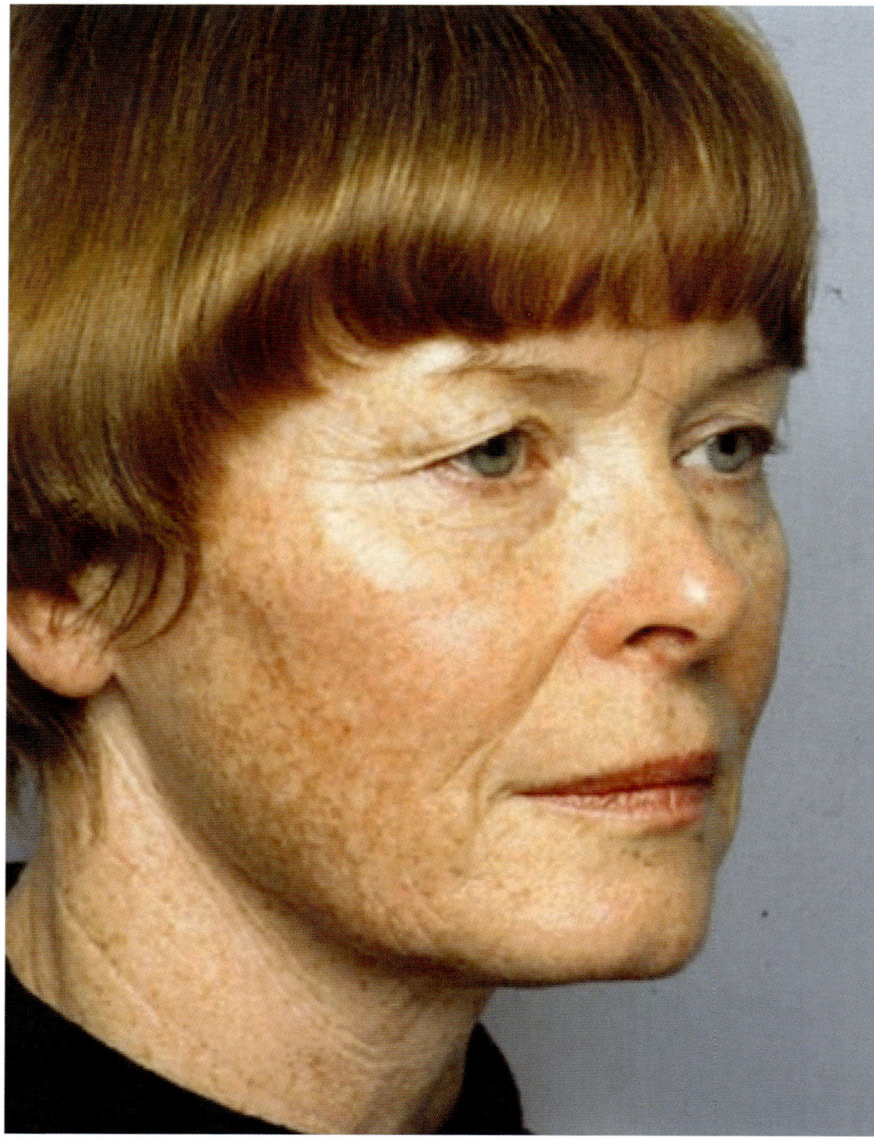

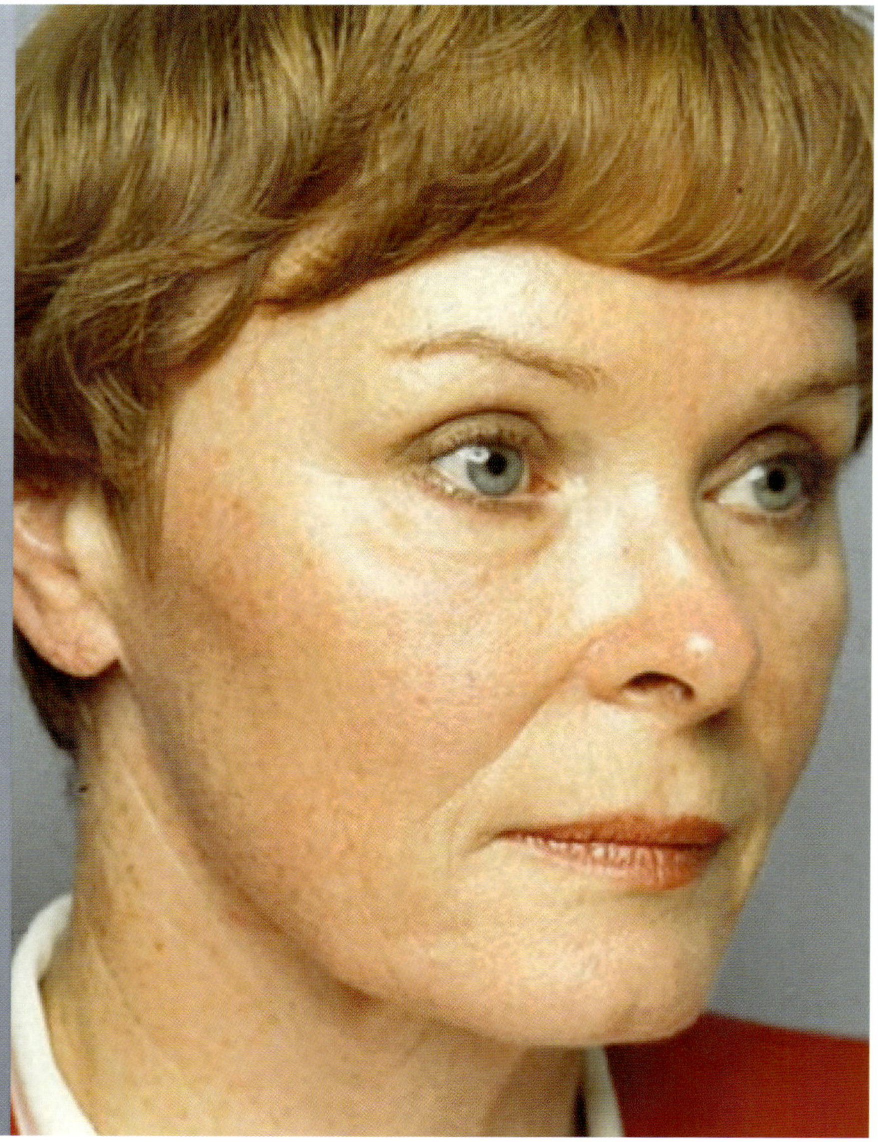

Results after 15 years.

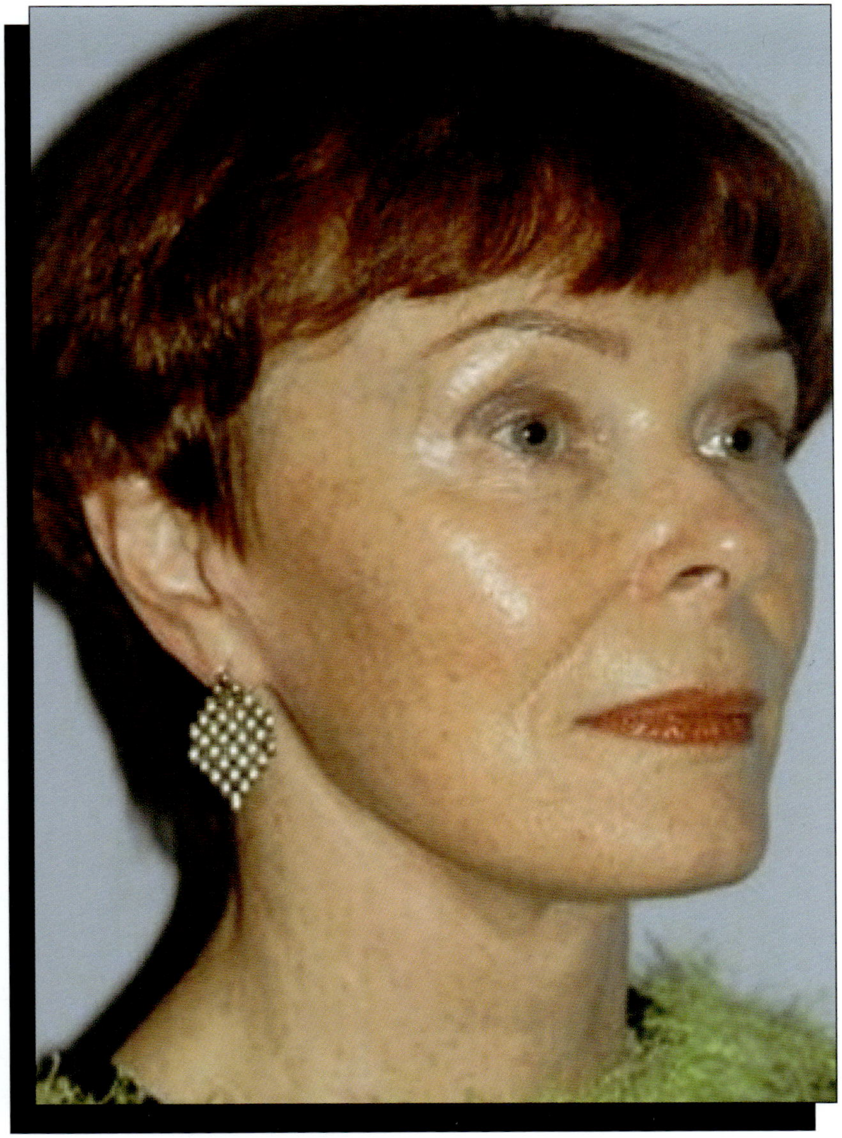

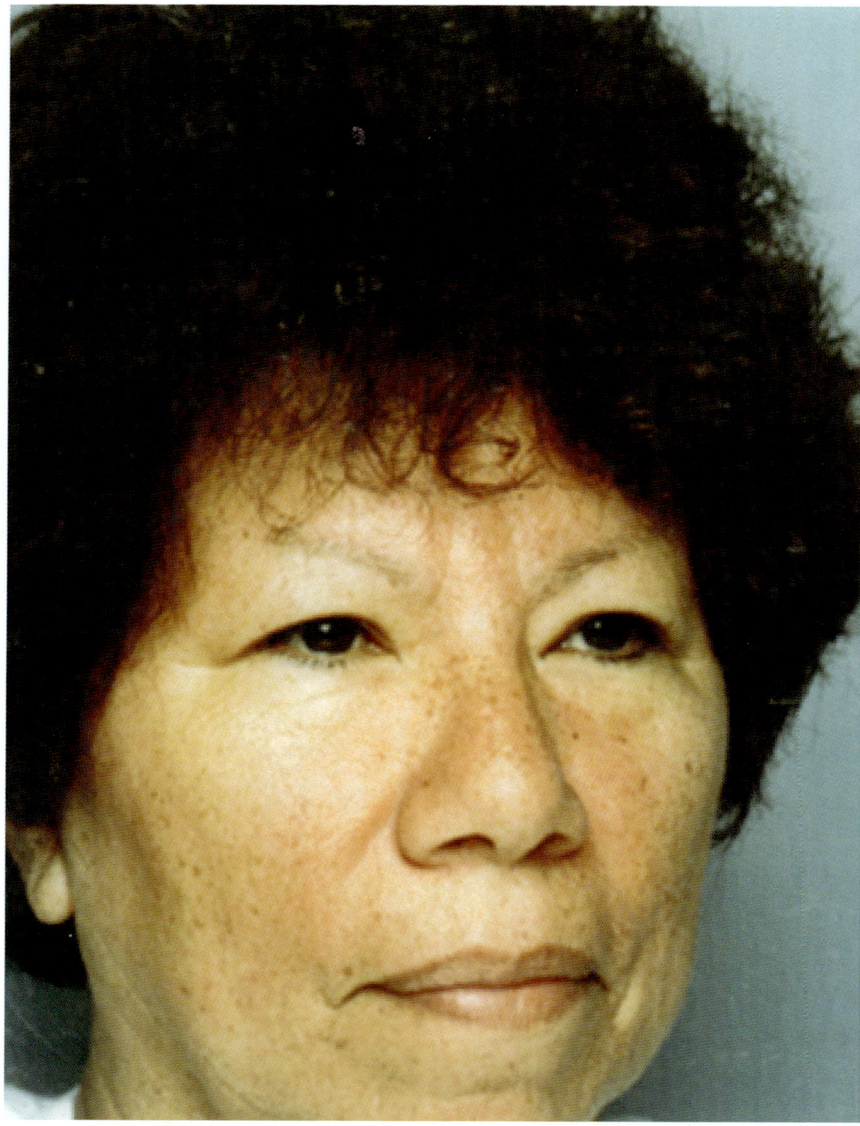
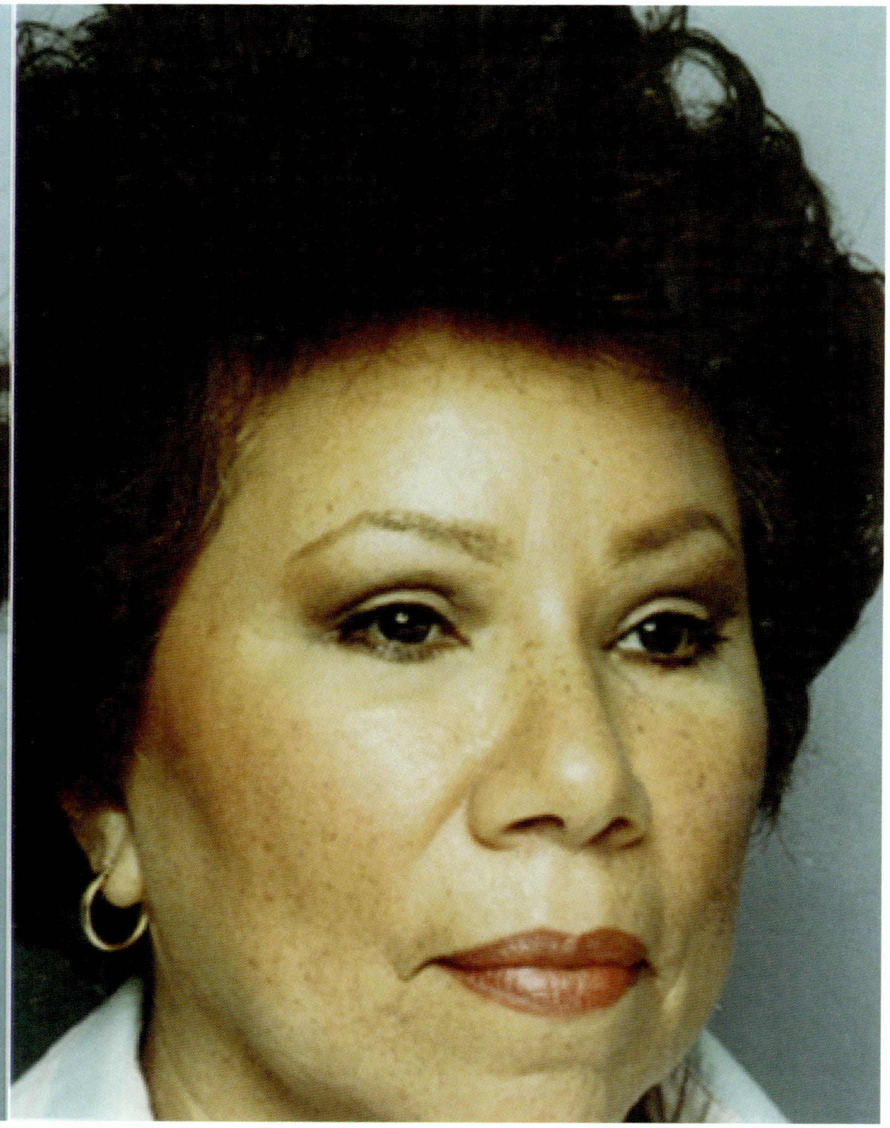

EYELID REJUVENATION

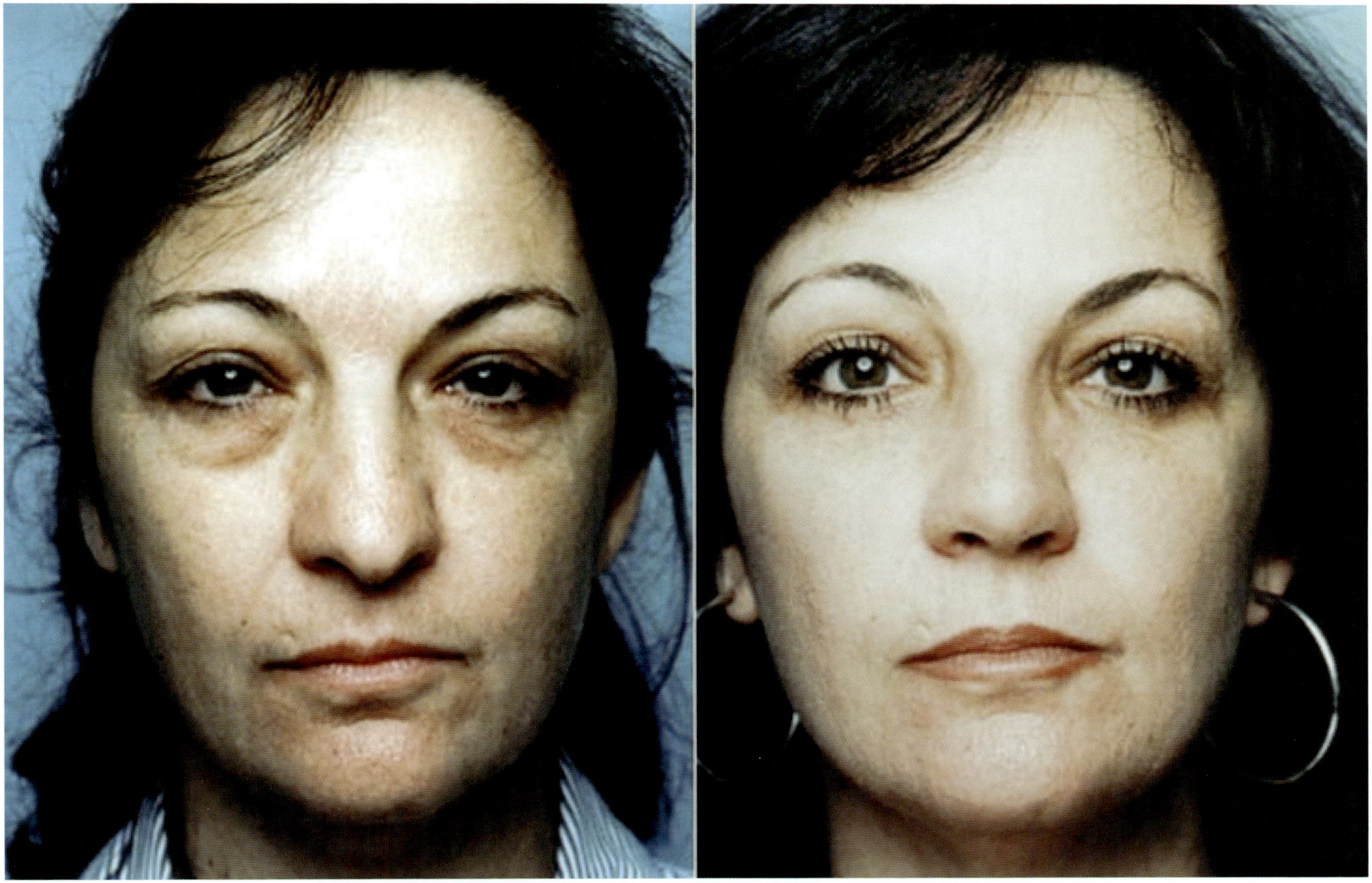

FACIAL REJUVENATION IN THE MALE

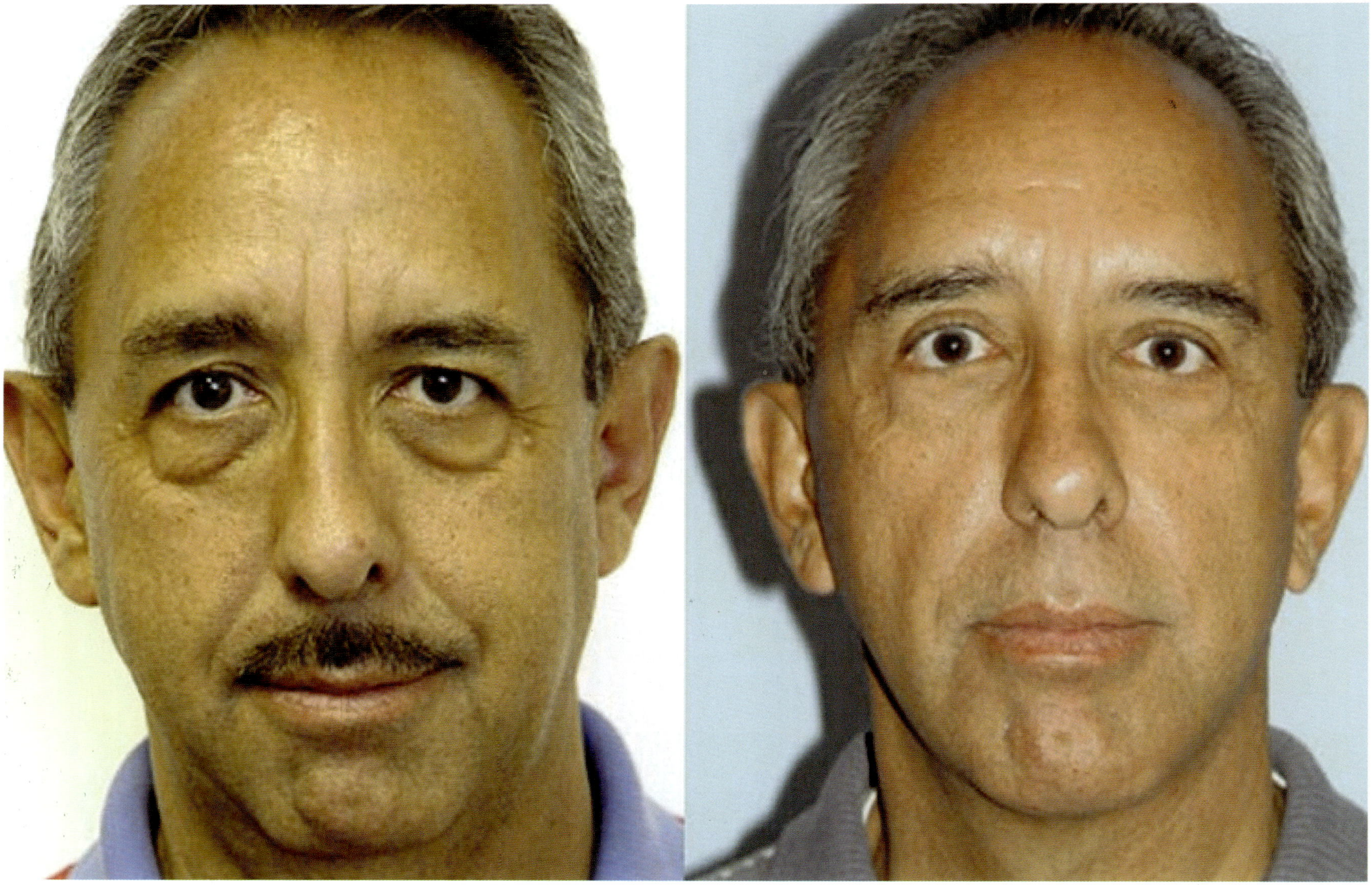

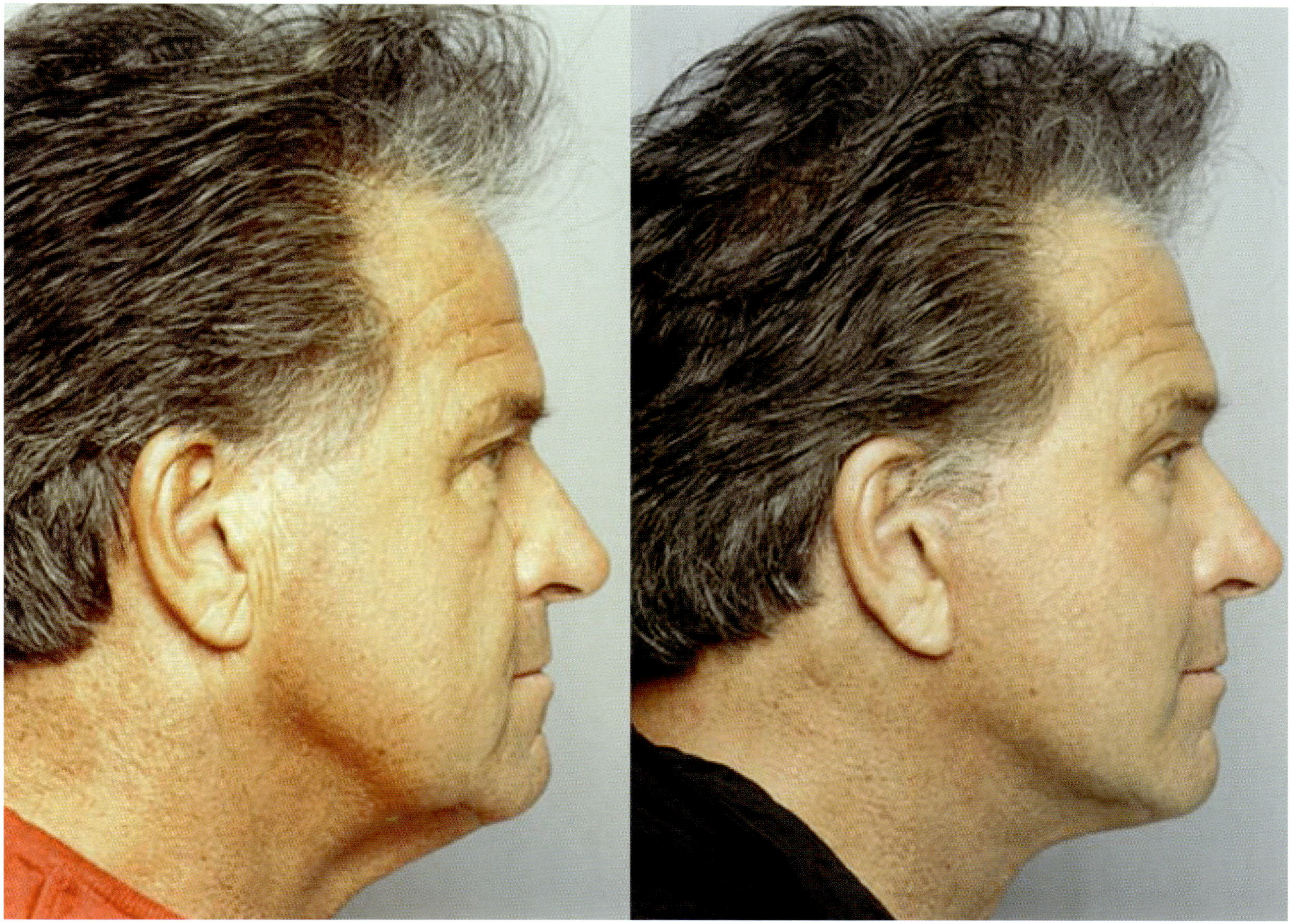

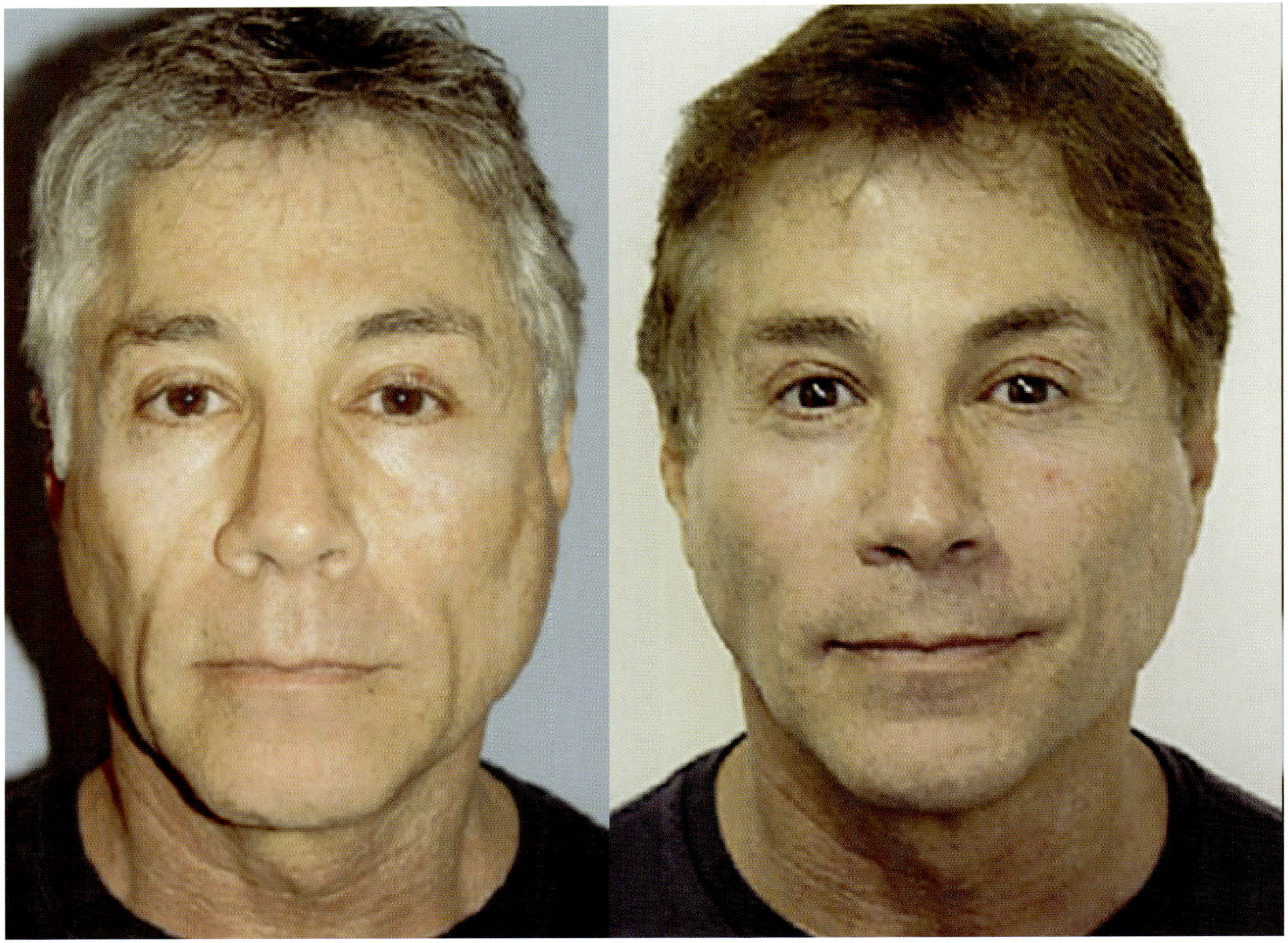

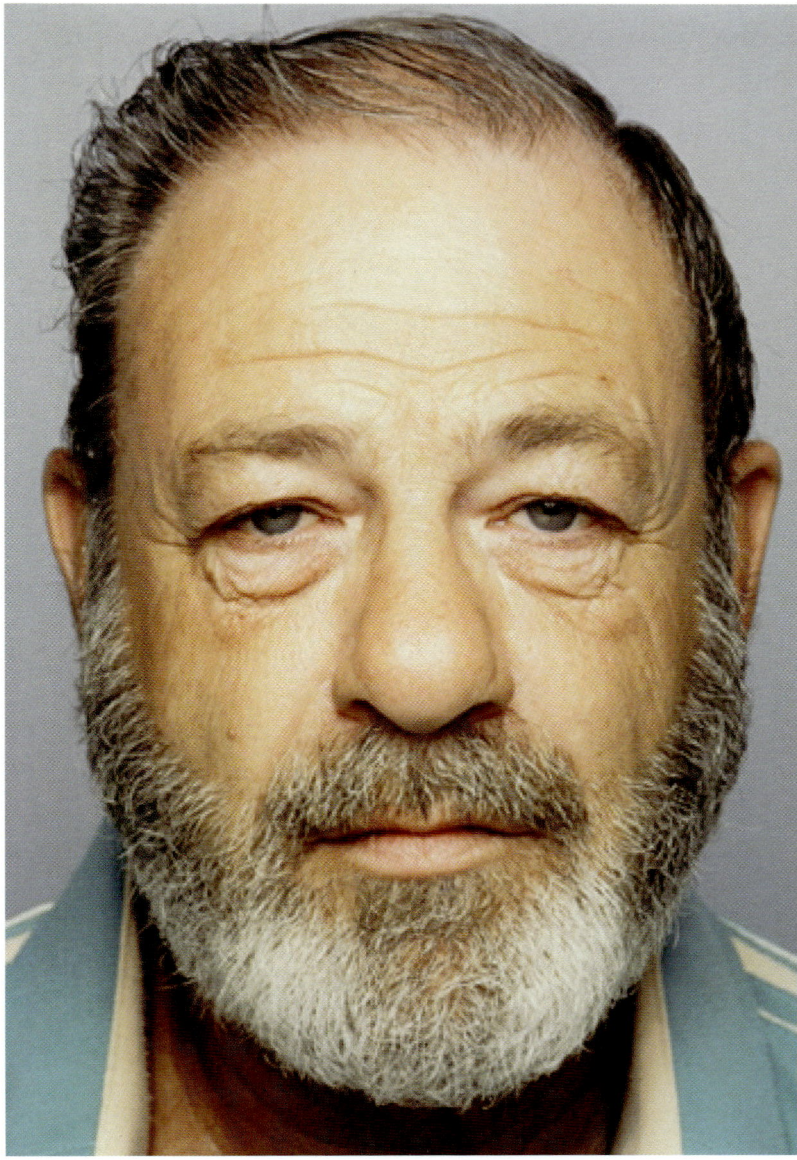
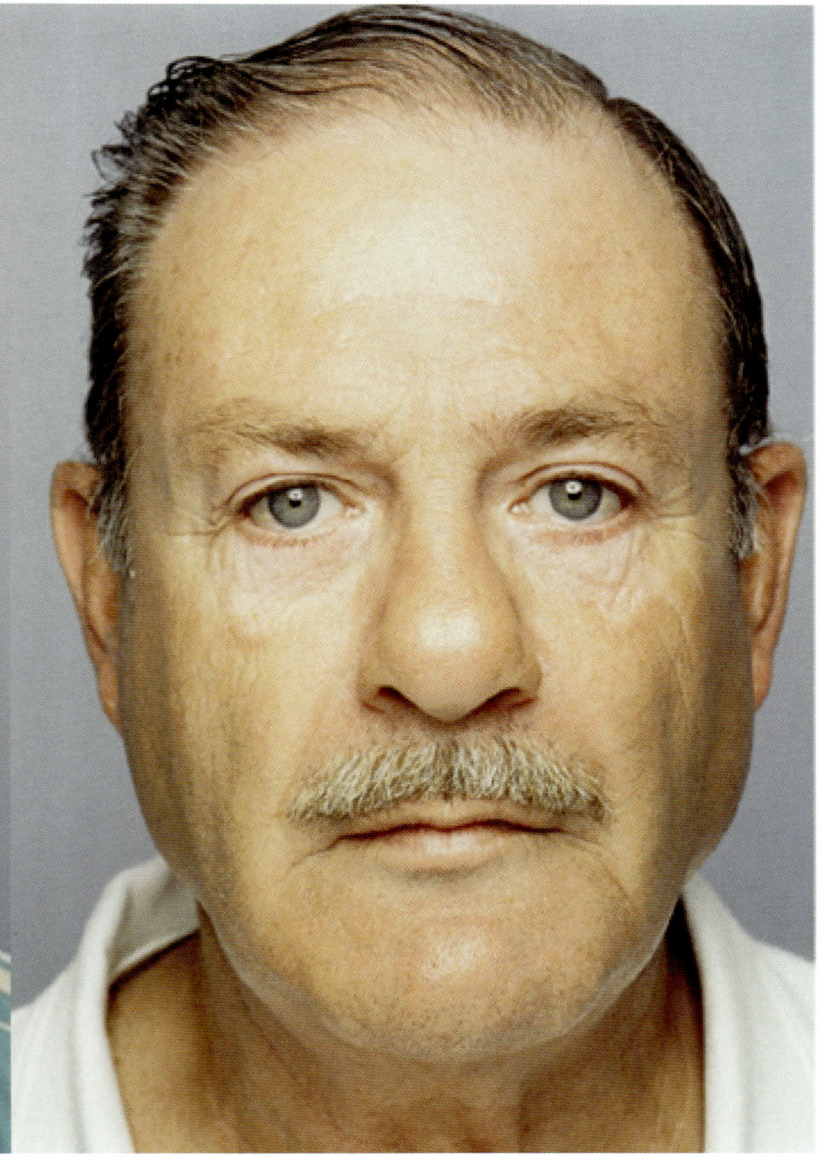

NOSE SURGERY

Rhinoplasty, or surgery to reshape the nose, is one of the most common of all plastic surgery procedures. Rhinoplasty can reduce or increase the size of the nose, change the shape of the tip or the bridge, narrow the span of the nostrils, or change the angle between your nose and the upper lip. It may also correct a birth defect or injury, or help relieve breathing problems.

Surgery of the nose is performed on an out-patient basis and involves virtually no pain, no packing and no external incisions.

RHINOPLASTY (NOSE RESHAPING)

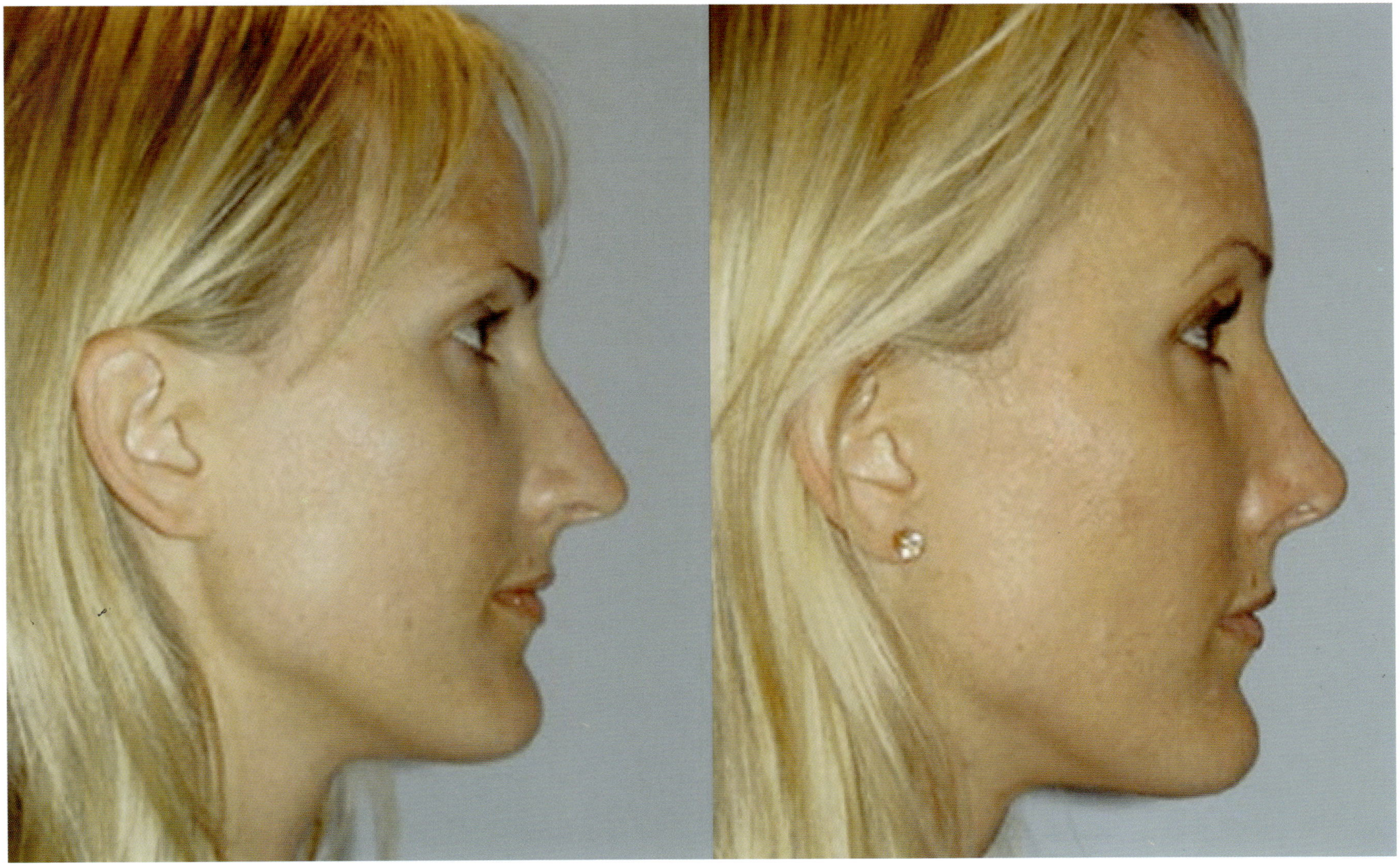

Some people want only a small change in their appearance

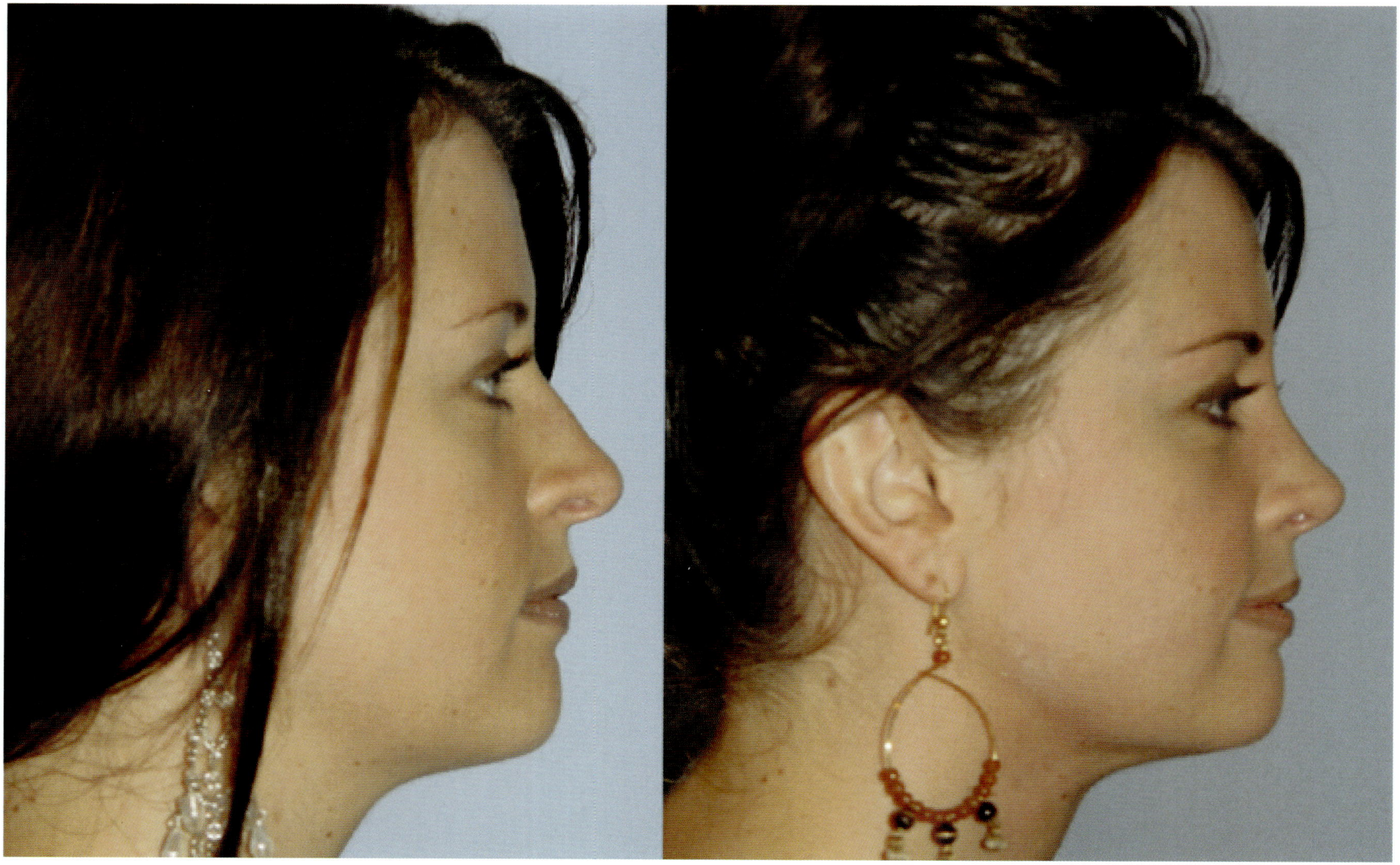

while others are seeking a more dramatic change.

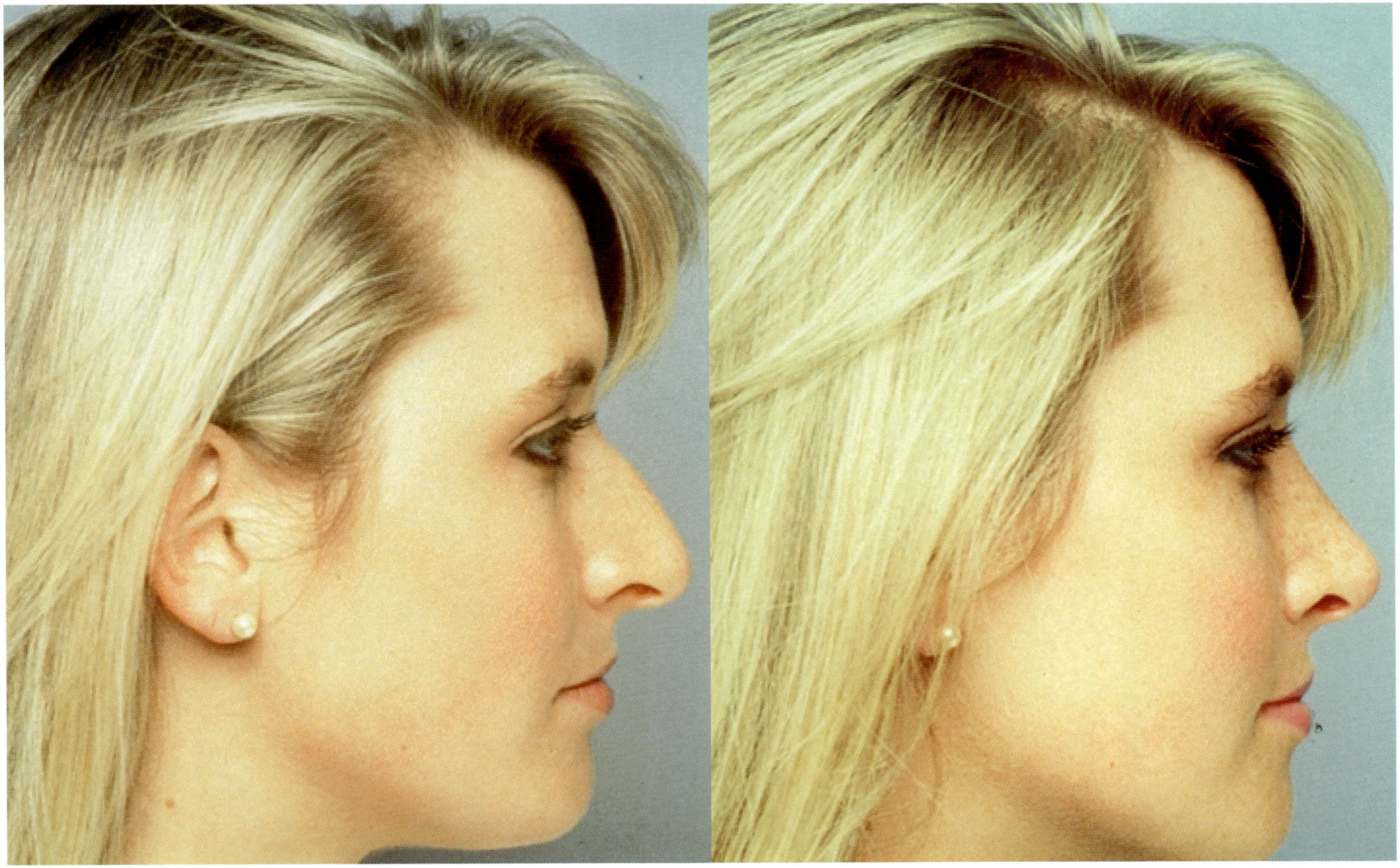

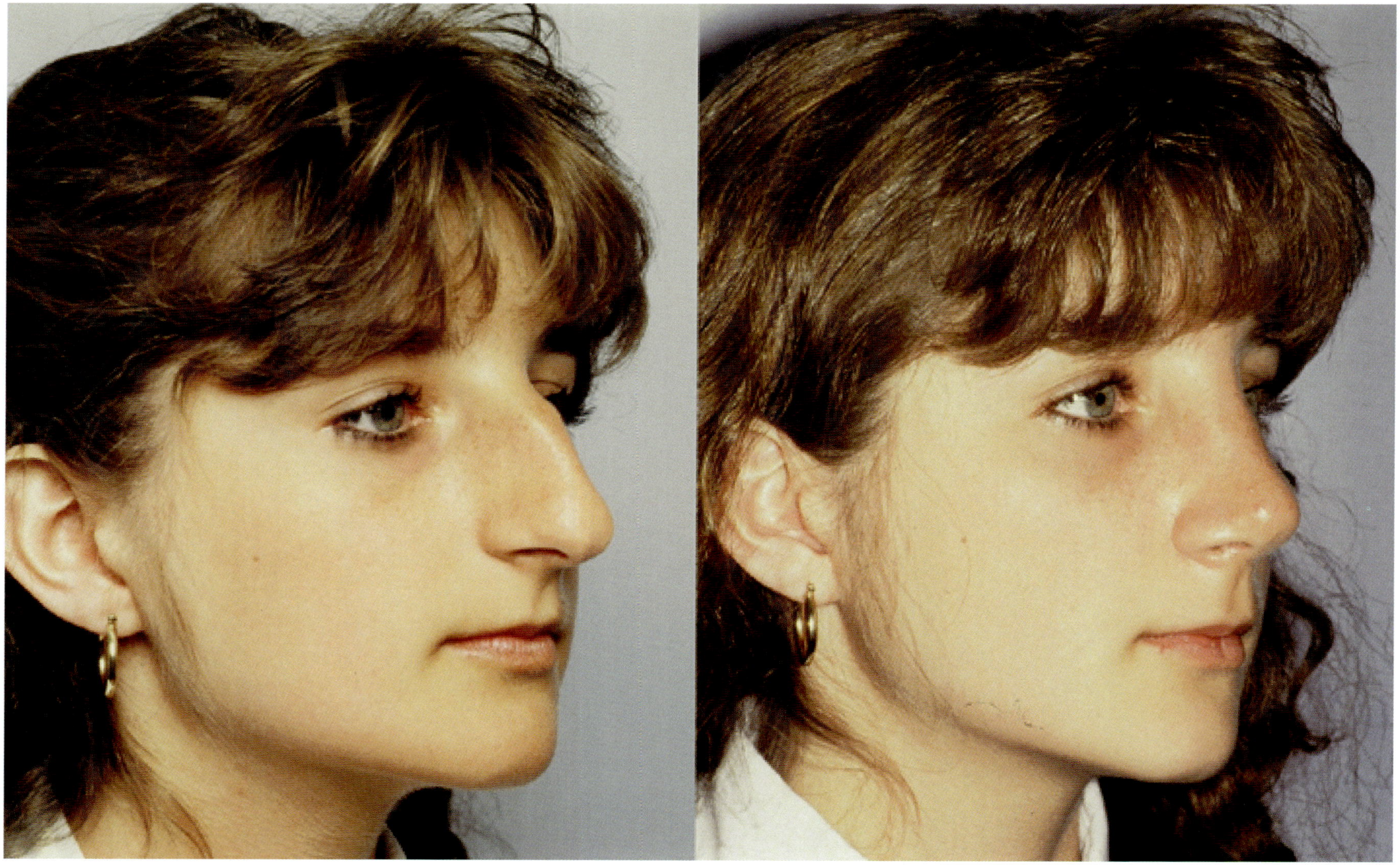

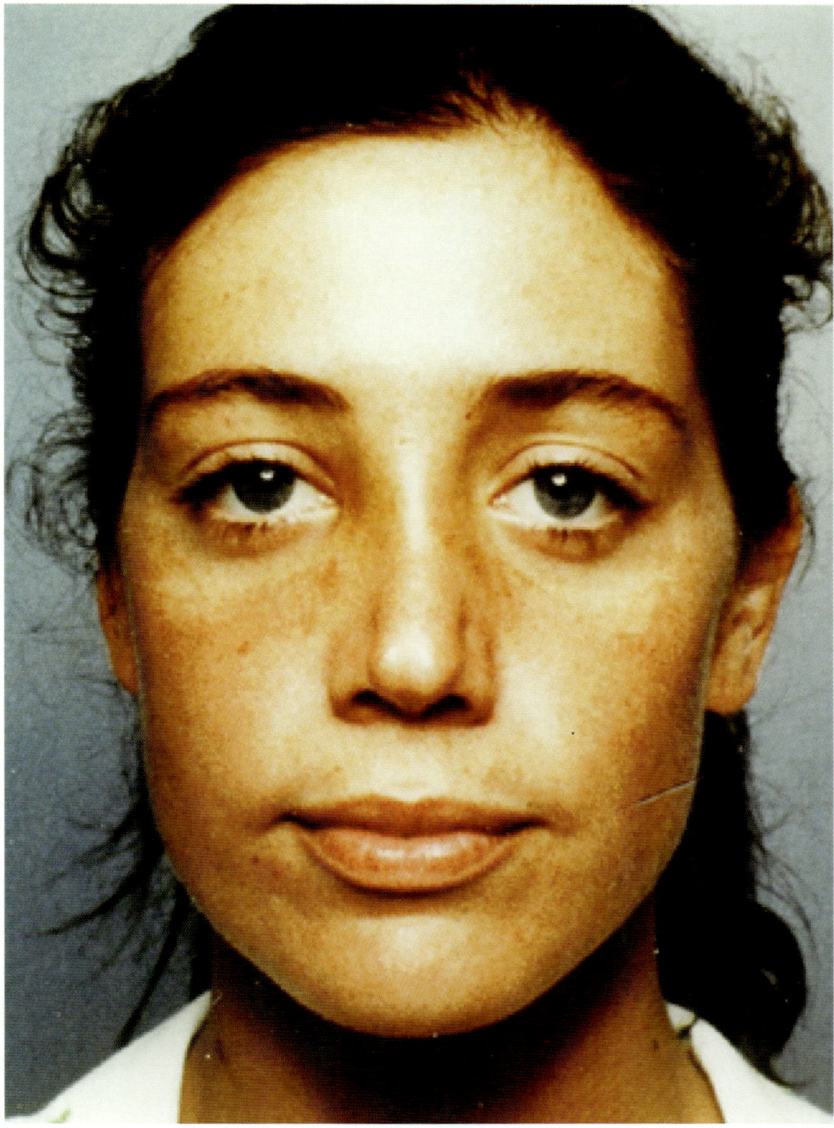

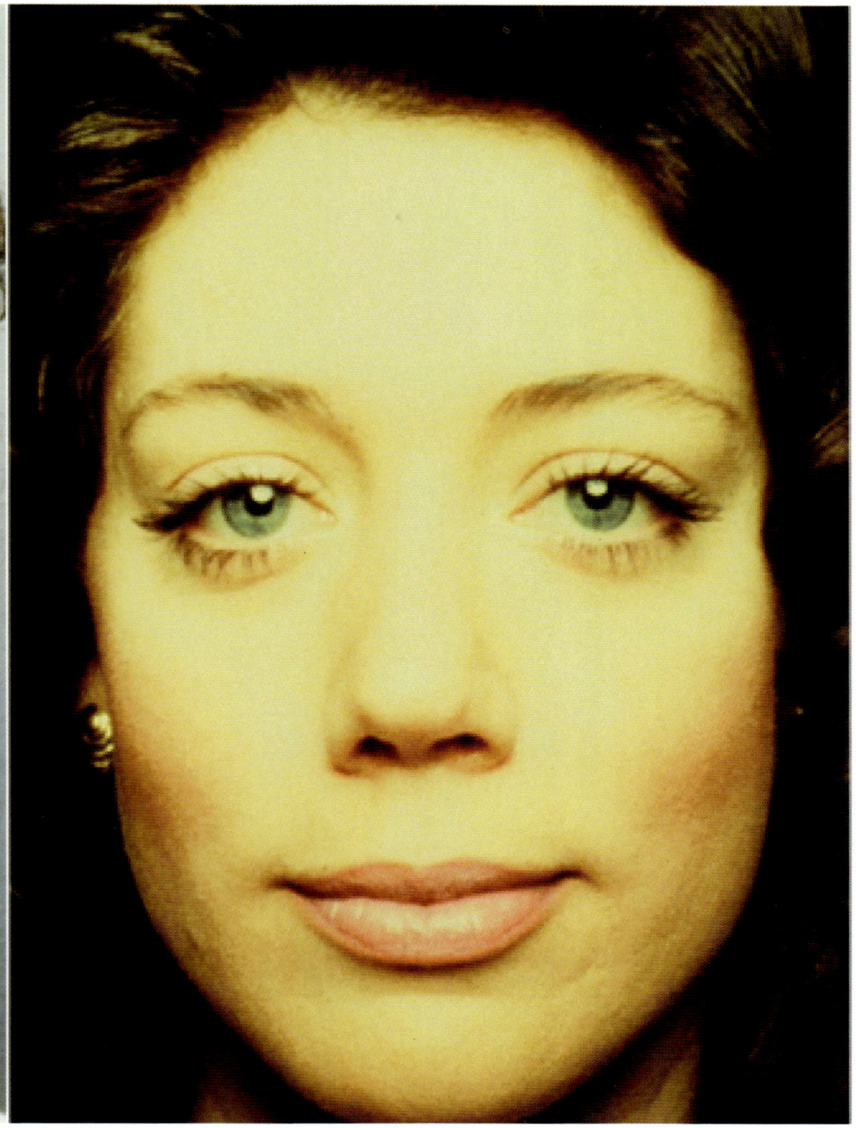

SHORTENING THE MALE NOSE

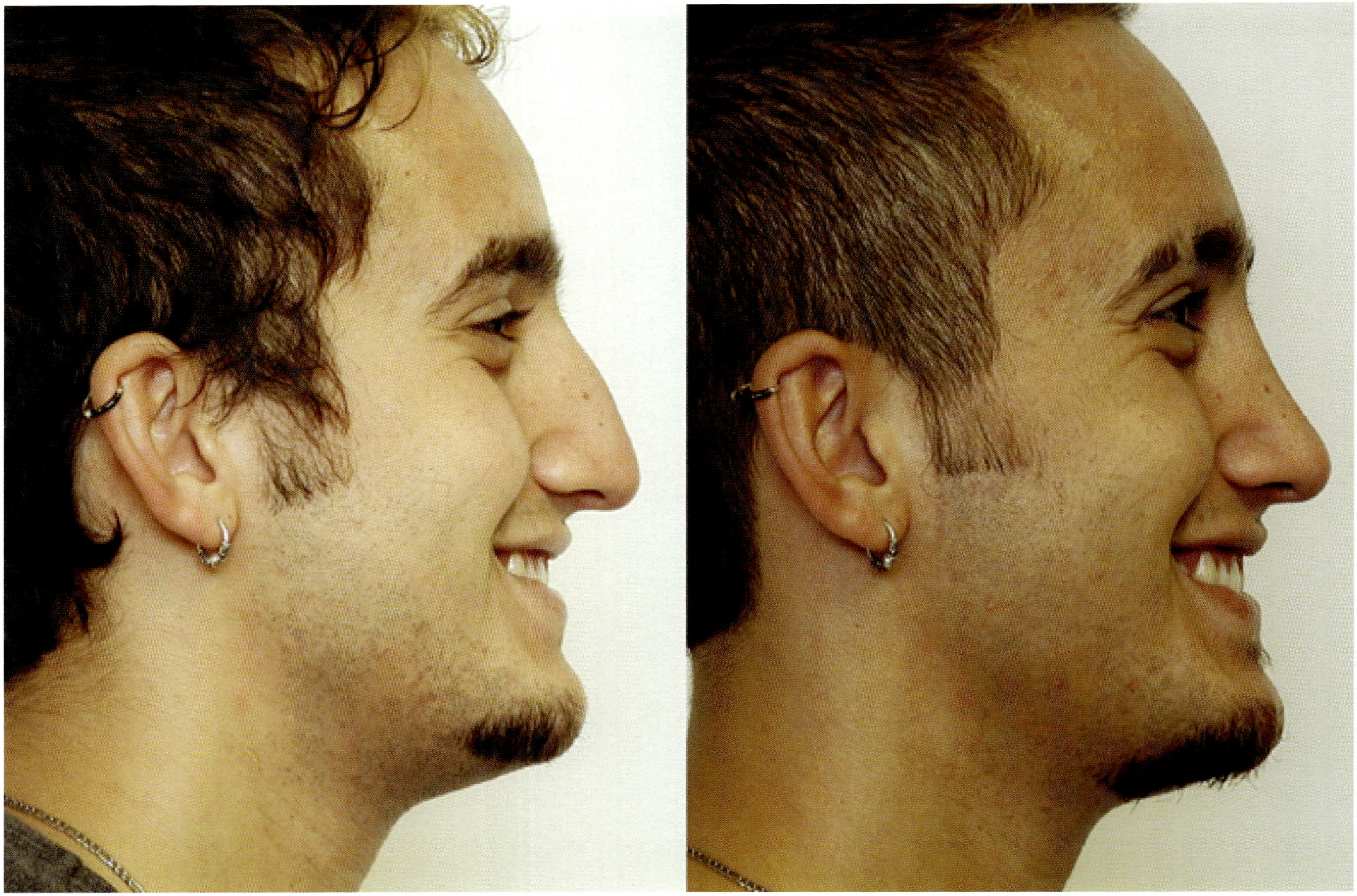

NARROWING THE ETHNIC NOSE

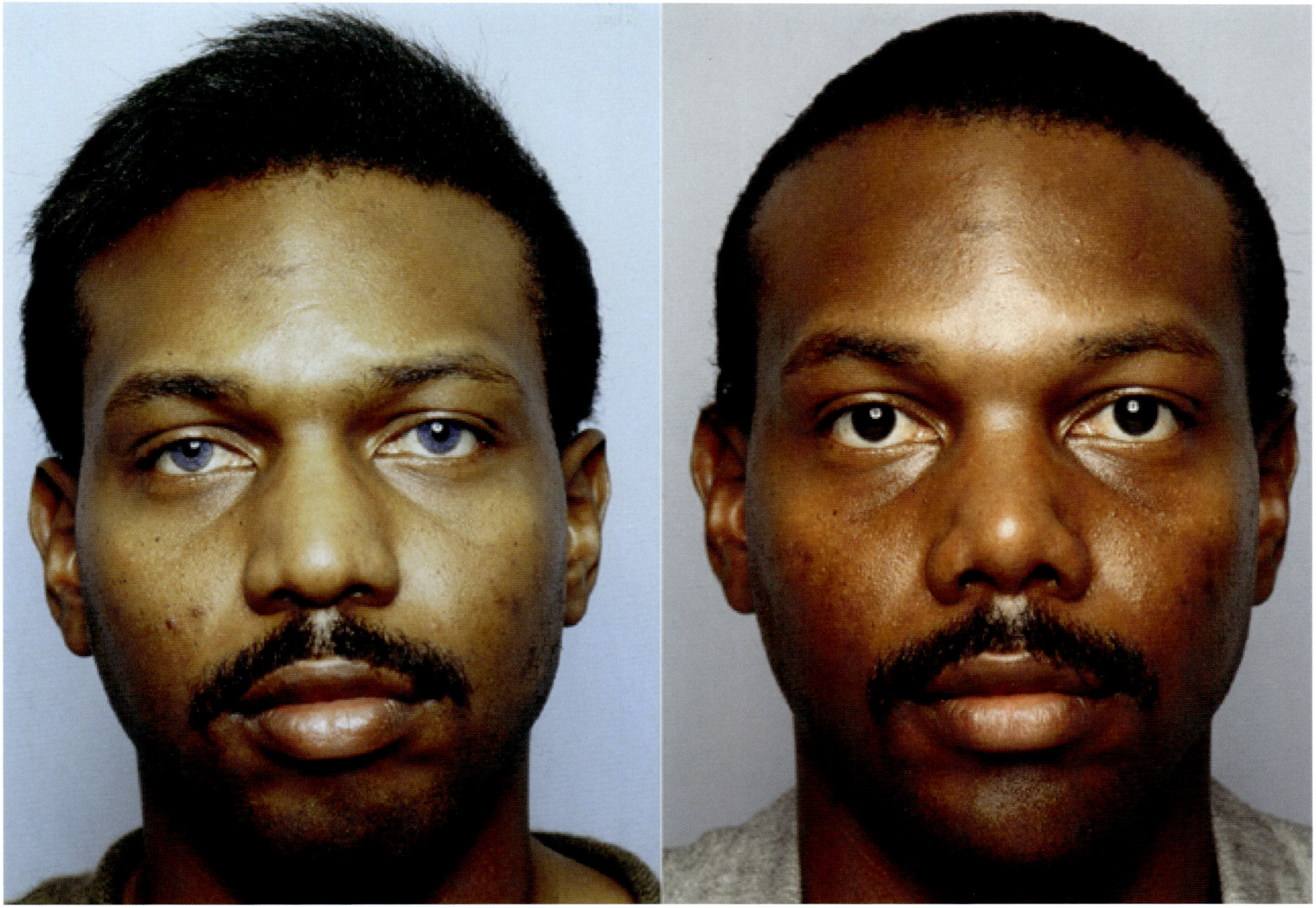

RAISING THE NASAL BRIDGE

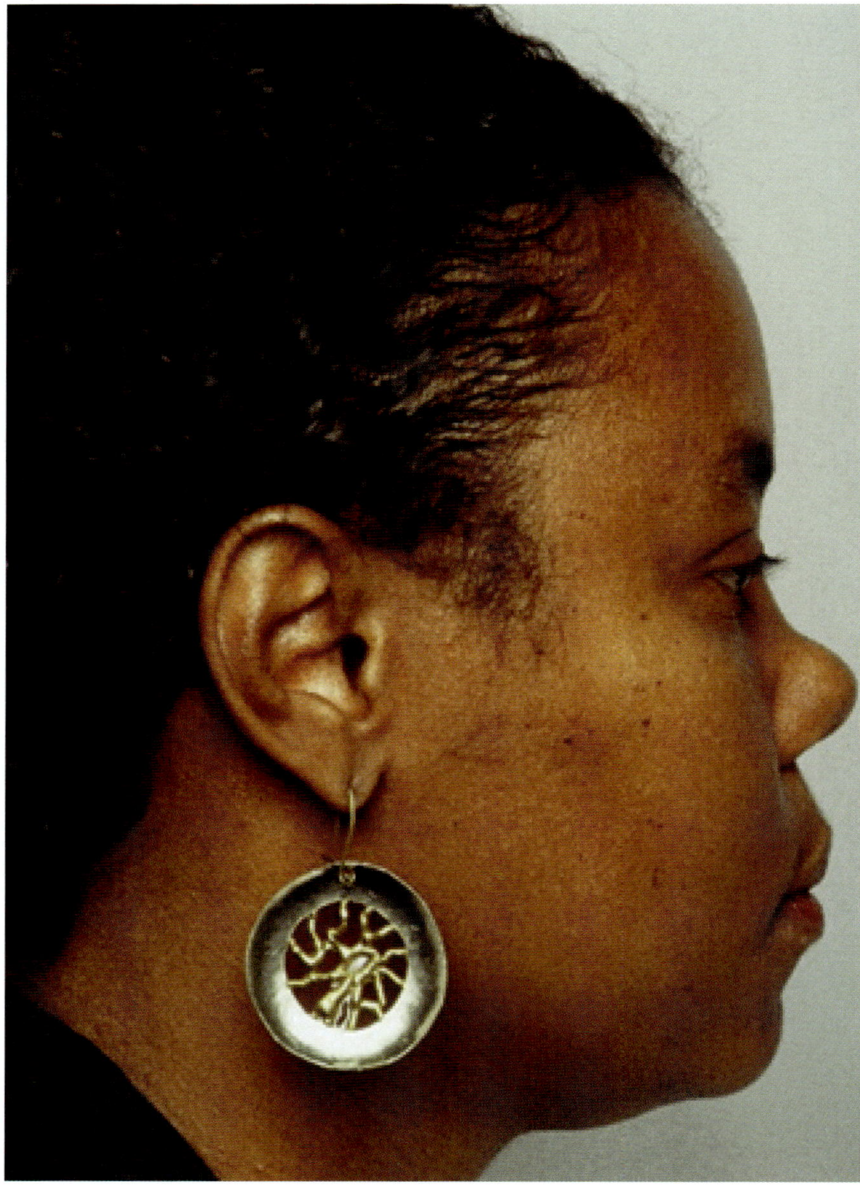

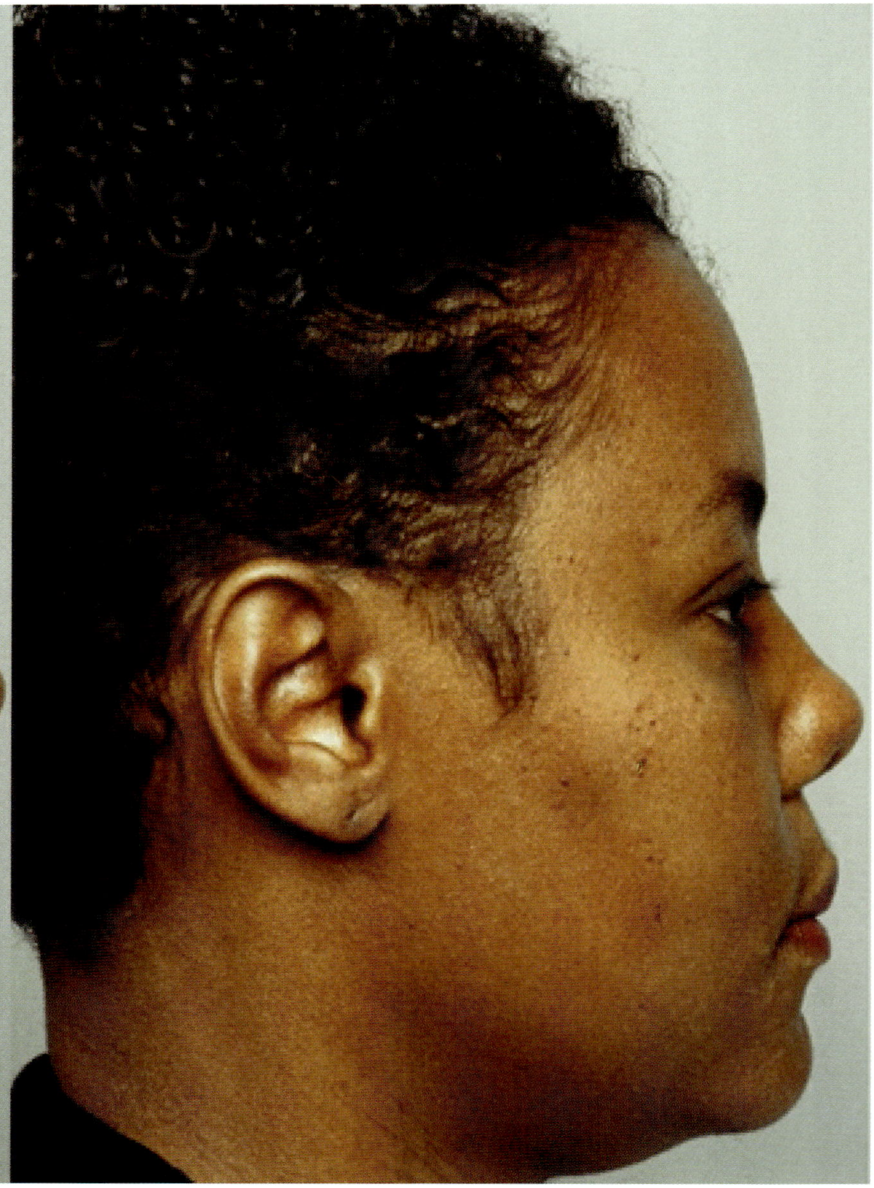

NOSE AND CHIN IMPLANT

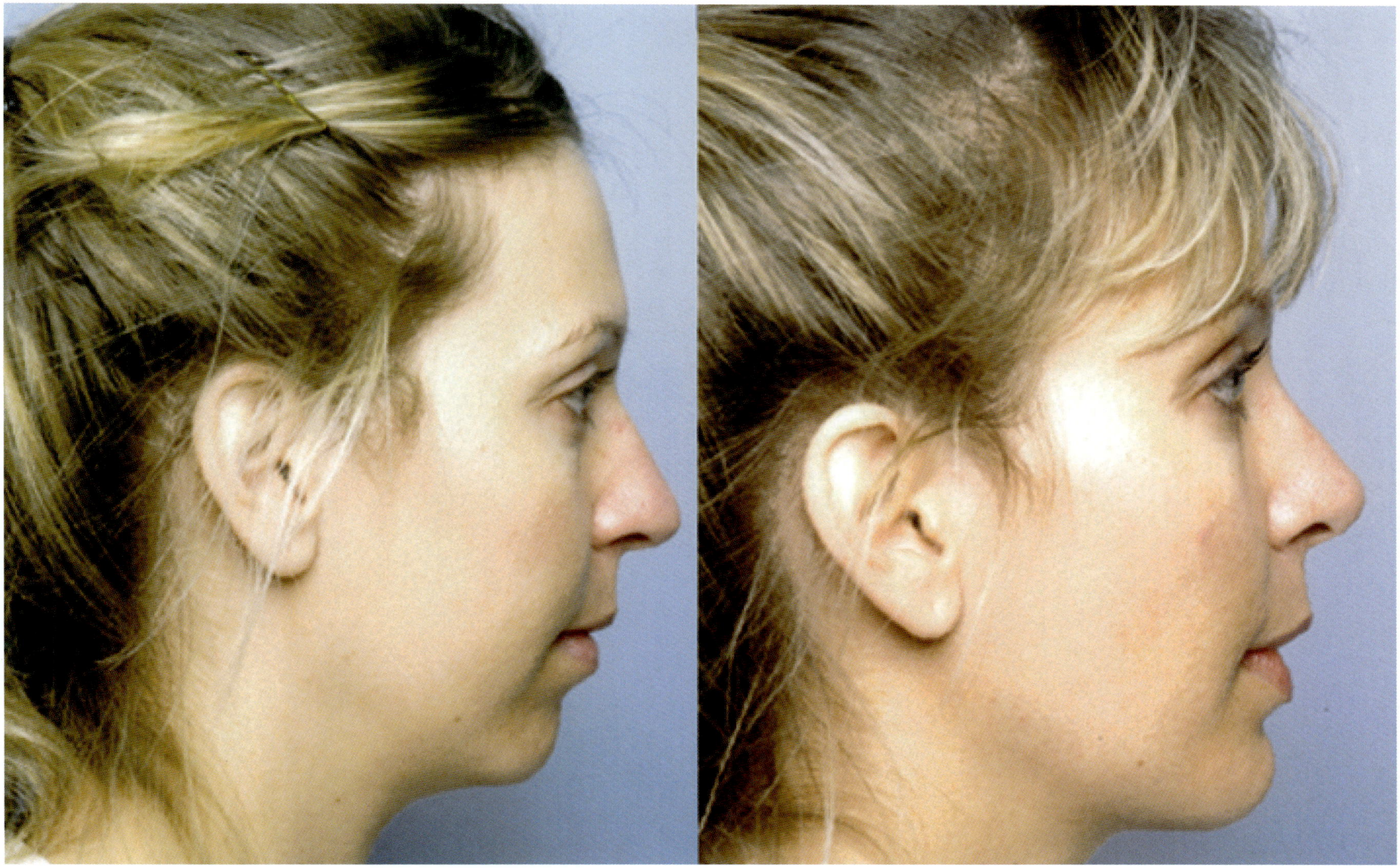

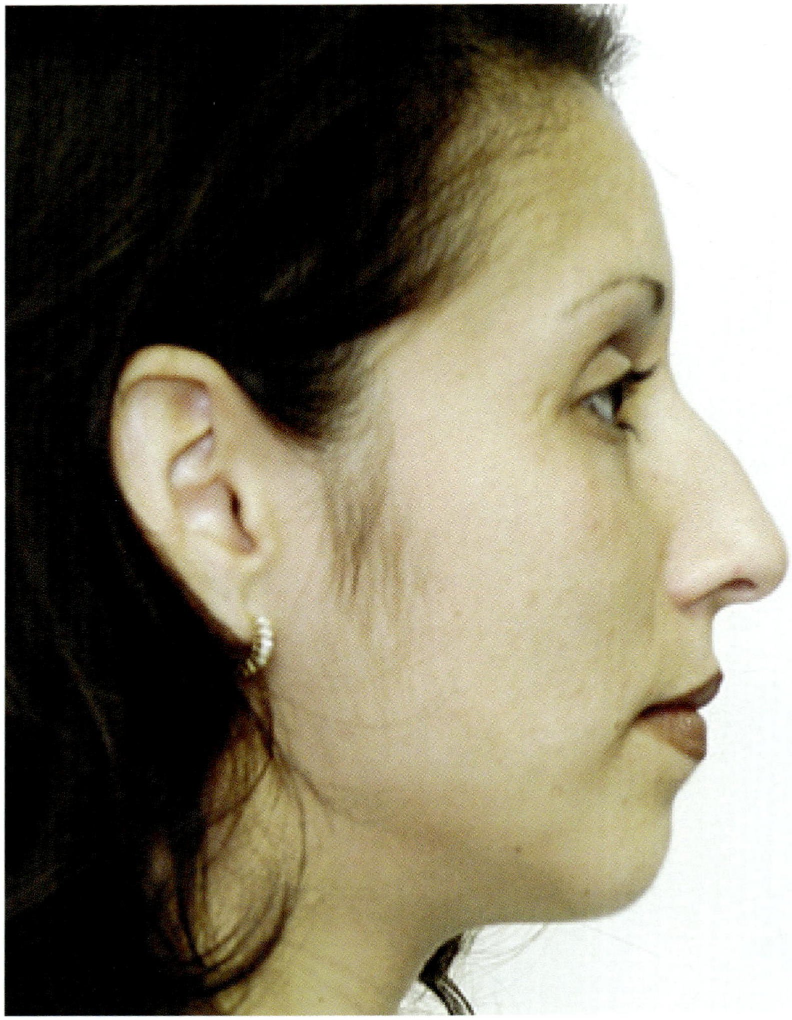 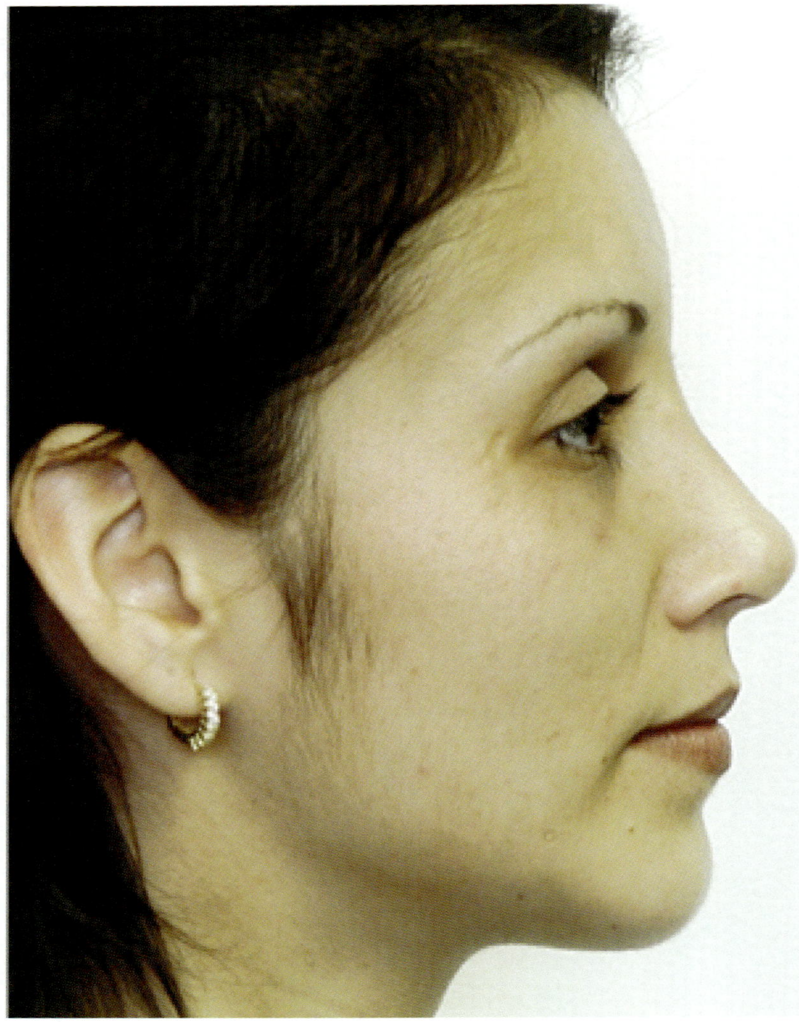

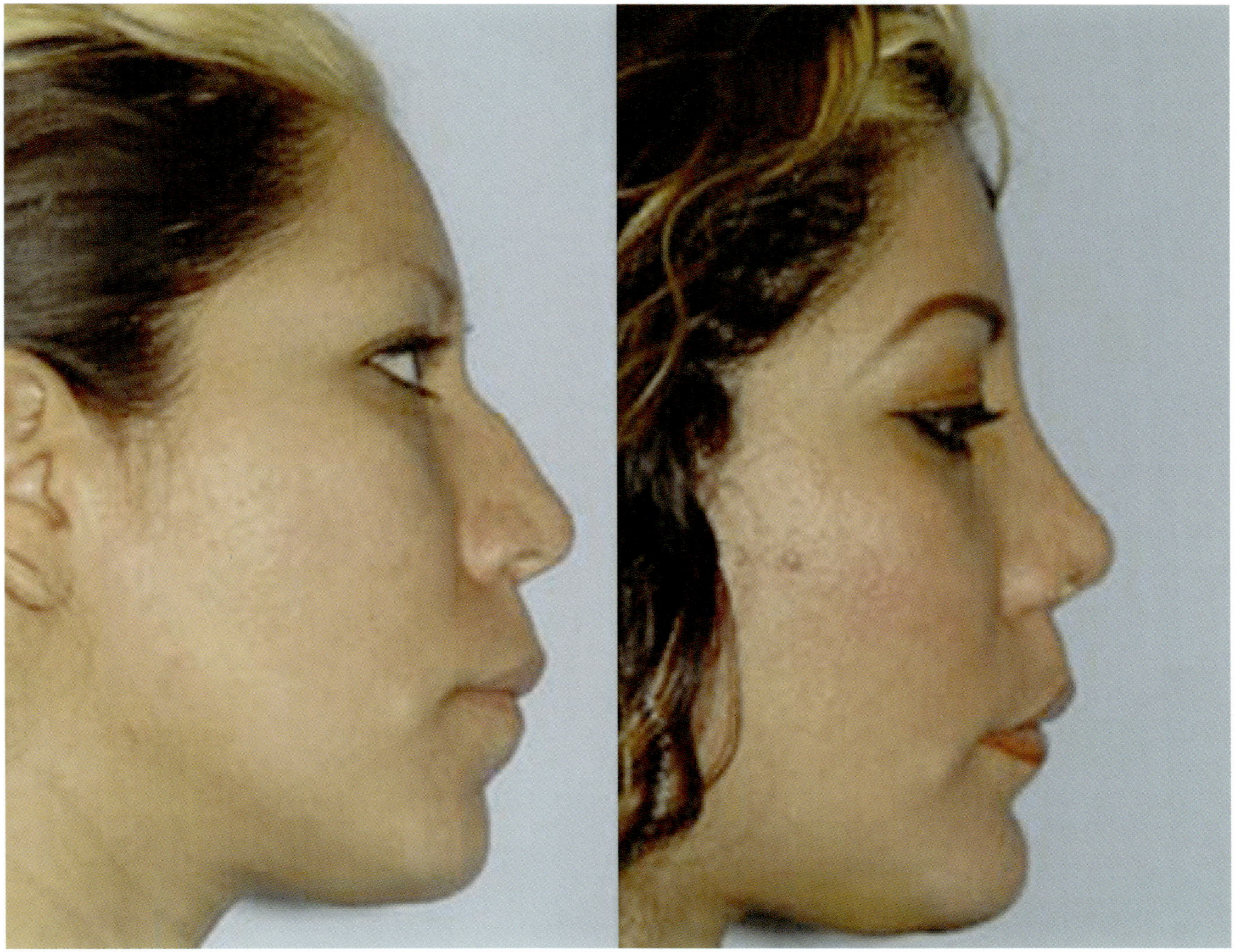

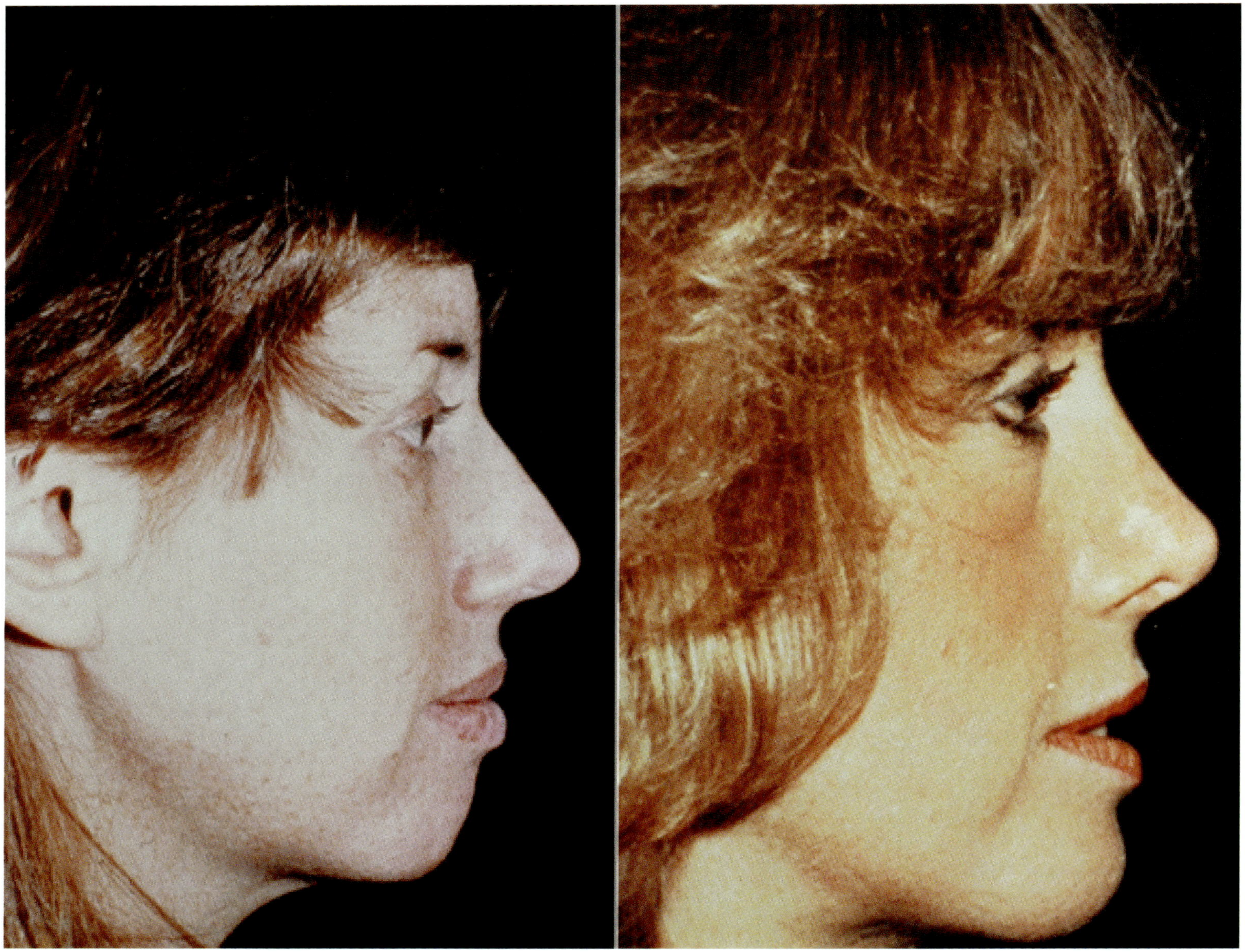

CHIN IMPLANT

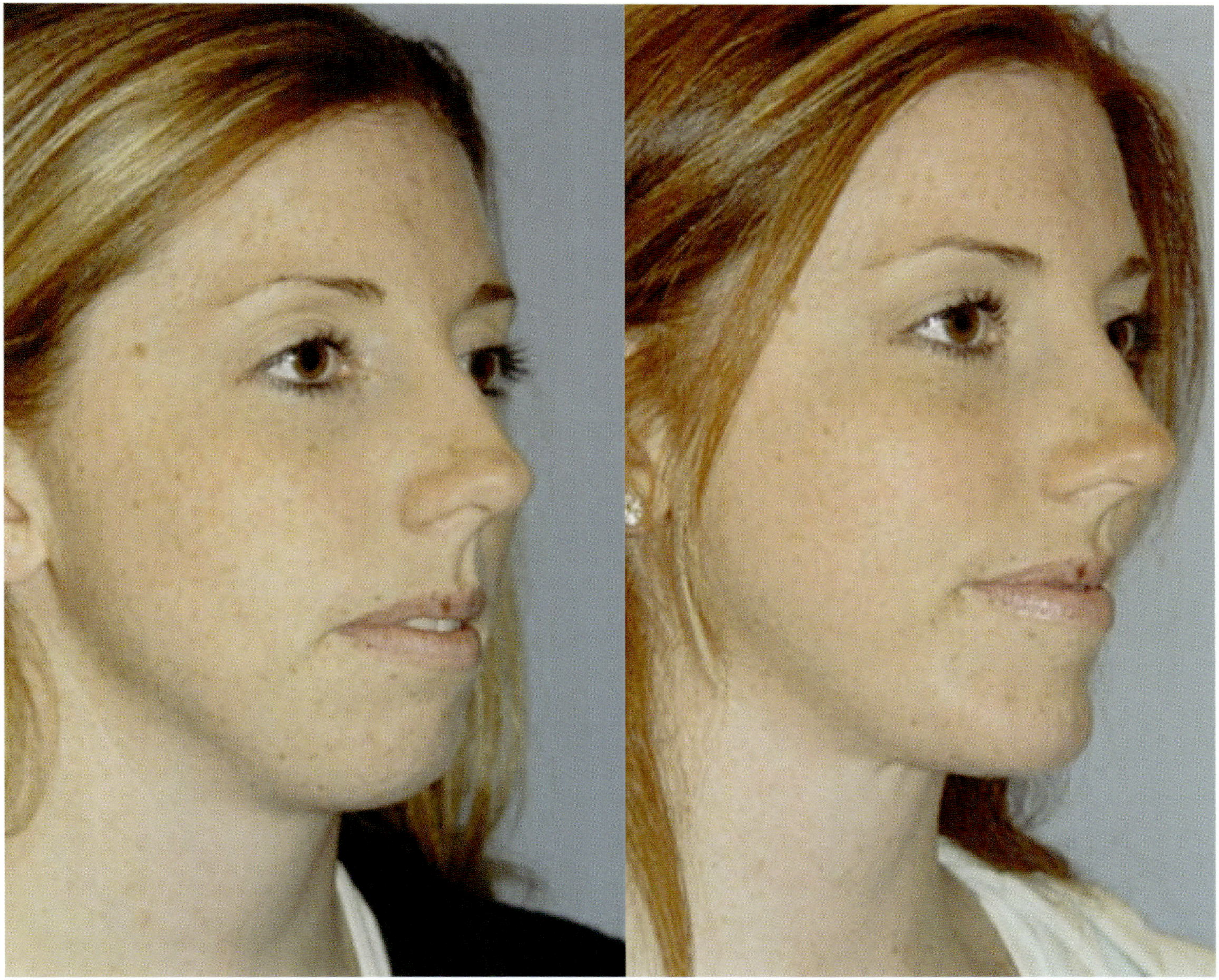

NOSE, CHIN IMPLANT AND NECK CONTOURING

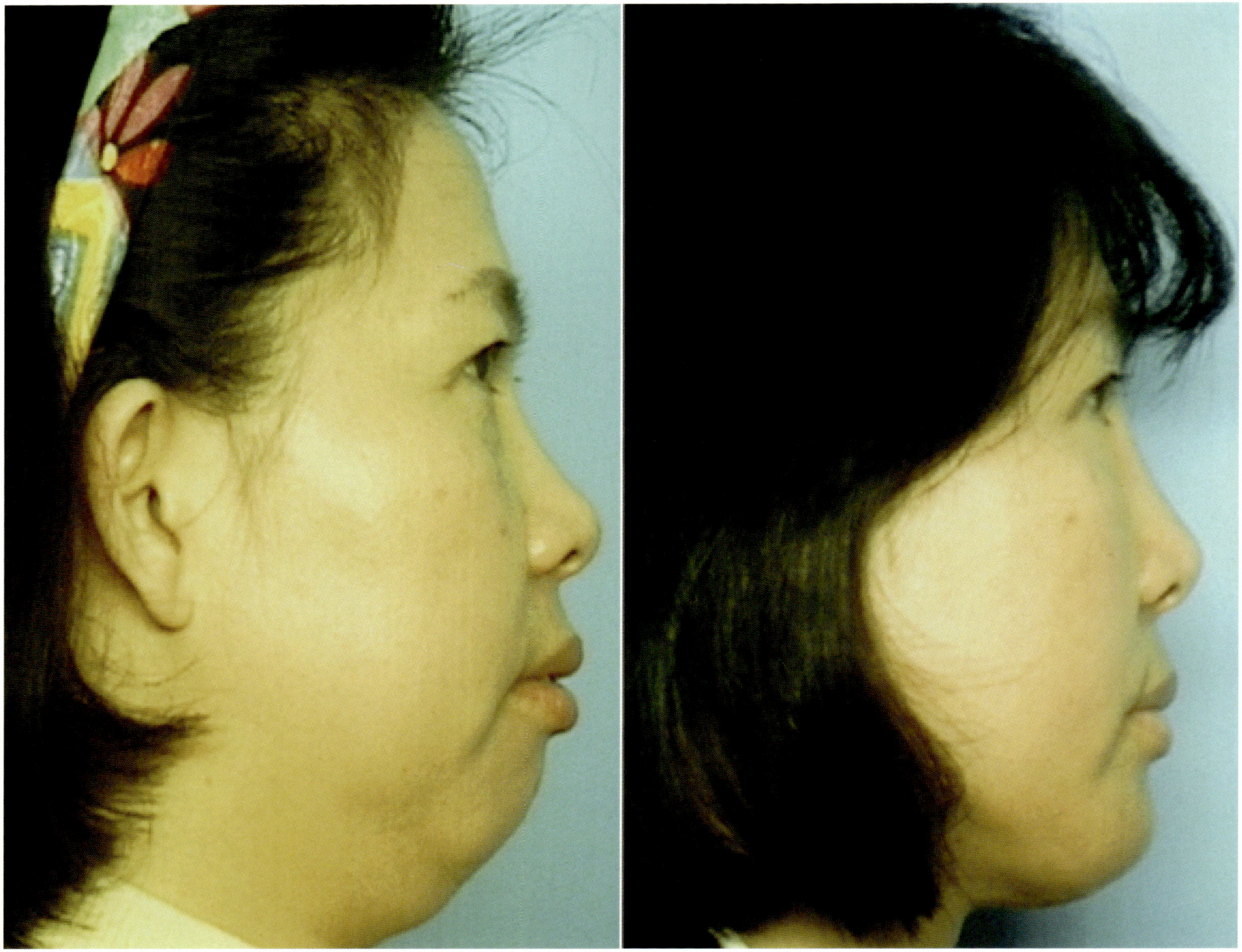

CONTOURING THE NECK

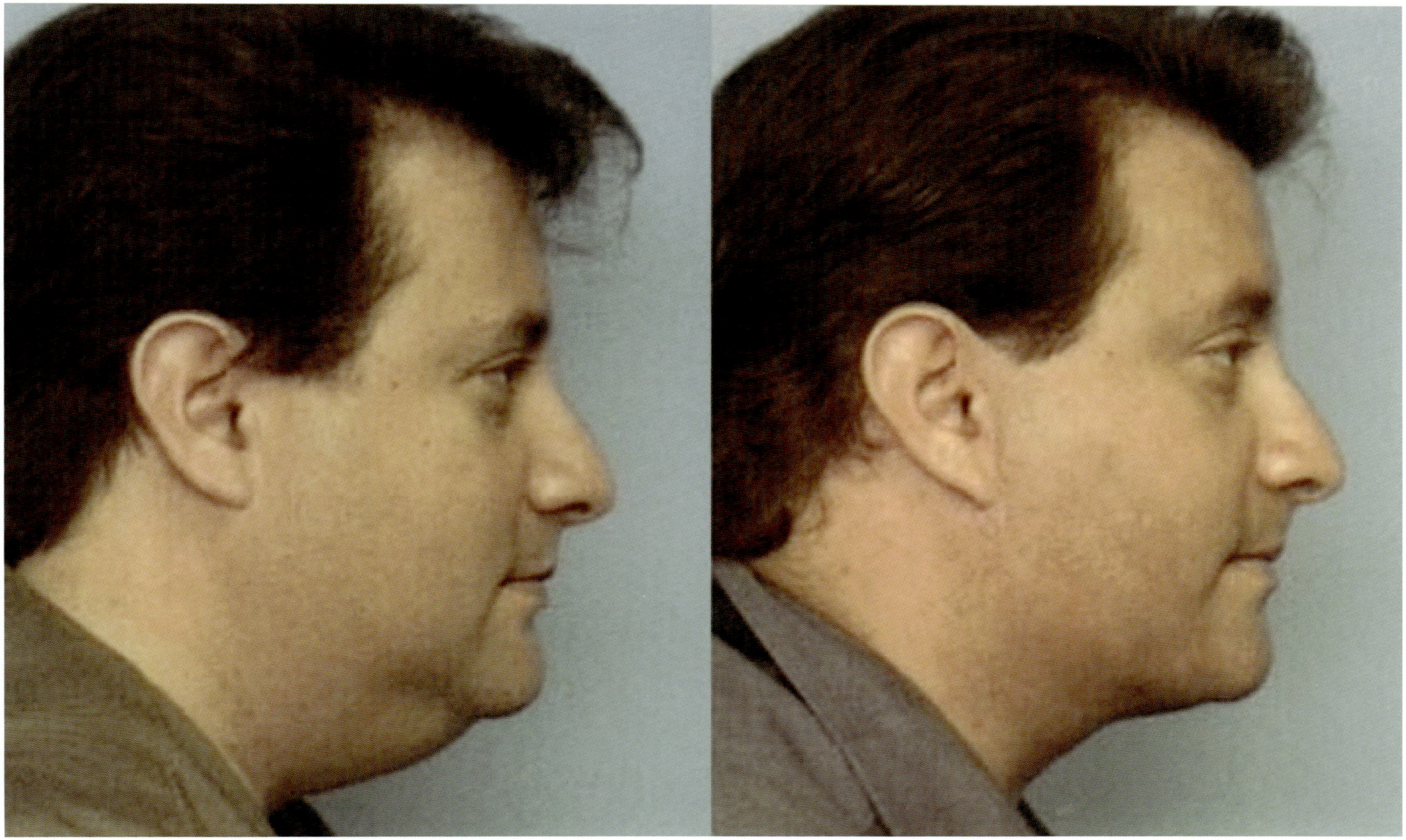

Injectable fillers can be used to replenish soft tissue loss of the cheek.

Available fillers today are:

1. Fat 2. Sculptra 3. Silikon

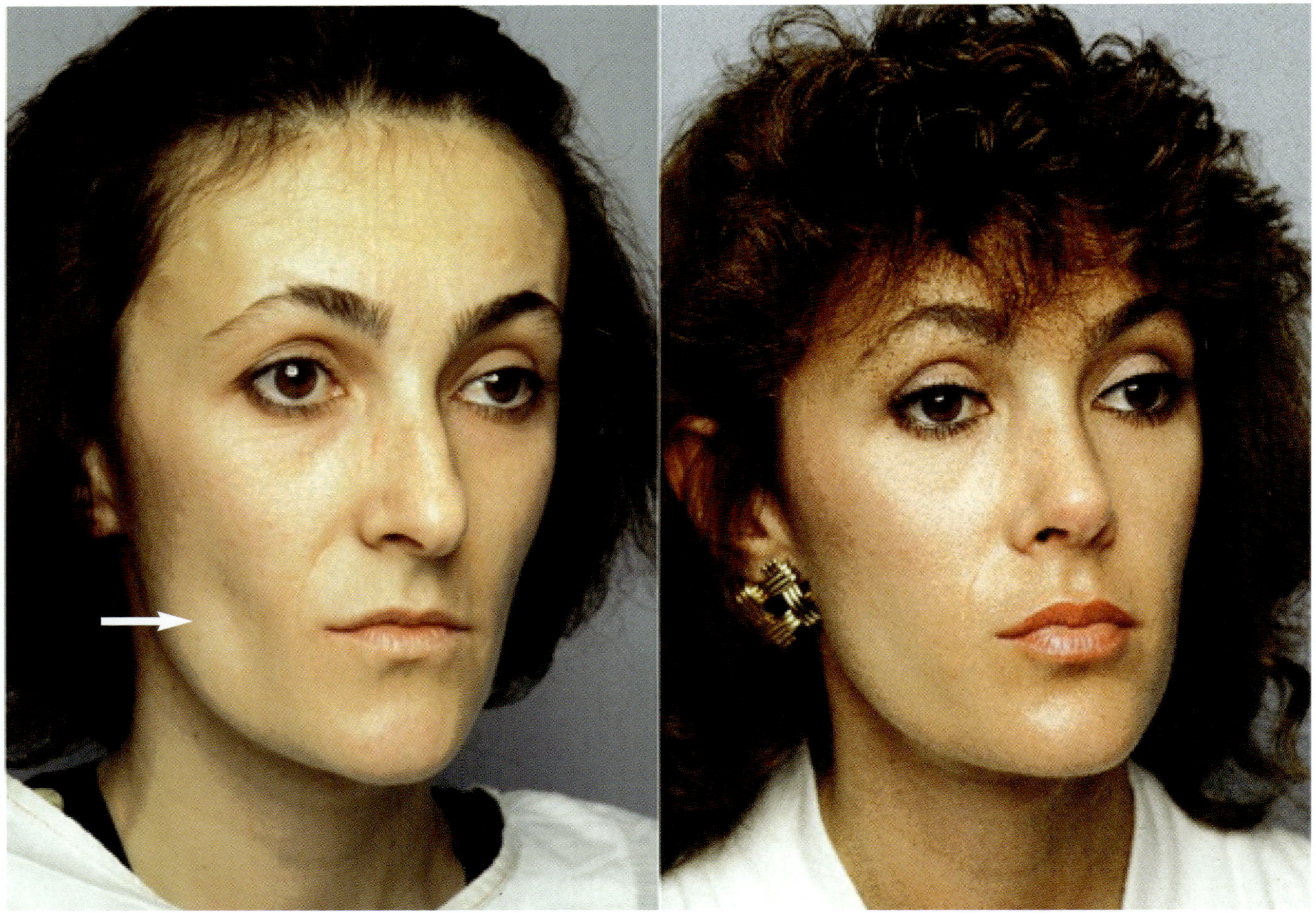

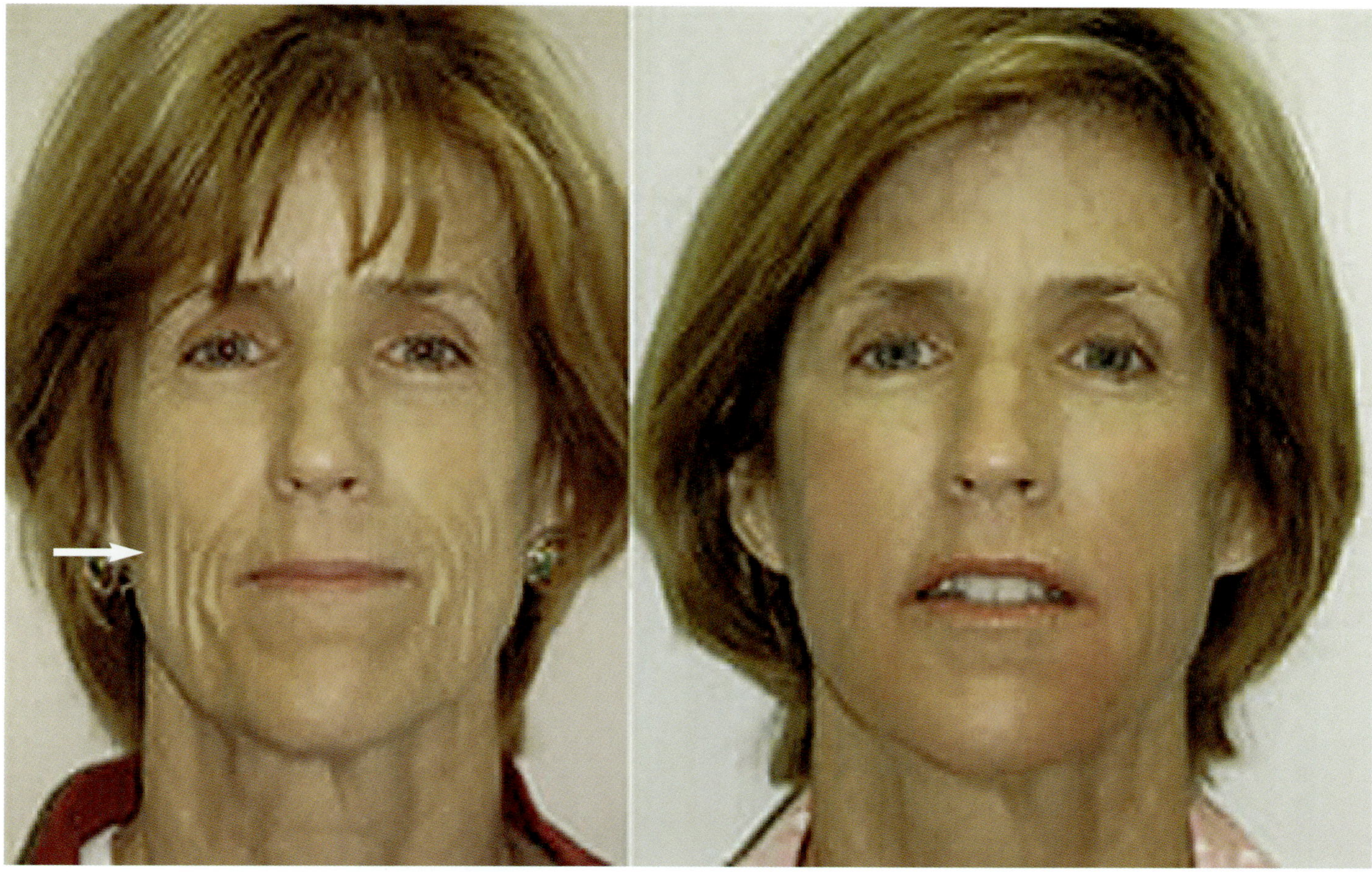

CHEEK IMPLANT

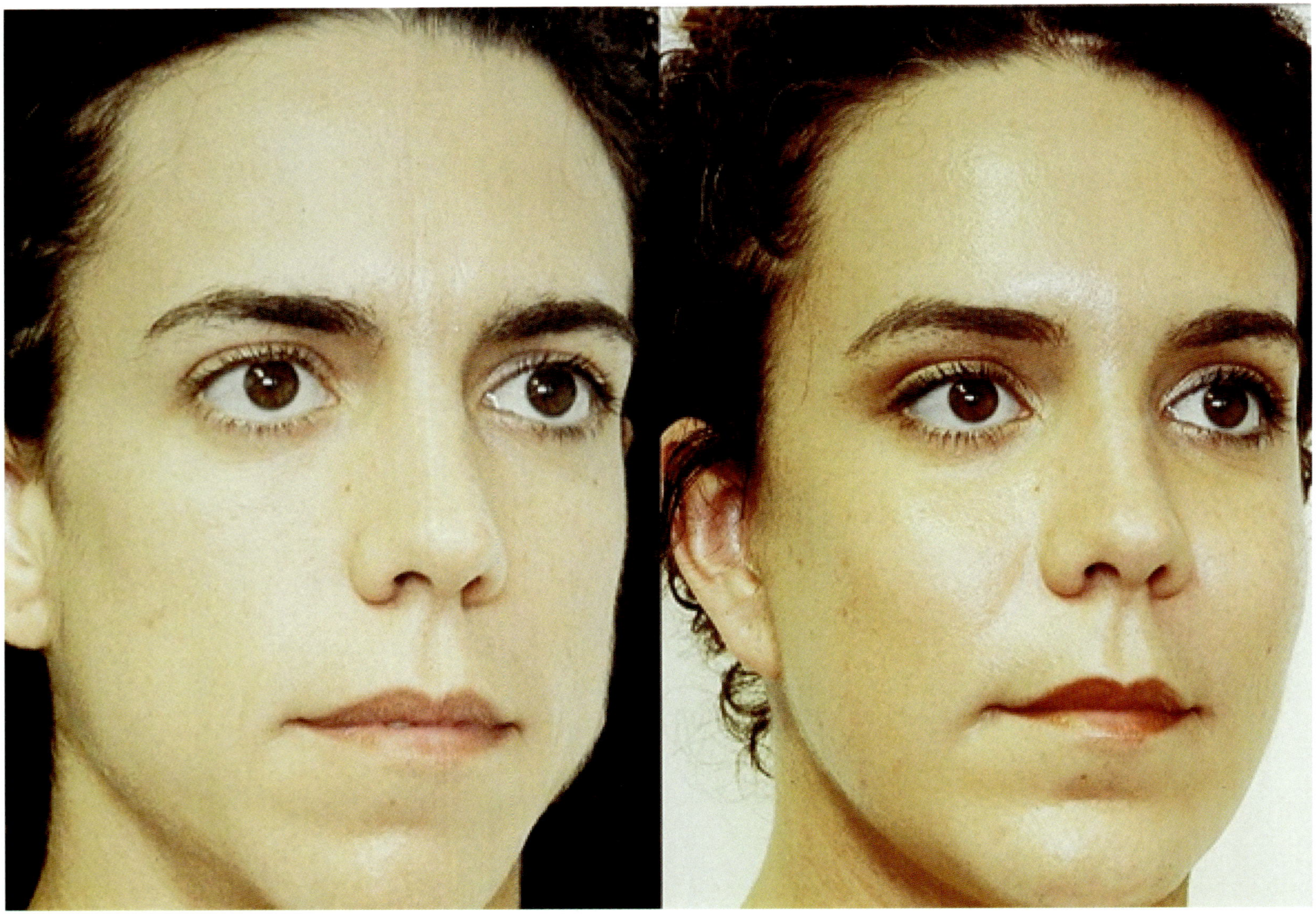

LIP ENHANCEMENT

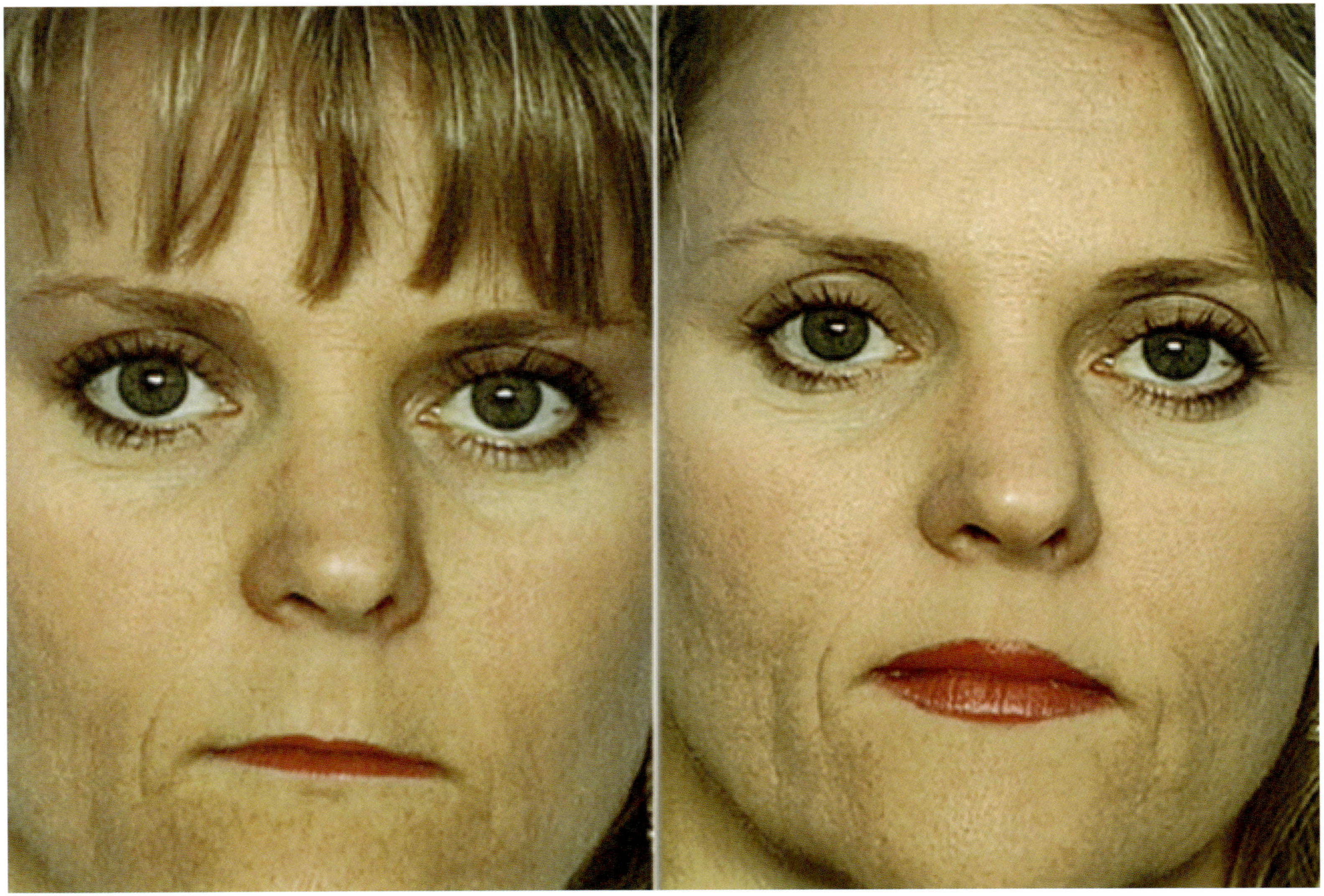

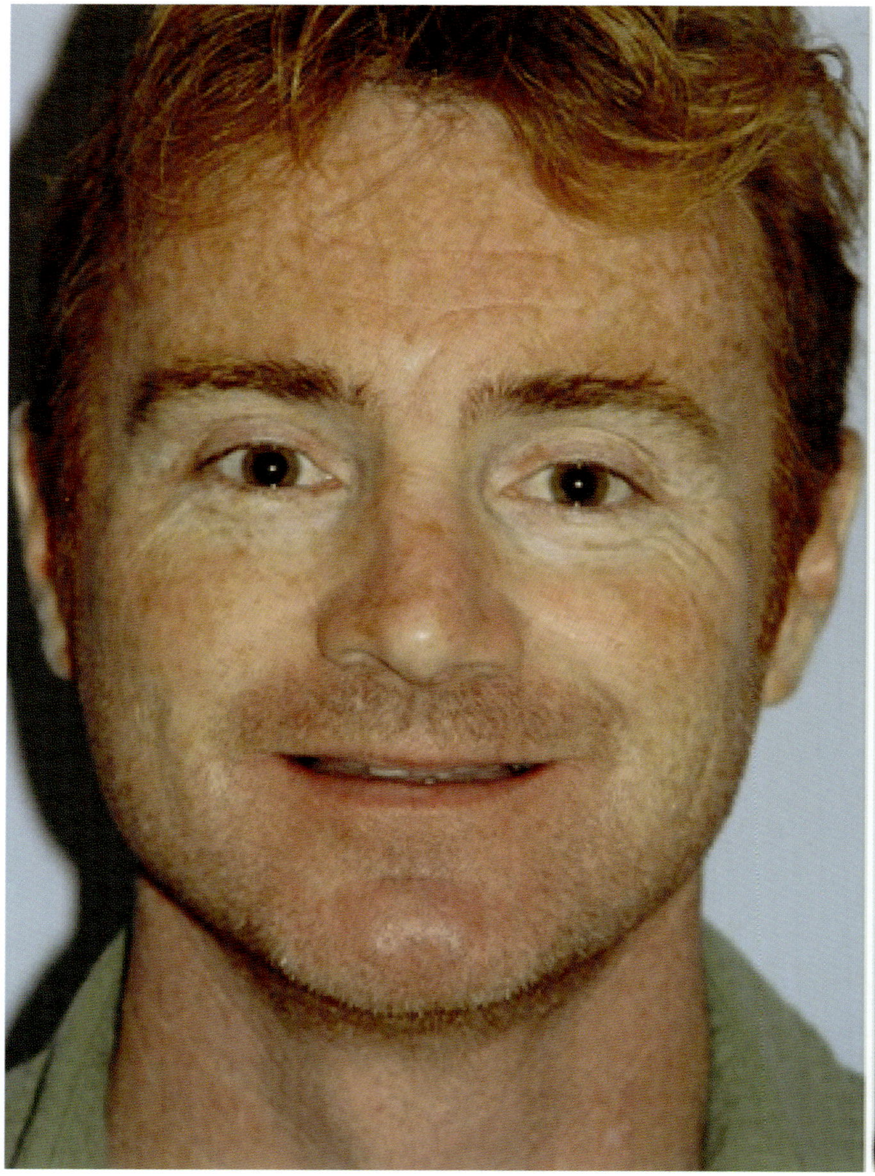

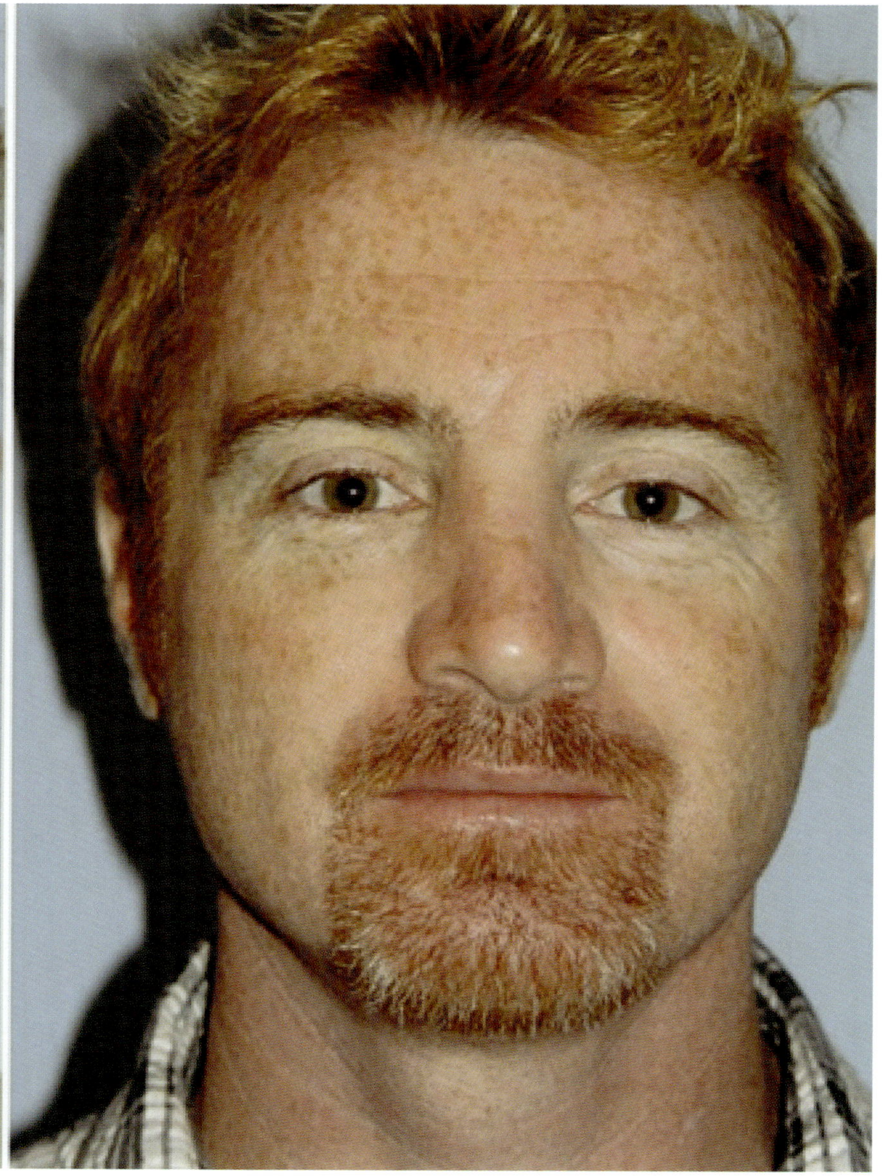

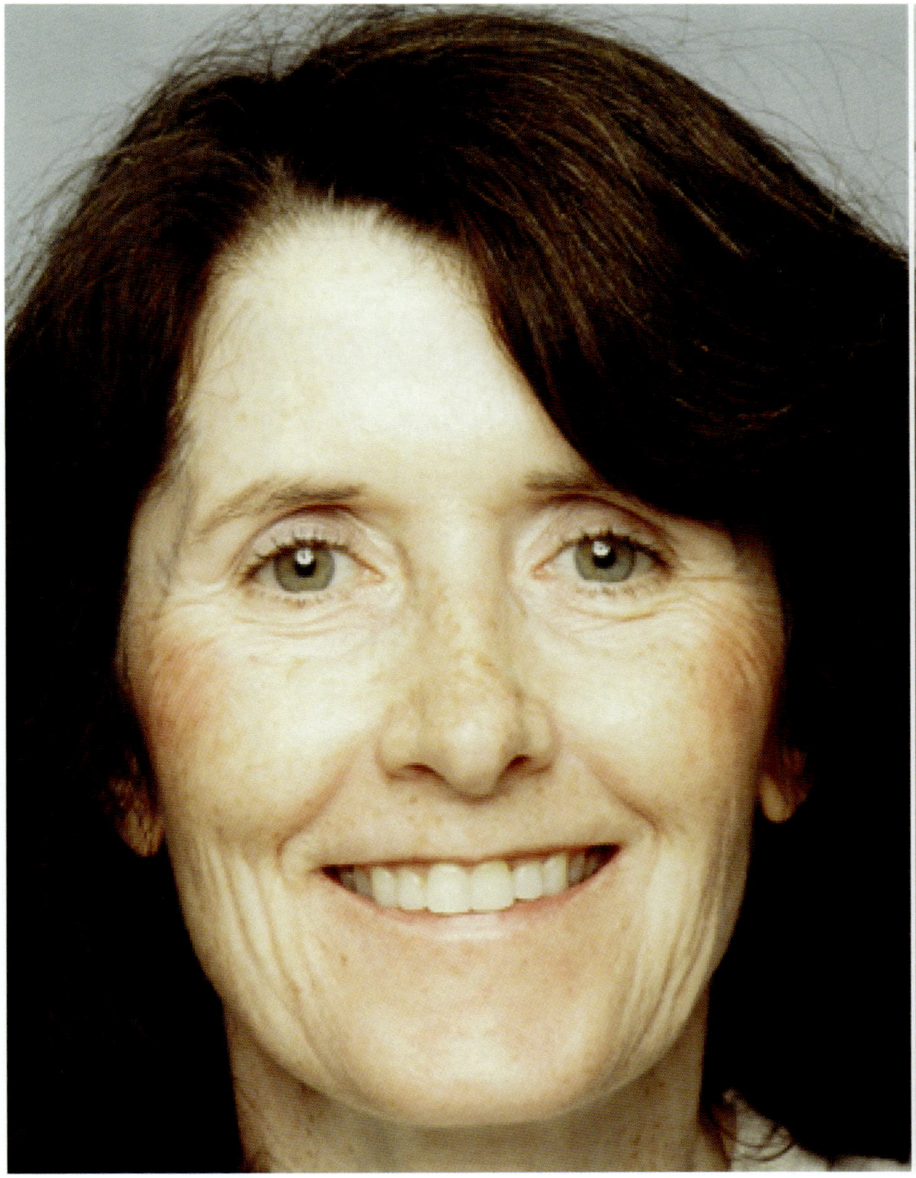

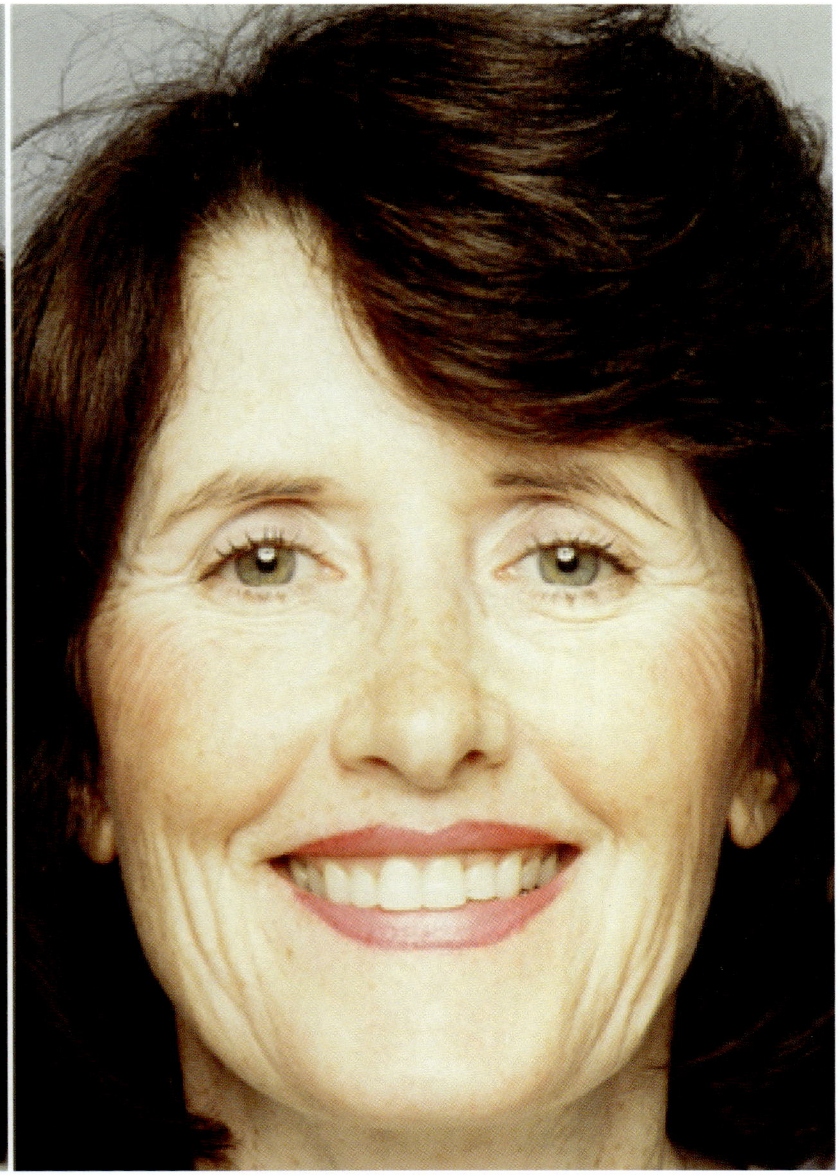

COSMETIC DENTISTRY

BLEACHING WITH BONDING

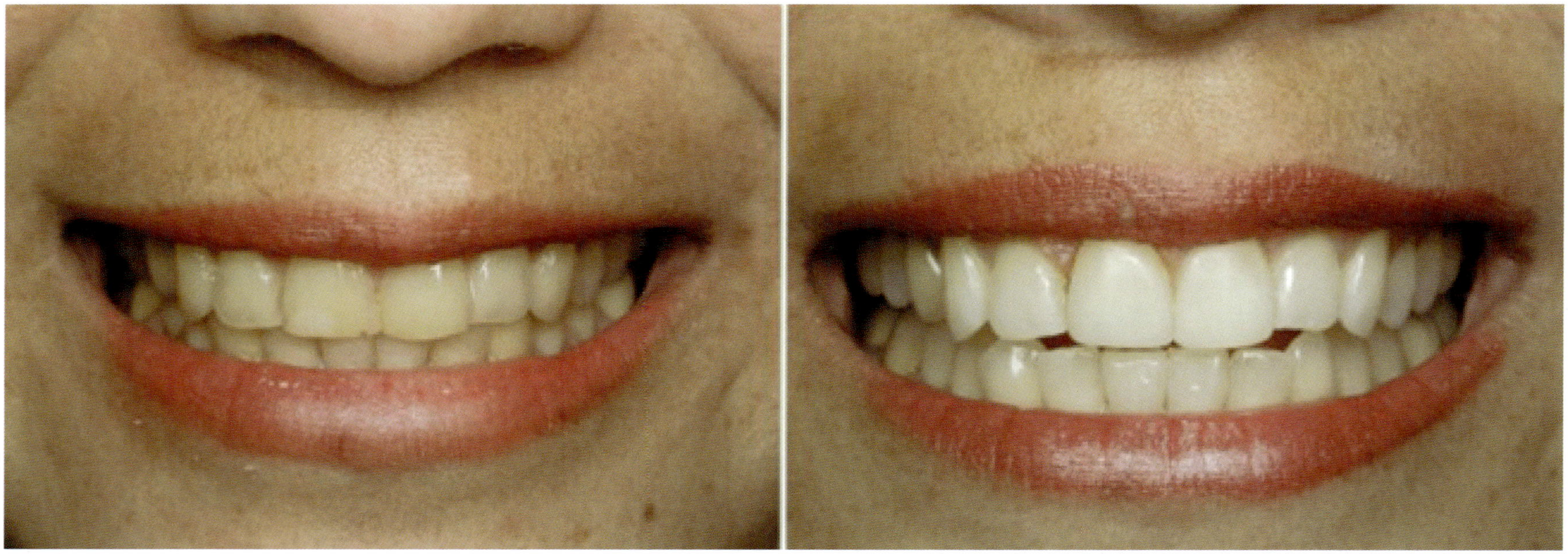

Courtesy of Dr. Arthur Helliwell, DDS
www.helliwelldds.com

DIRECT BONDING

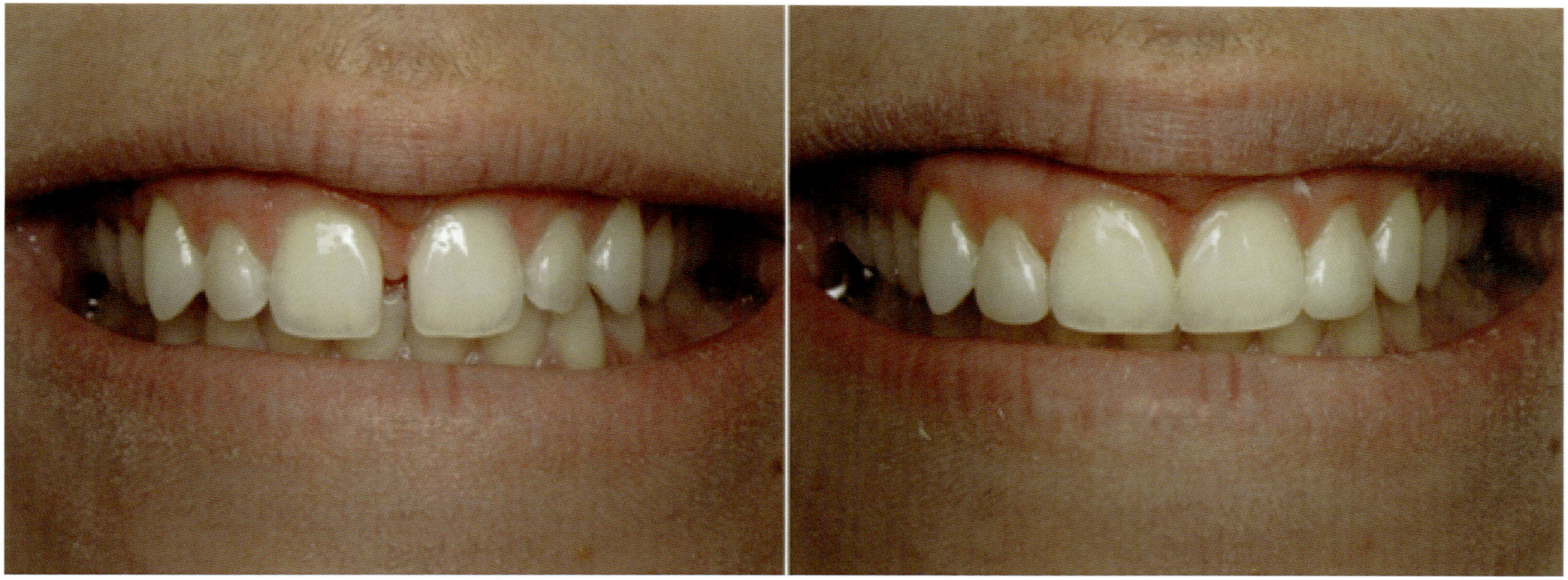

Courtesy of Dr. Arthur Helliwell, DDS
www.helliwelldds.com

BONDING WITH RECONTOUR

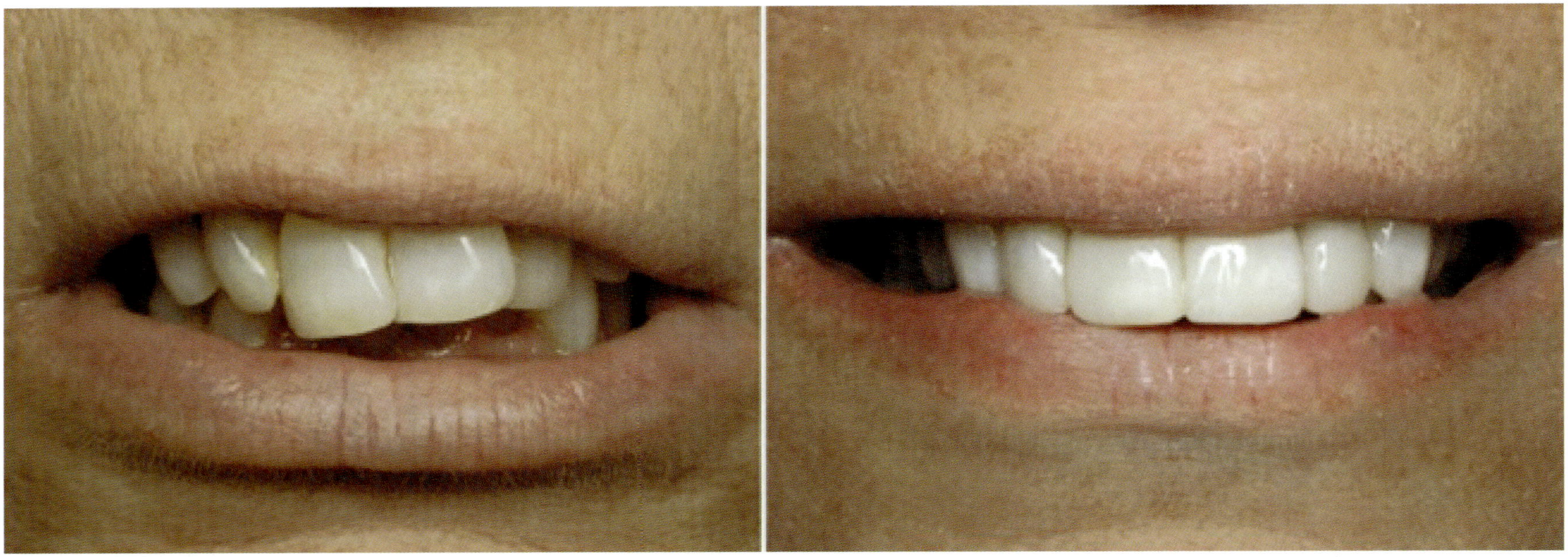

Courtesy of Dr. Arthur Helliwell, DDS
www.helliwelldds.com

STRAIGHTENING OF THE TEETH

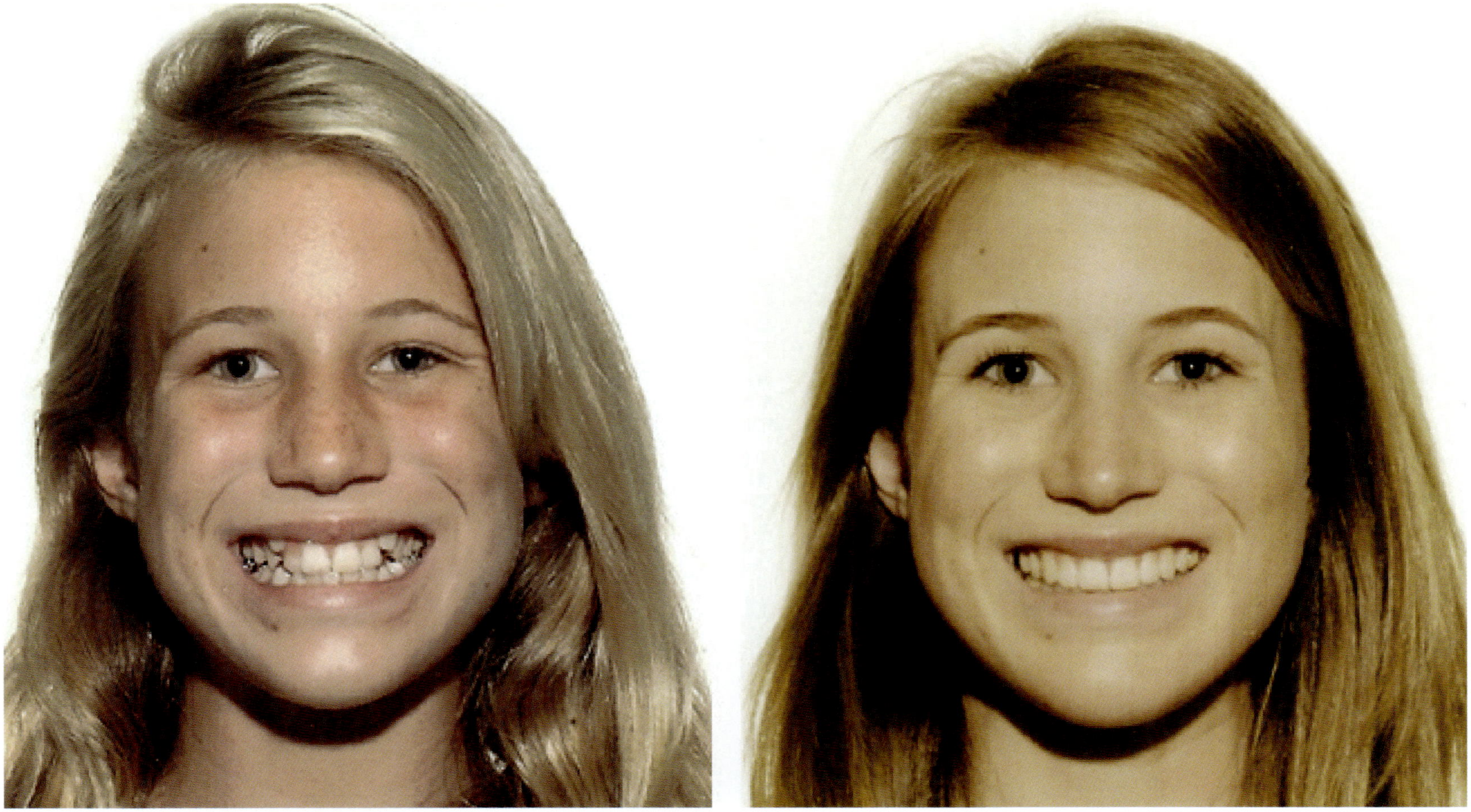

Courtesy of Dr. Todd Walkow, DDS
www.walkowortho.com

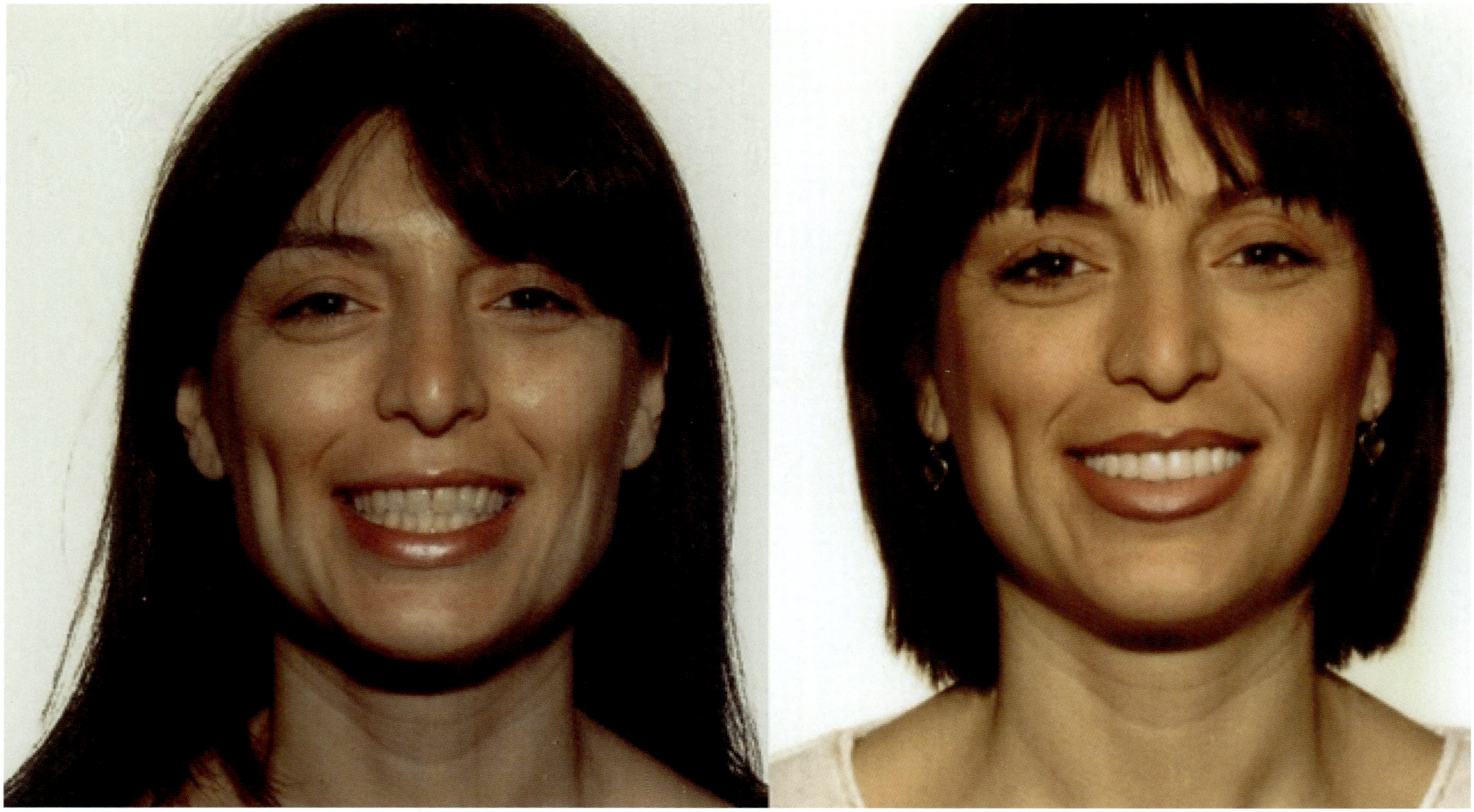

Courtesy of Dr. Todd Walkow, DDS
www.walkowortho.com

LOWER FACIAL REJUVENATION

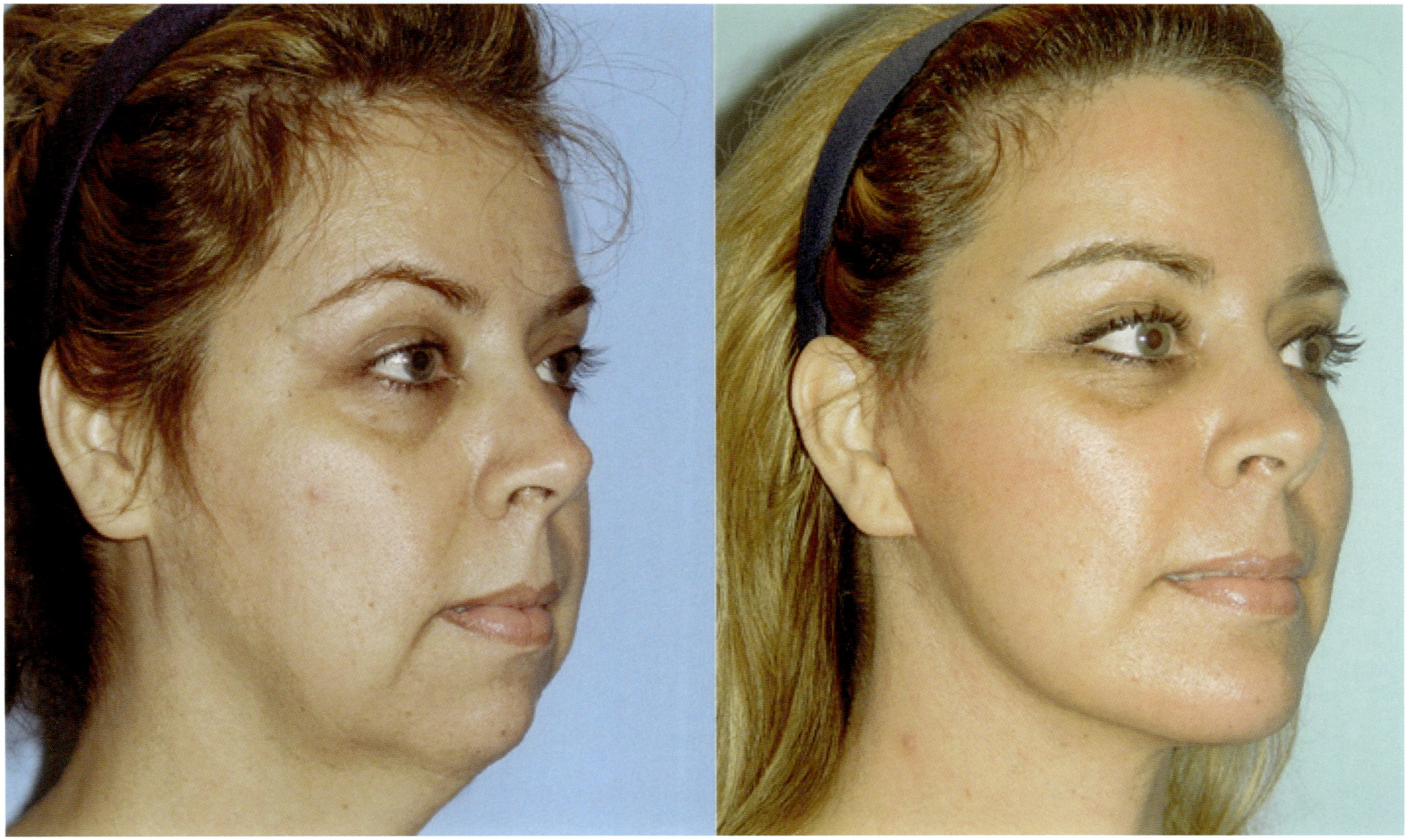

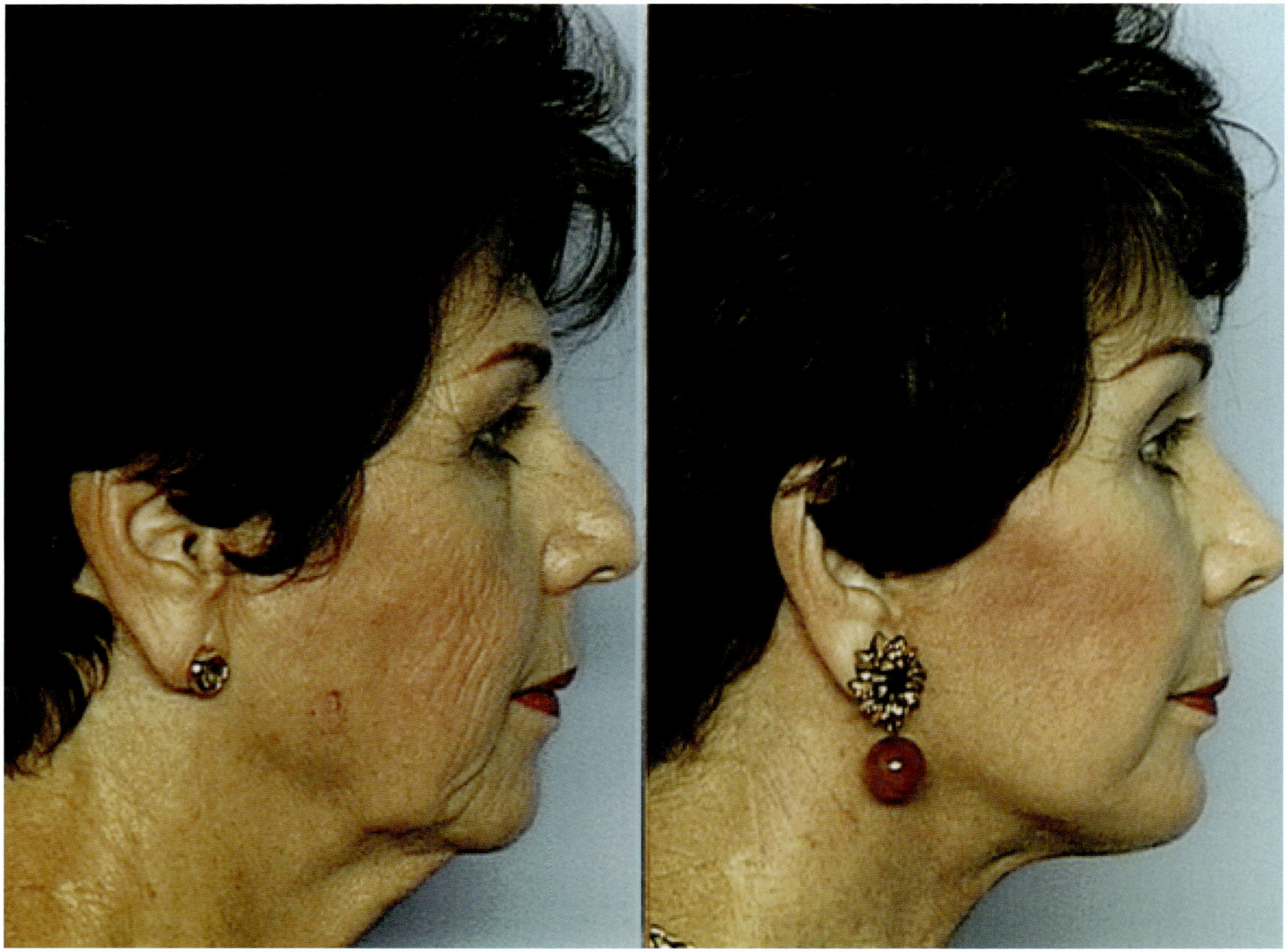

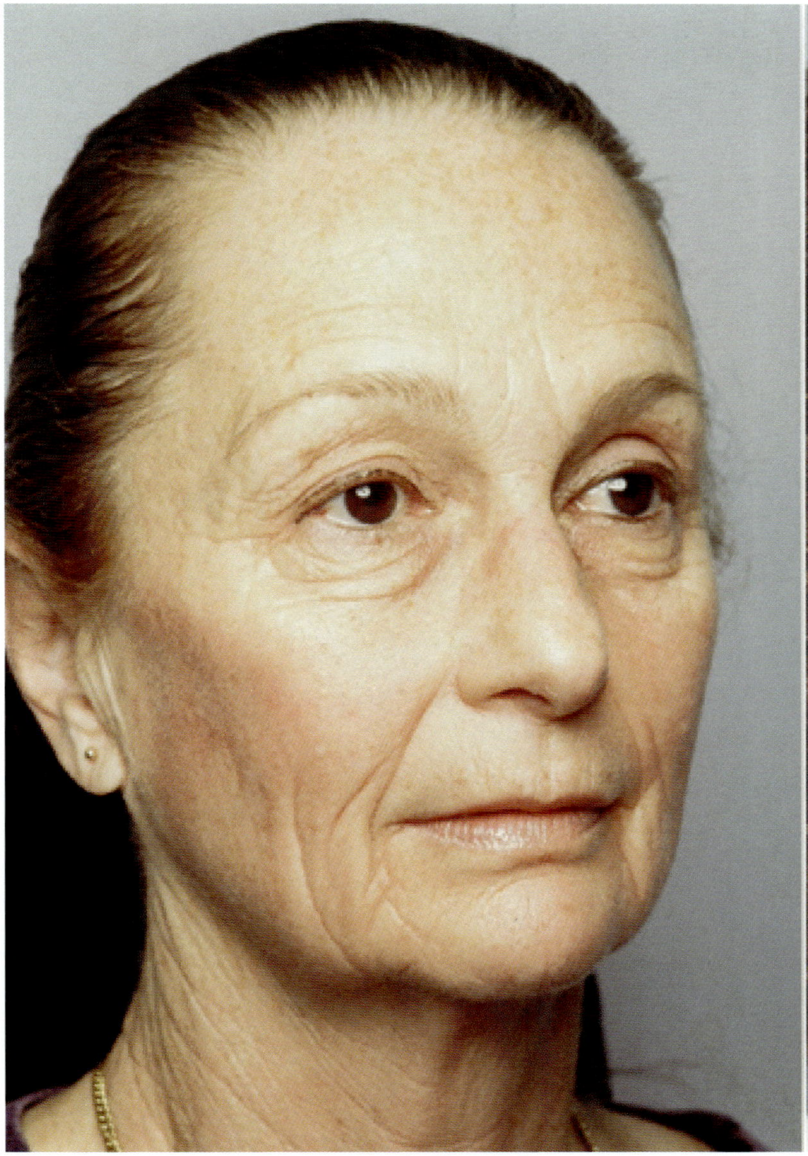

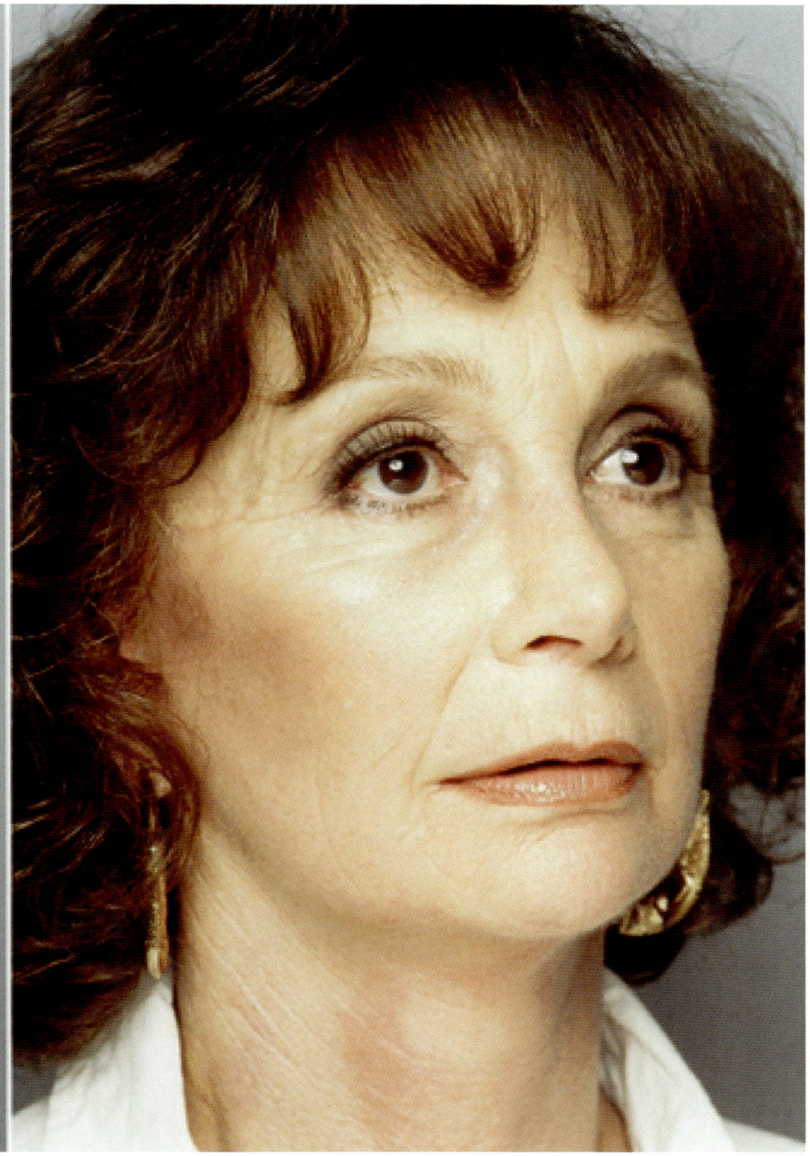

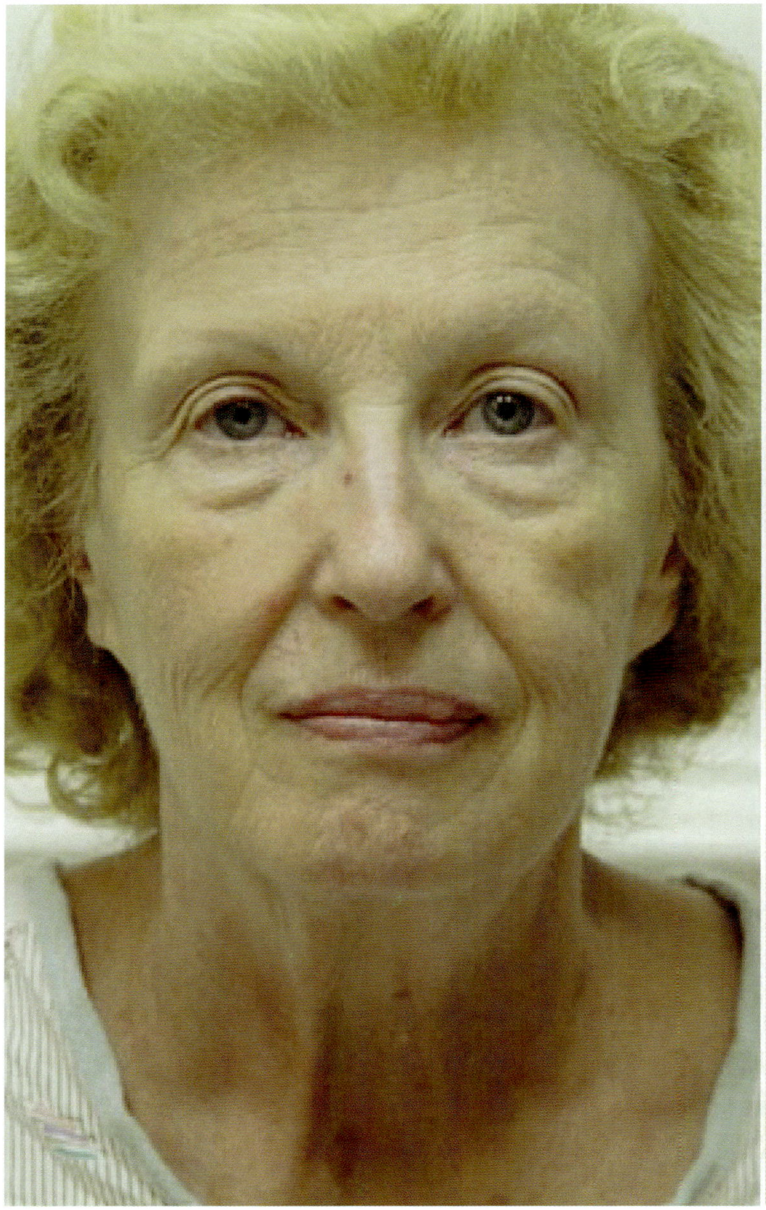

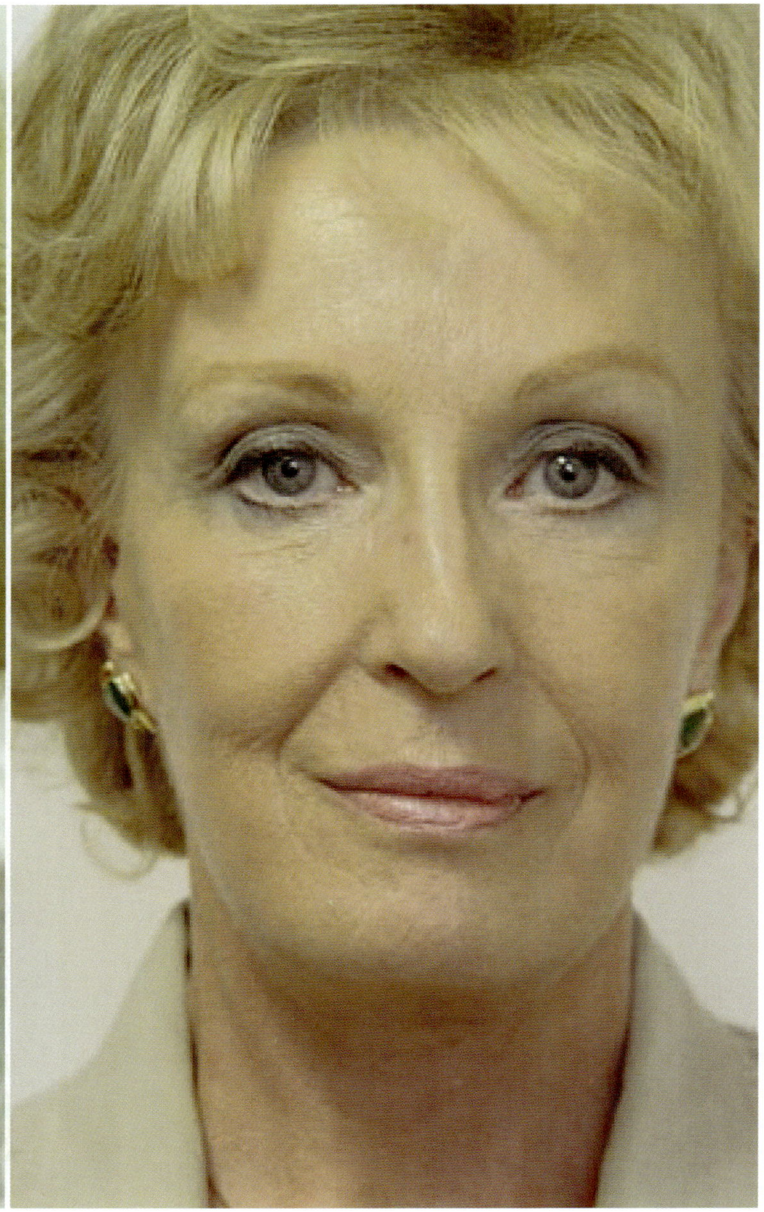

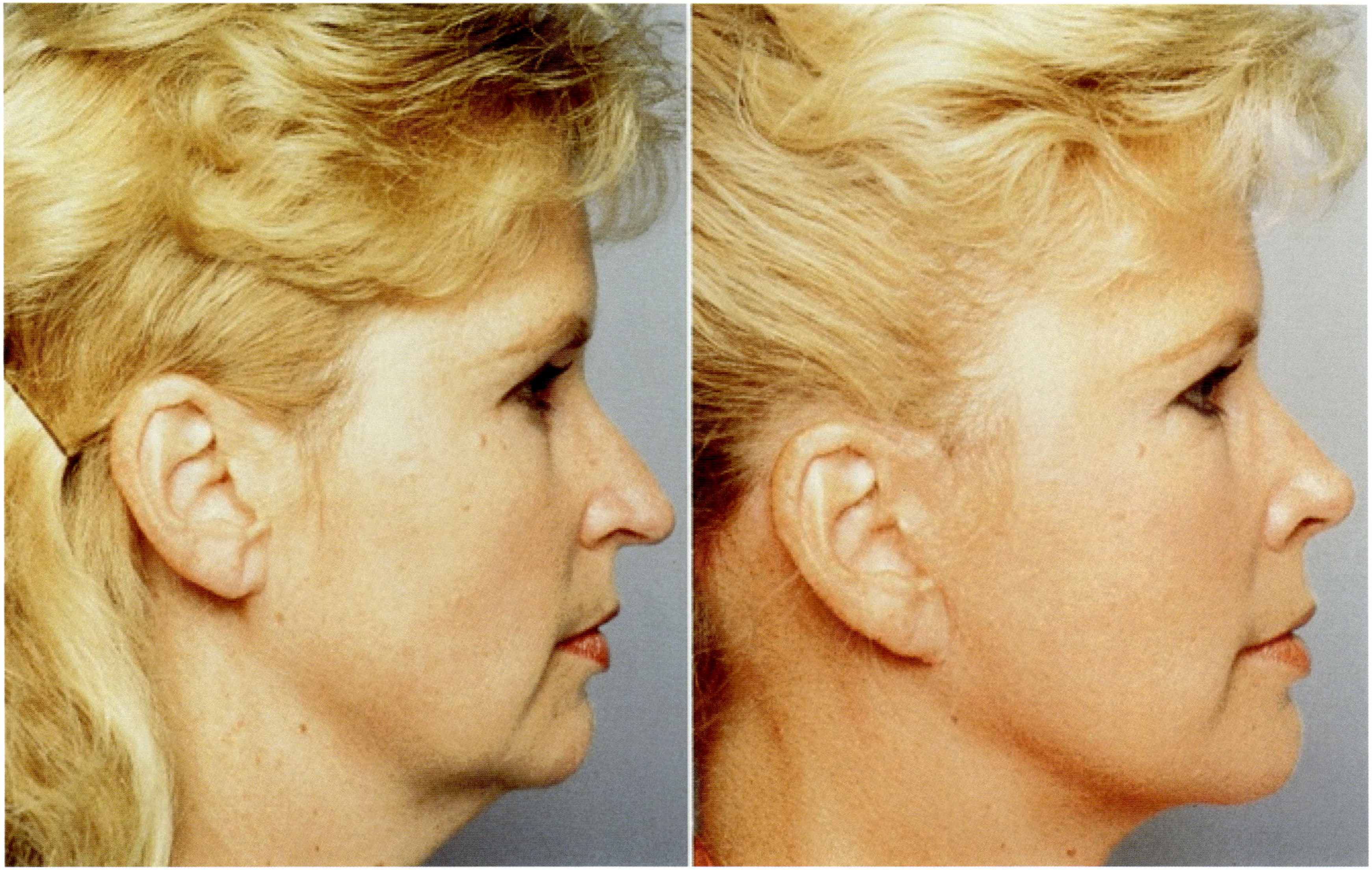

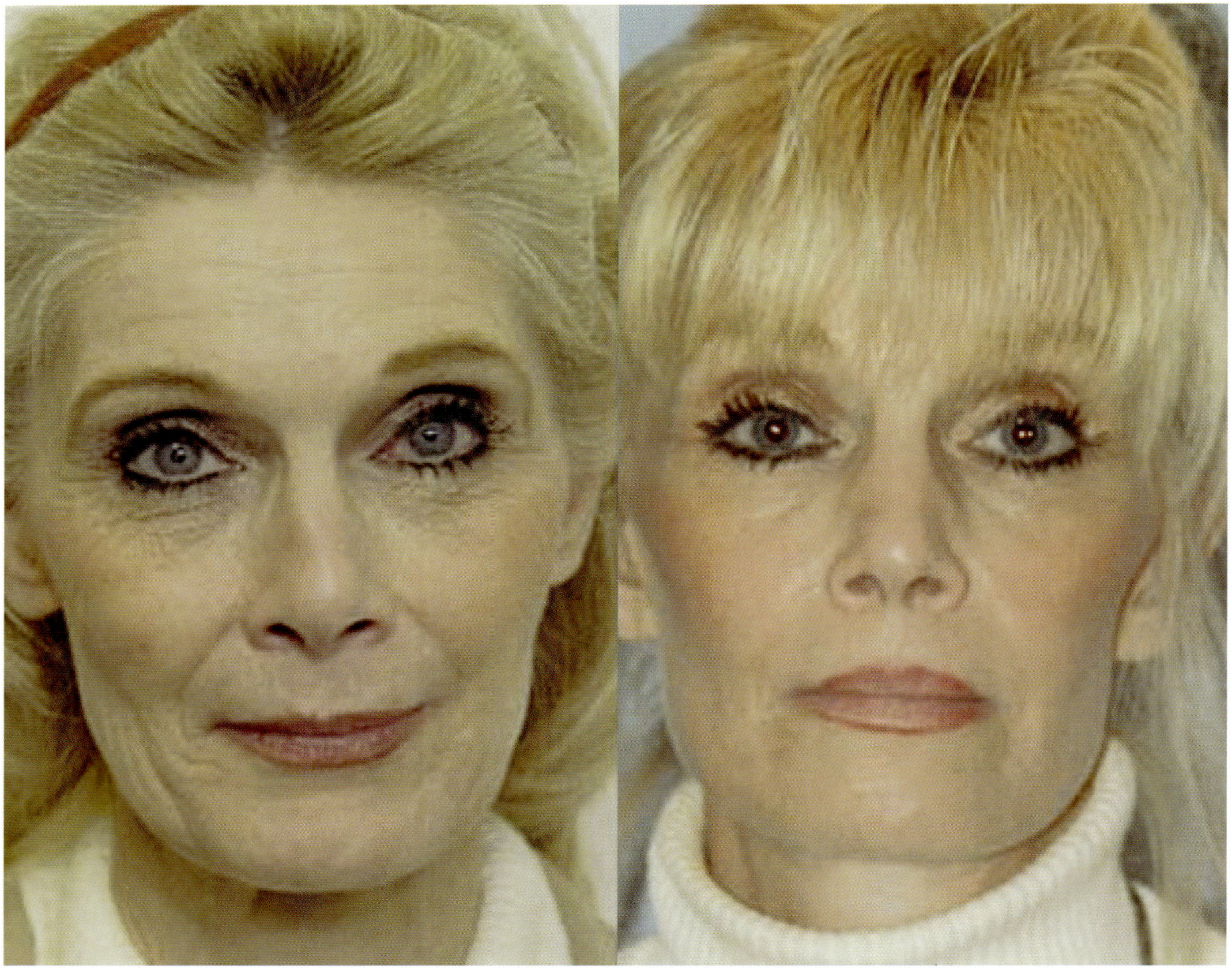

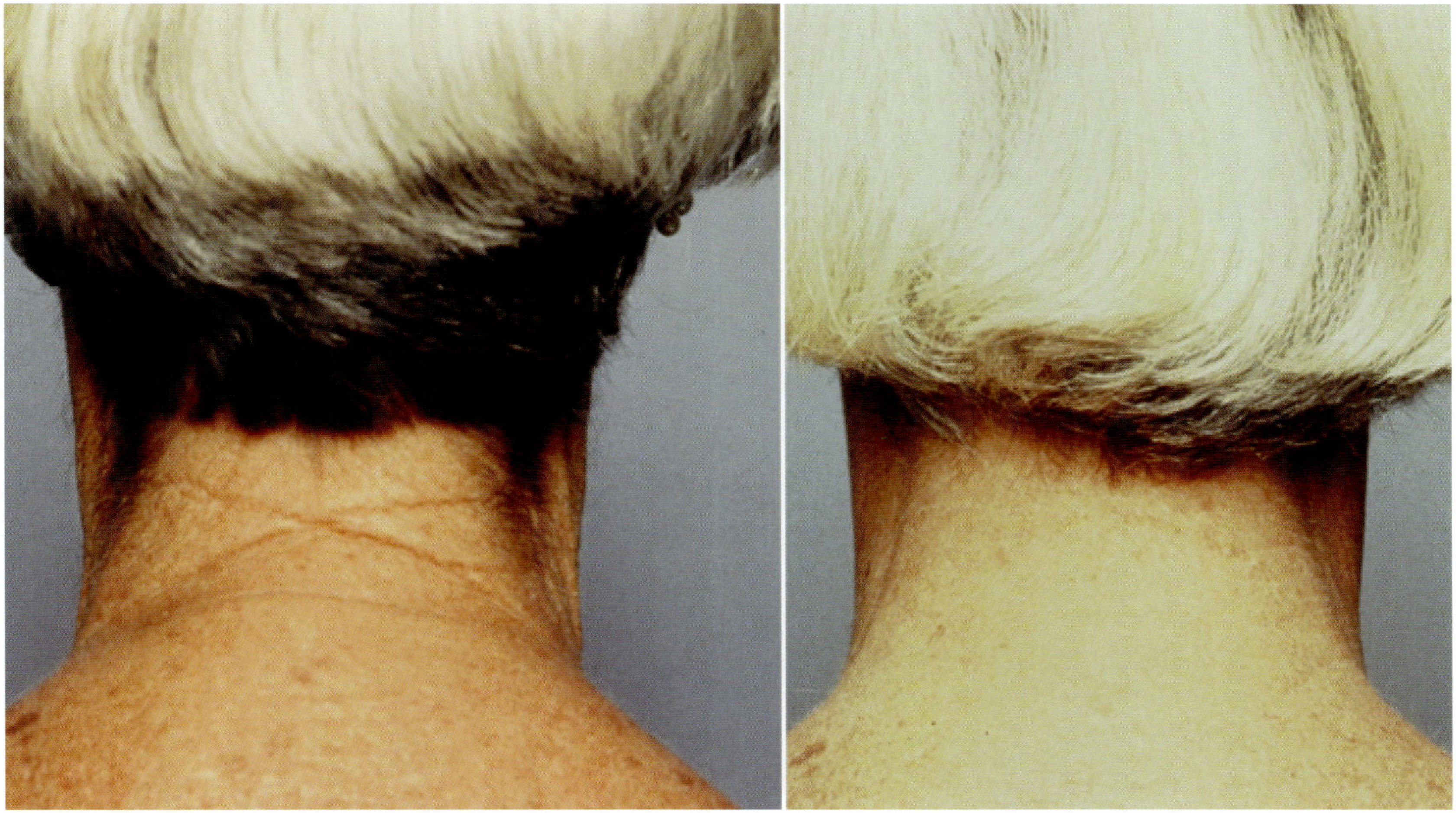

REJUVENATION OF THE BACK OF THE NECK

THE QUEST FOR BEAUTIFUL SKIN

Written by Joyce Scherer

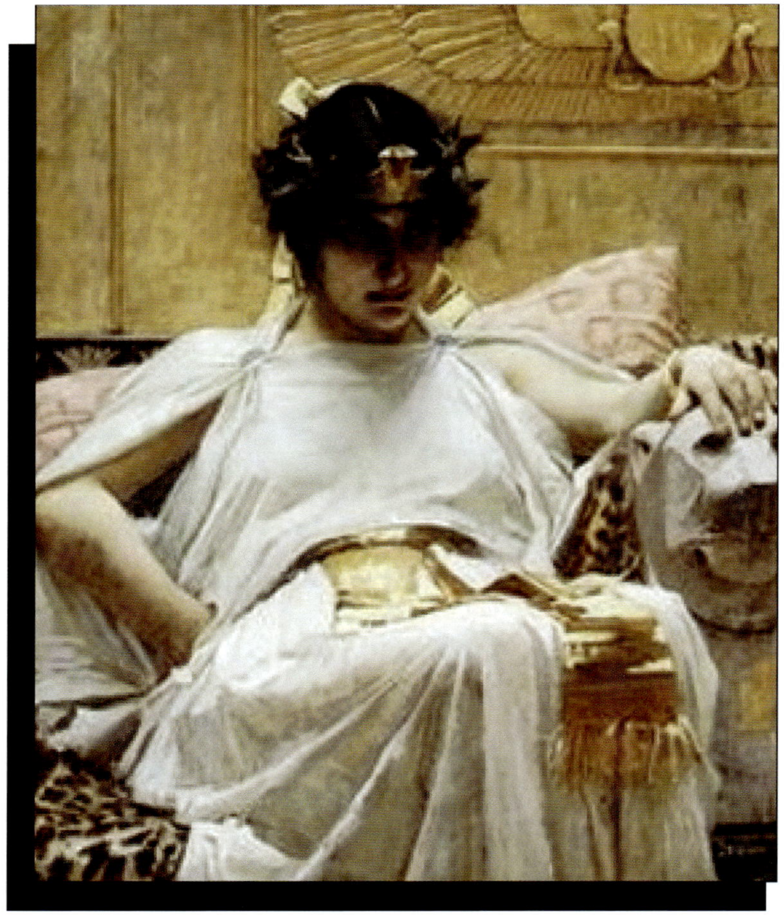

Cleopatra, the queen of Egypt, seduced Marc Anthony and Julius Caesar with her flawless beauty. Or did she? Early first century Roman writers lauded her enticing charm, alluring voice and eloquent speech. Missing, it appears, are comments on her exquisite loveliness. Relics, such as a coin dating from 32 B.C., depict the queen with a pointed chin, thin lips and a hooked nose. Maybe Elizabeth Taylor's glamorous movie portrayal of Cleopatra has skewed reality? Regardless of truth or lore, what does have substantial merit is how skin care practices, derived from ancient Egypt, have transcended time, gender, and status.

Cleopatra, said to have pretty skin, bathed in milk and honey for the smooth results of natural alpha hydroxy acid. Moisturizing oils were liberally applied by men and women to protect their skins from Egypt's hot and arid climate.

One familiar chant, "Ding Dong, Avon calling," is still heard nearly 120 years after David Hall McConnell, a book salesman, founded the company which would eventually be called Avon Products Inc. By 1906, the company - originally called the California Perfume Co. - had nationally recruited about 10,000 ladies to ring doorbells pitching the *Famous Tula Water for the Complexion*. Today, 4.9 million Avon representatives are scattered worldwide generating about $7.7 billion annually.

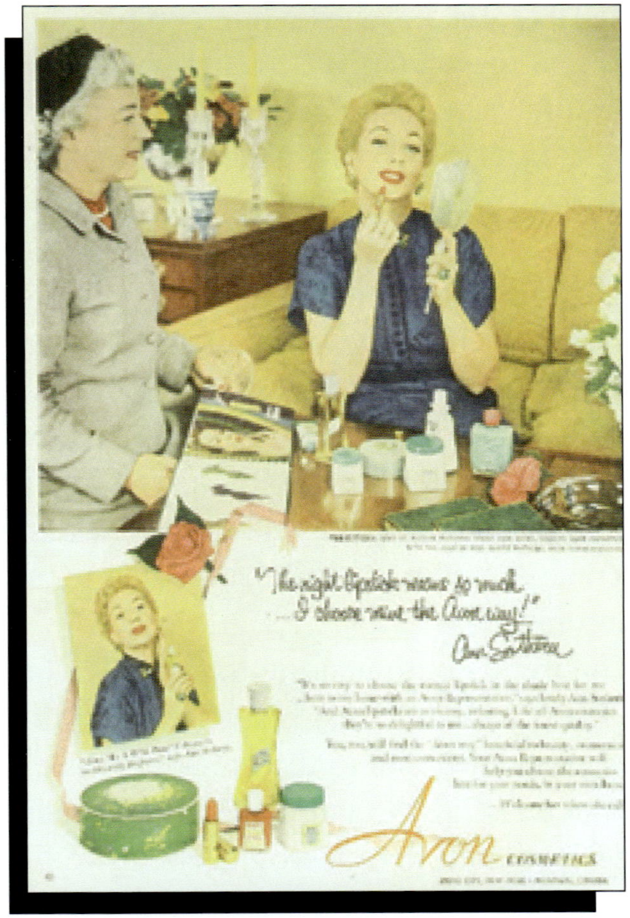

In 1922, the envious white complexion fizzled after fashion maven Coco Channel went sailing on the Duke of Westminster's yacht and inadvertently tanned her face. Suddenly, Channel's tea-colored face was looked upon with new eyes. A few years later, manufacturers were peddling sunless tanning products. The momentum continued drawing into its bronzed fold such Hollywood beauties as bathing suit pinups Betty Grable and Rita Hayworth. By the 1940s, women's magazines touted the benefits of sun-kissed skin. Homemade mixtures of baby oil and iodine became popular as both genders smeared on the concoction and baked sunny-side up under damaging rays.

The trend continued into the 1950s, '60s, and '70s as surfers loaded long boards atop stylin' woodies and steered the cars to the breaking waves. Beach movies, Gidget, and tanned bodies continued to be the rage until dermatologists bellowed long and hard about the sun's damage to skin and health.

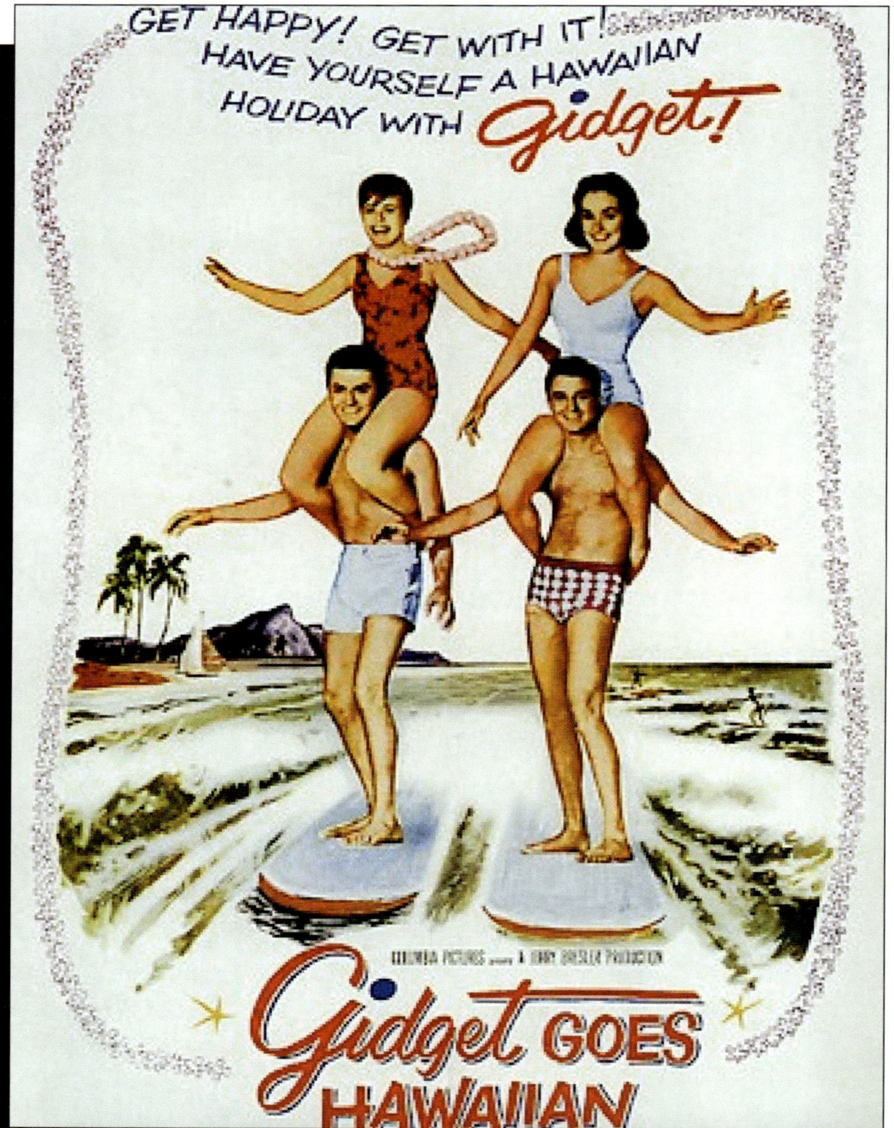

Reportedly, medical and skin care professionals have eased the burden of choice by helping people recognize the biggest detriment to the pursuit of great skin. The major factor, all say, is sun exposure. According to the Mayo Clinic, the skin protects itself from the sun by increasing production of melanocytes. These cells produce the dark brown pigment called melanin. Extra melanin is what darkens the skin. The results from sun damage can be brown spots, mottled red appearance, and sagging, wrinkled skin. Diligent, daily use of sunscreen – formulated with specific ingredients to block both UVA and UVB rays – is the recommended protection path.

While 21st century skin care continues to be explored, Cleopatra and her gang seem to have correctly set the bar for generations to come. The avoidance of sun and use of naturally-made products for anti-aging and rejuvenation were valued then as our range of rituals and products are today. Perhaps, the modern saying, "If it ain't broke, don't fix it," is more relevant than presumed when seeking out ways to attain beautiful skin.

SKIN REJUVENATION – THE SPECTRUM CONCEPT

We are all born with virgin skin – Depending on heredity and sun exposure we have a varying degree of sun damage.

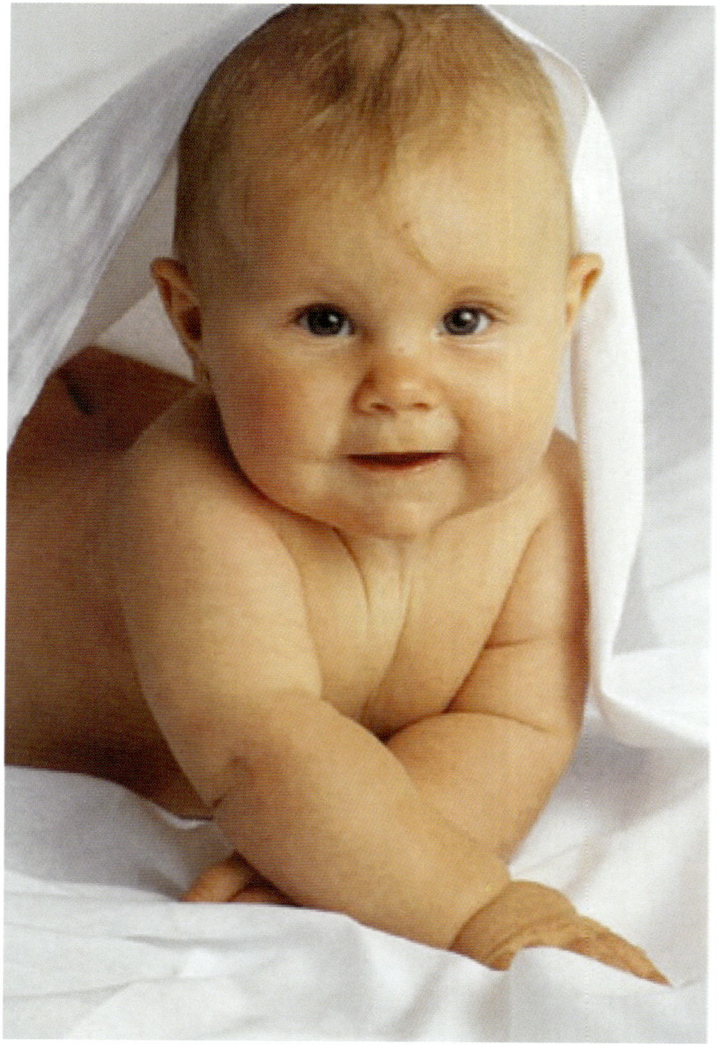

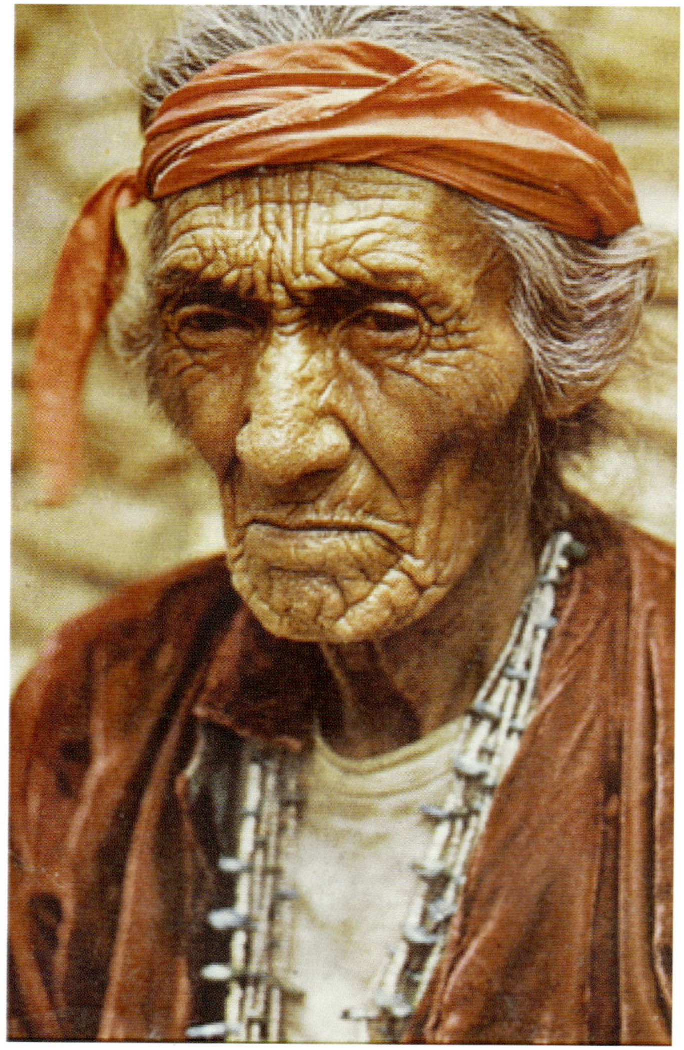

Normal skin consists of two basic layers; the outer layer called the epidermis which contains the cells that shed daily (exfoliation) and pigment cells. And the deeper layer of the skin called the dermis containing collagen, elastic fibers, hair follicles,oil and sweat glands and a network of blood vessels.

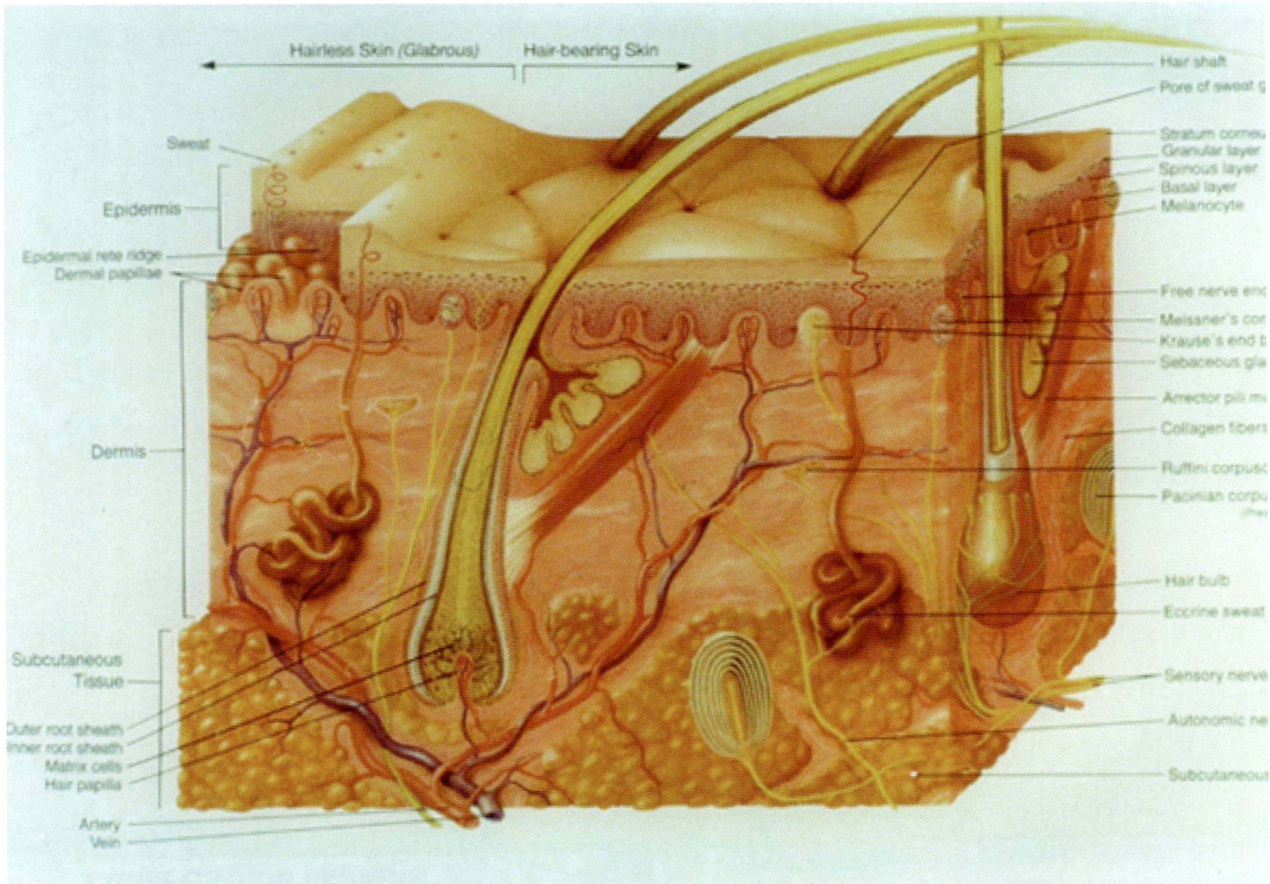

Everyone is on the diagnostic spectrum and everyone should be on the therapeutic spectrum.

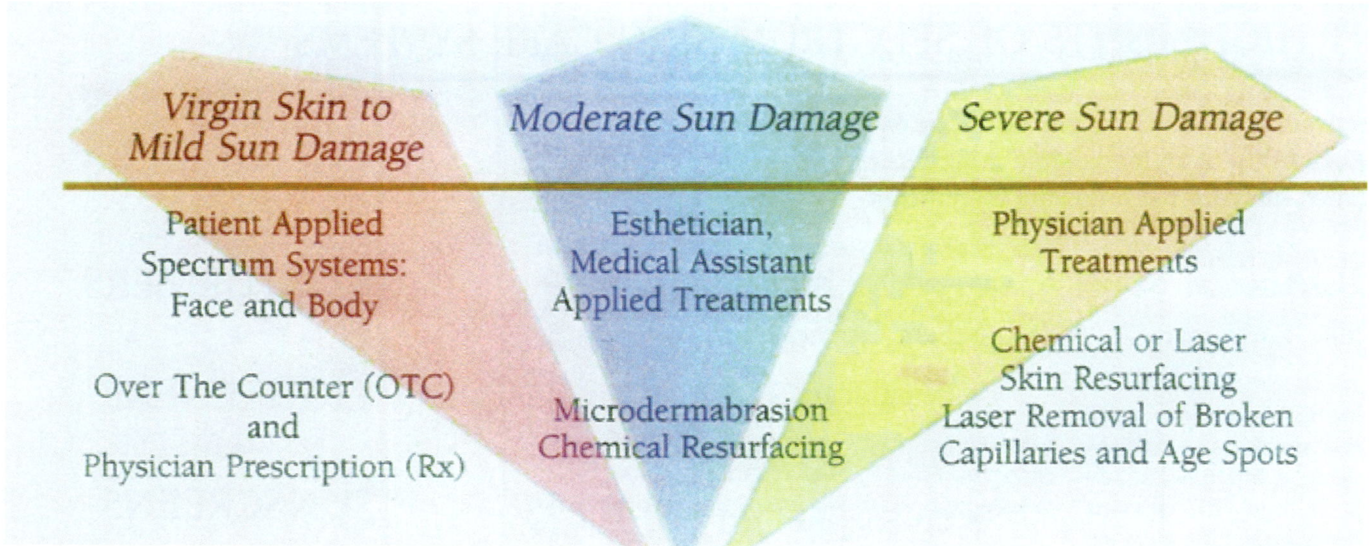

At one end of the spectrum is virgin or mildly sun damaged skin and the therapeutic concept is a patient applied system. The most mild form is an over-the-counter non-prescription strength. There is a more concentrated formula, which is prescription strength, but is also patient applied.

The middle range of the spectrum is moderate sun damage – these conditions are best treated by first pre-conditioning the skin with the patient applied system for several weeks and then followed by an esthetician applied series of systems that will serve to resurface the skin and reverse sun damage to re-establish youthful skin.

In the far end of the spectrum we see severe sun damage, which requires a patient applied system to pre-condition the skin and to start the exfoliation and rejuvenation process and then this is followed by a physician applied method of resurfacing the skin either by chemicals or lasers.

Sun damage is visible to the naked eye and we see this very commonly in people who work or play outdoors. The front part of a women's chest can exhibit severe sun damage due to that exposed skin. Here are just two examples of sun damage that is visible to the naked eye.

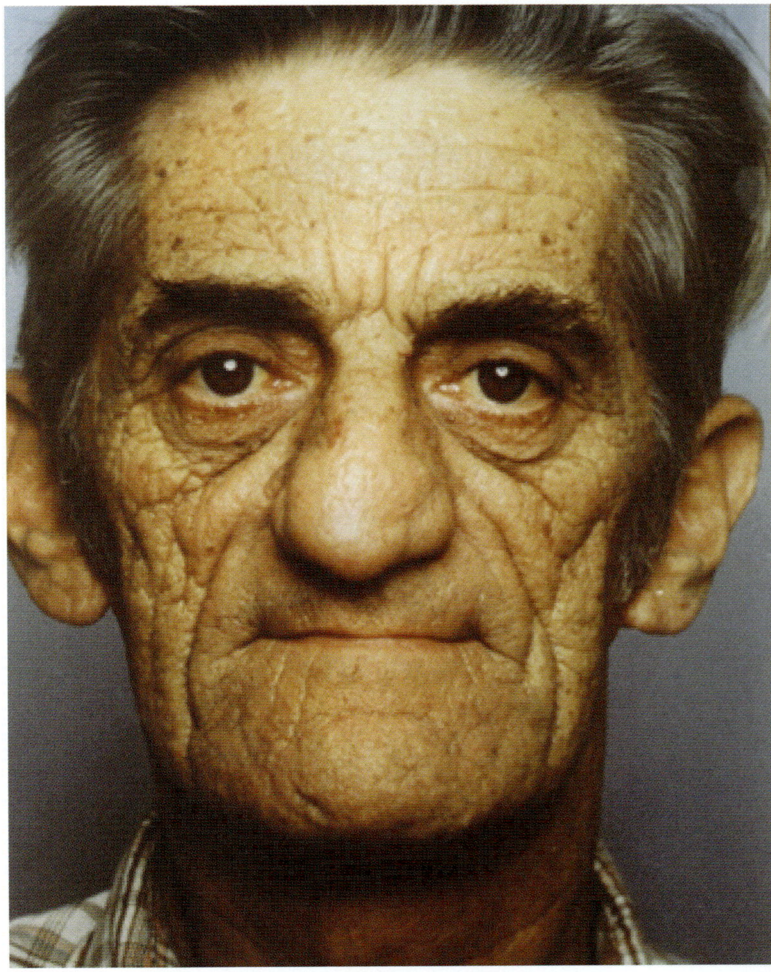

Facial Sun Damage.

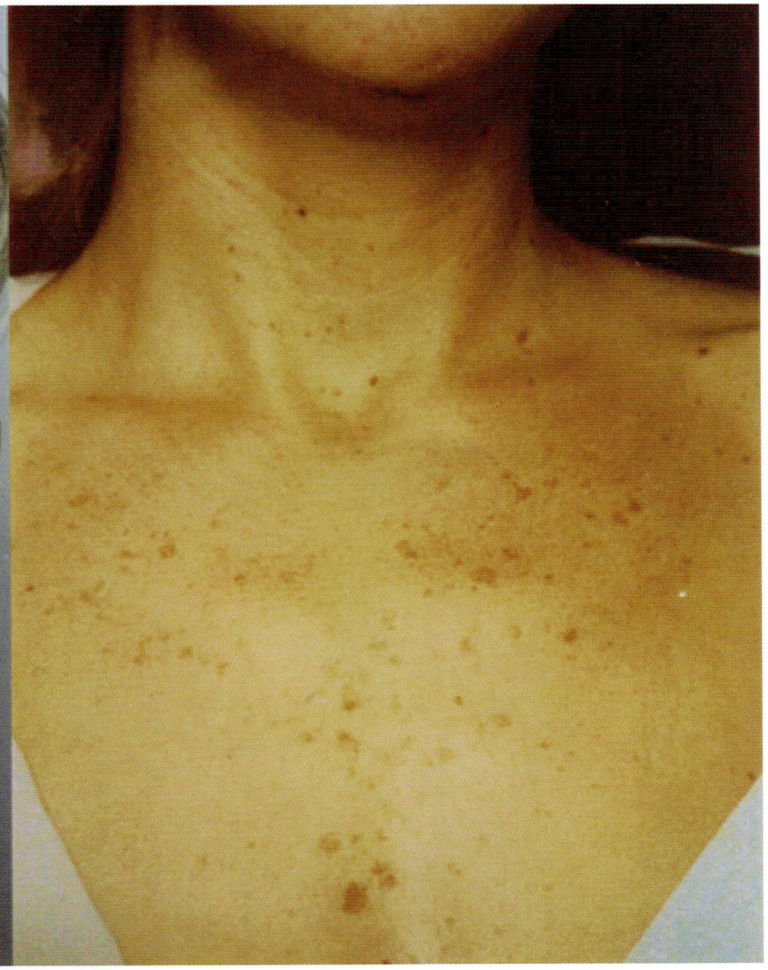

Sun damage to the decollate of a young women's chest.

The most common disease is sun damaged skin and the most common form of cancer is skin cancer. Sun damaged skin can develop thickening (solar keratosis) and pigmentation. Any and all of these can undergo what we call malignant degeneration, which may then develop into cancer, either basal, squamous or malignant melanoma. Here is an example of a young person who had early skin cancer requiring extensive surgery.

Although reconstructive surgery is successful, it is more prudent to prevent sun related skin cancer.

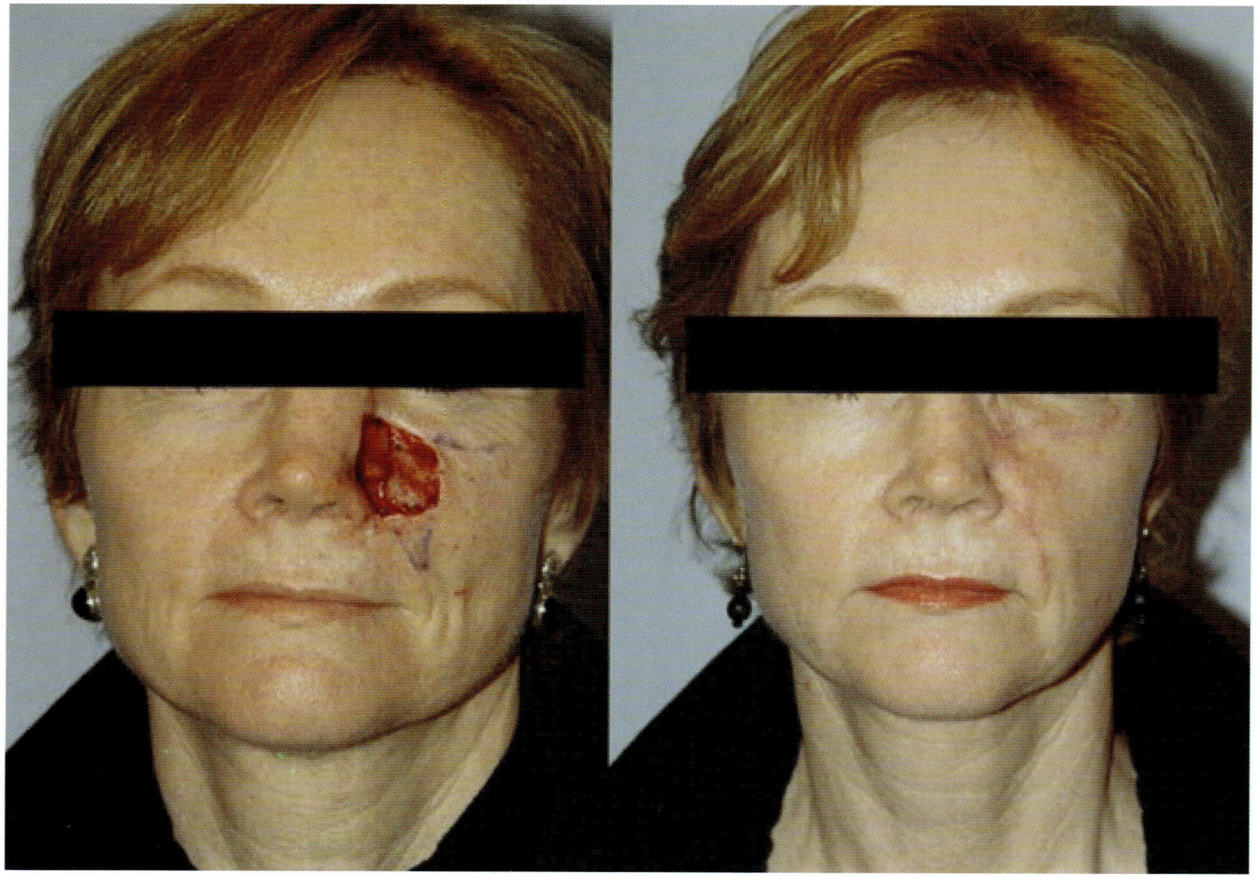

The UV camera shows us things that we cannot see with the naked eye. The UV camera serves as a warning system because it is a preview of the future.

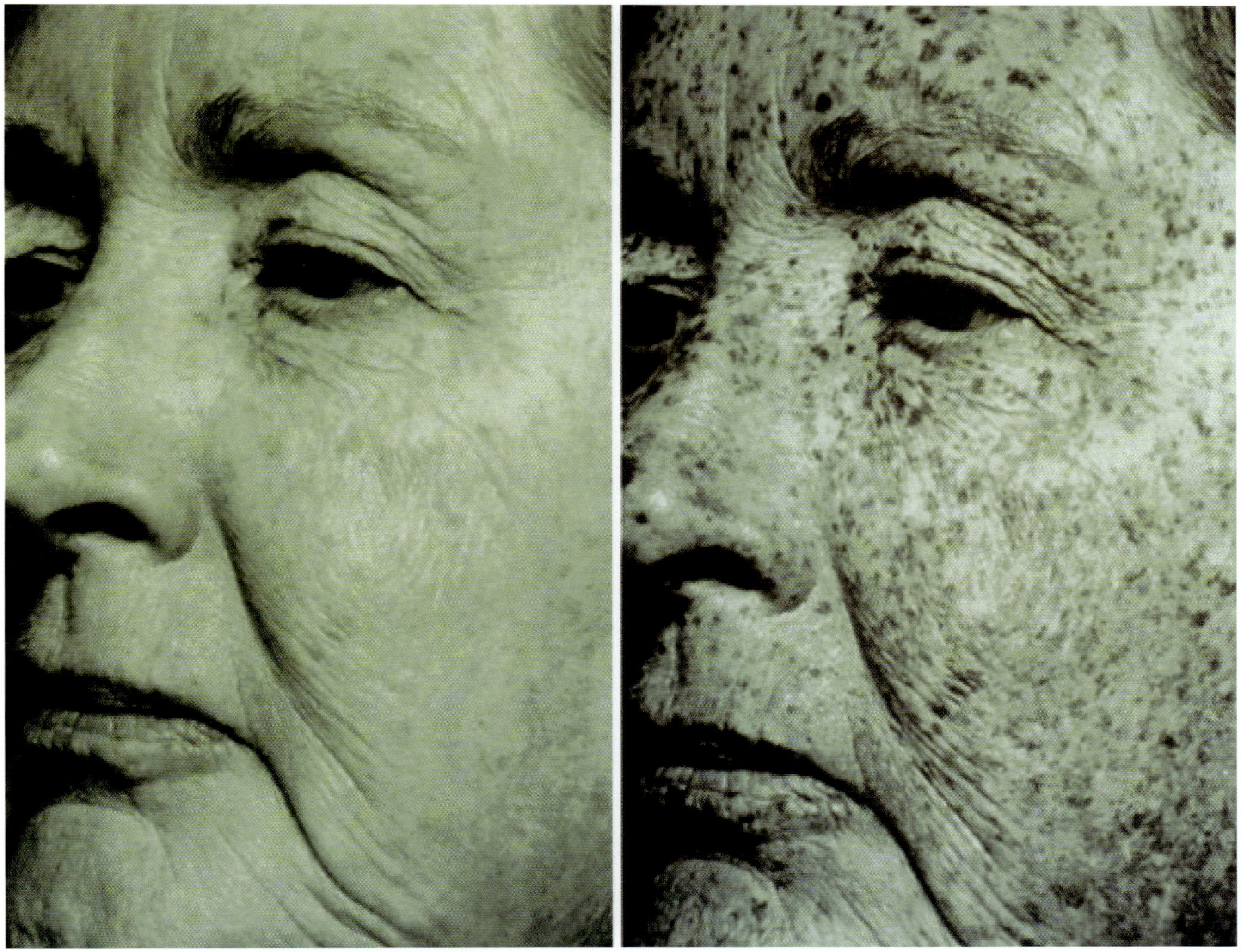

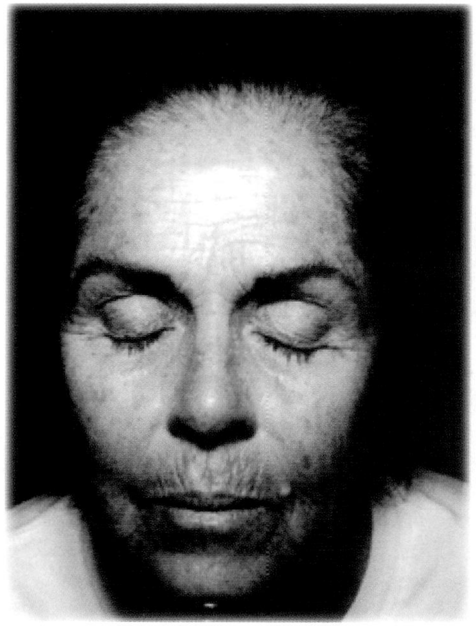

Photo of skin seen by the naked eye.

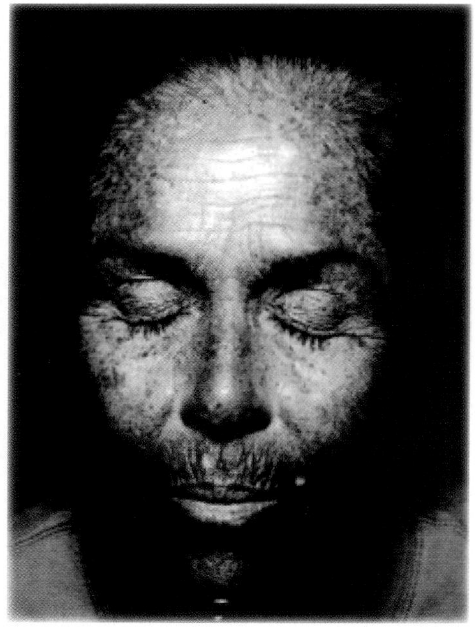

Photo of skin seen by UV camera prior to skin care system.

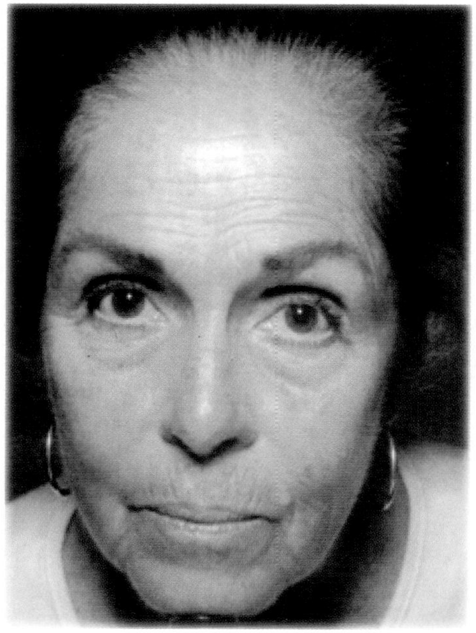

Photo of skin seen by the naked eye after 6 weeks of the skin care system.

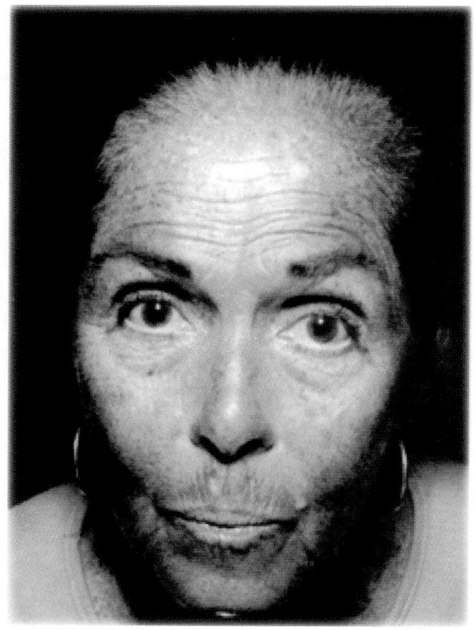

UV photo after 6 weeks patient applied skin care system.

MILD SUN DAMAGE

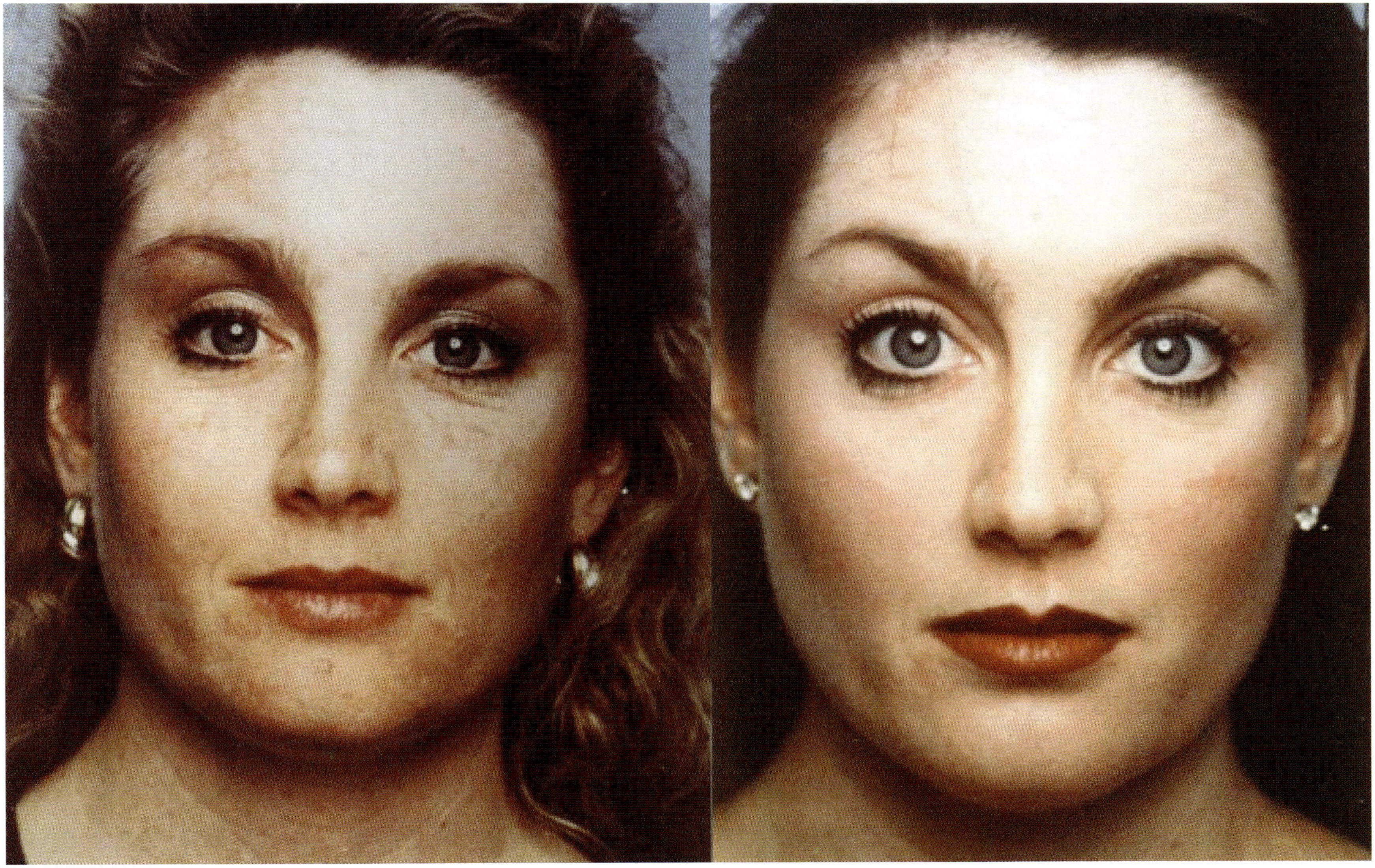

Result of patient applied system.

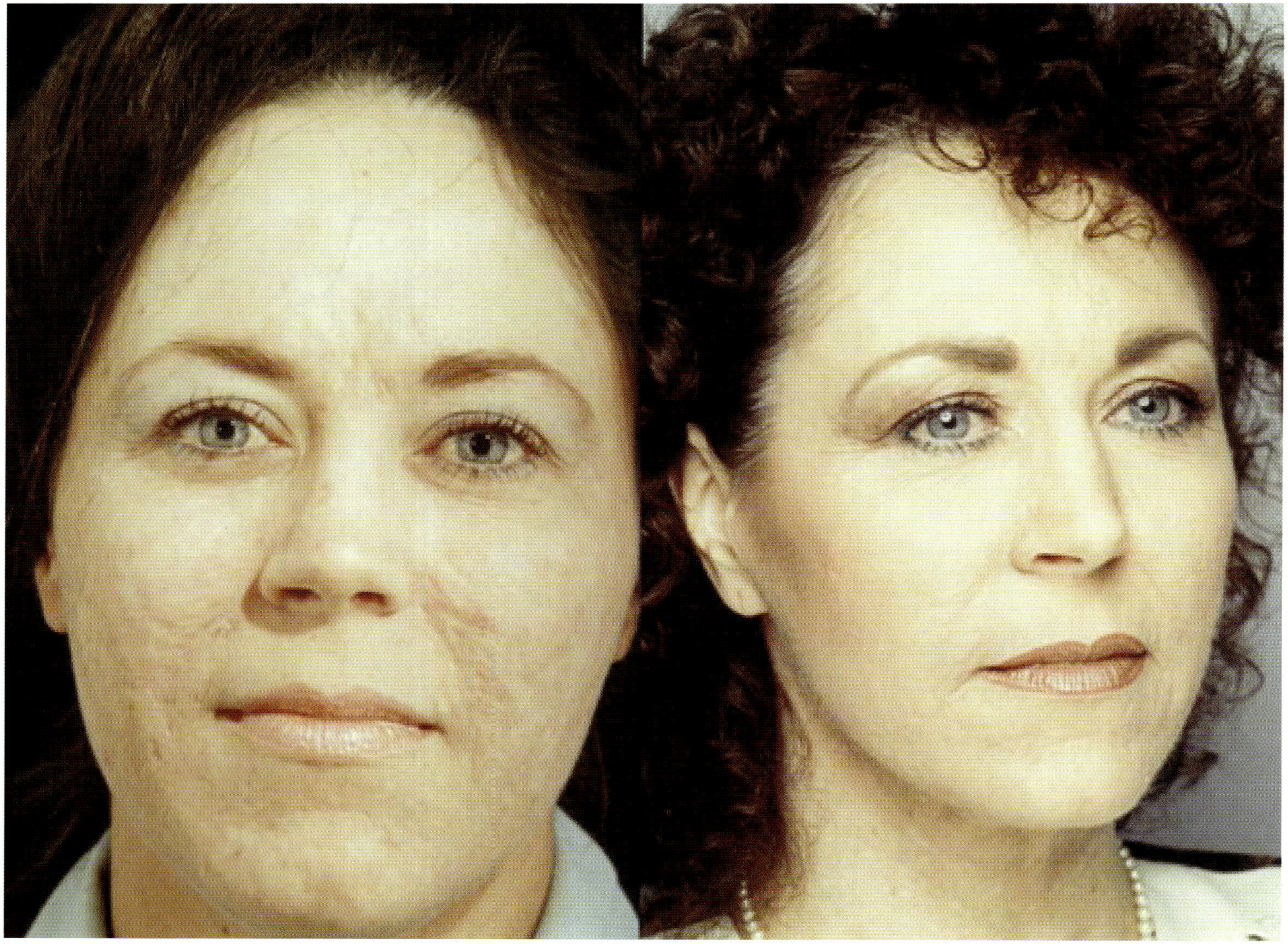

Result of combination of patient applied system and physician applied system.

SEVERE SUN DAMAGE

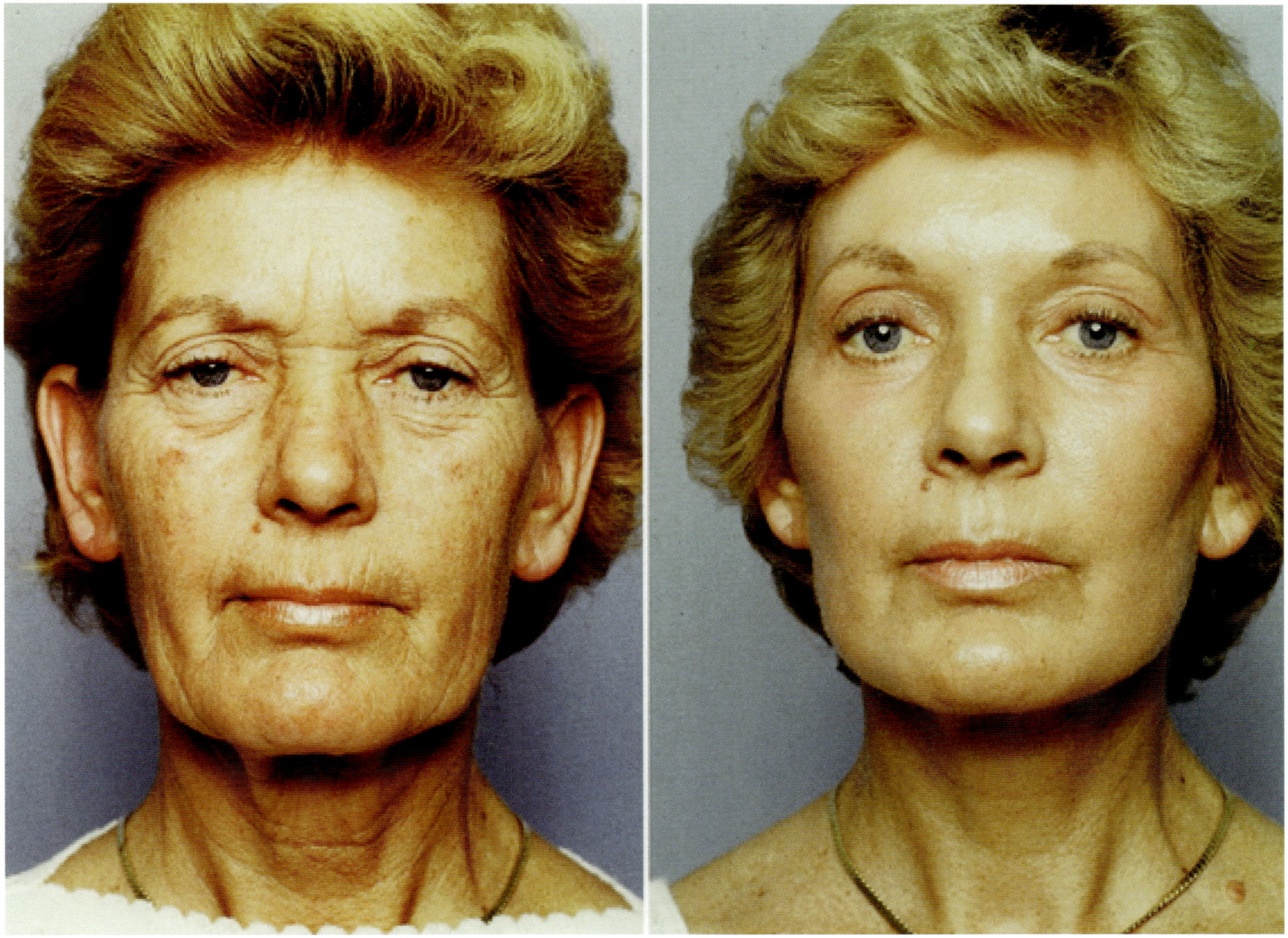

Result of rejuvenation surgery, patient applied system and physician applied skin care system.

SEVERE SUN DAMAGE

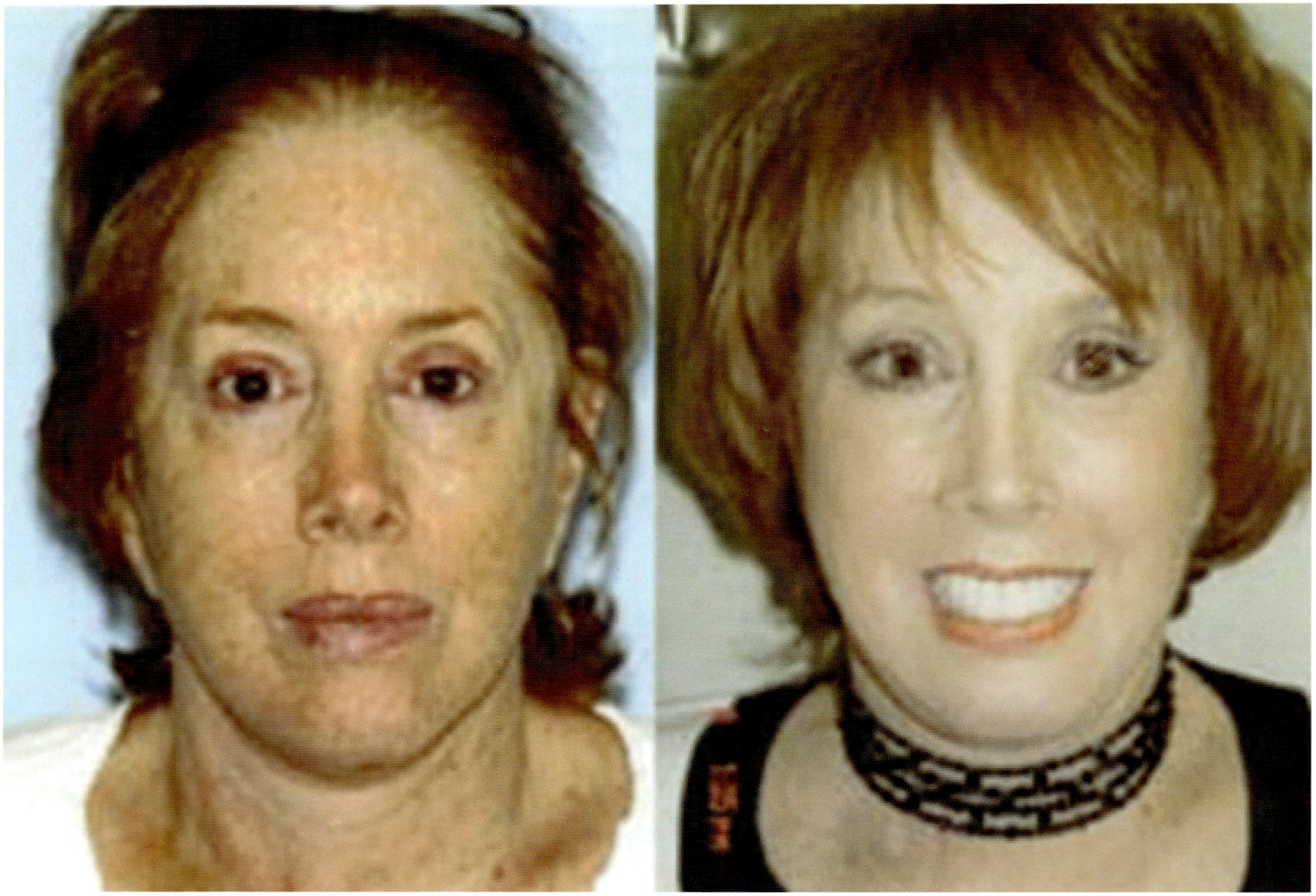

Result of rejuvenation surgery, patient applied system and physician applied skin care system.

ADOLESCENT ACNE

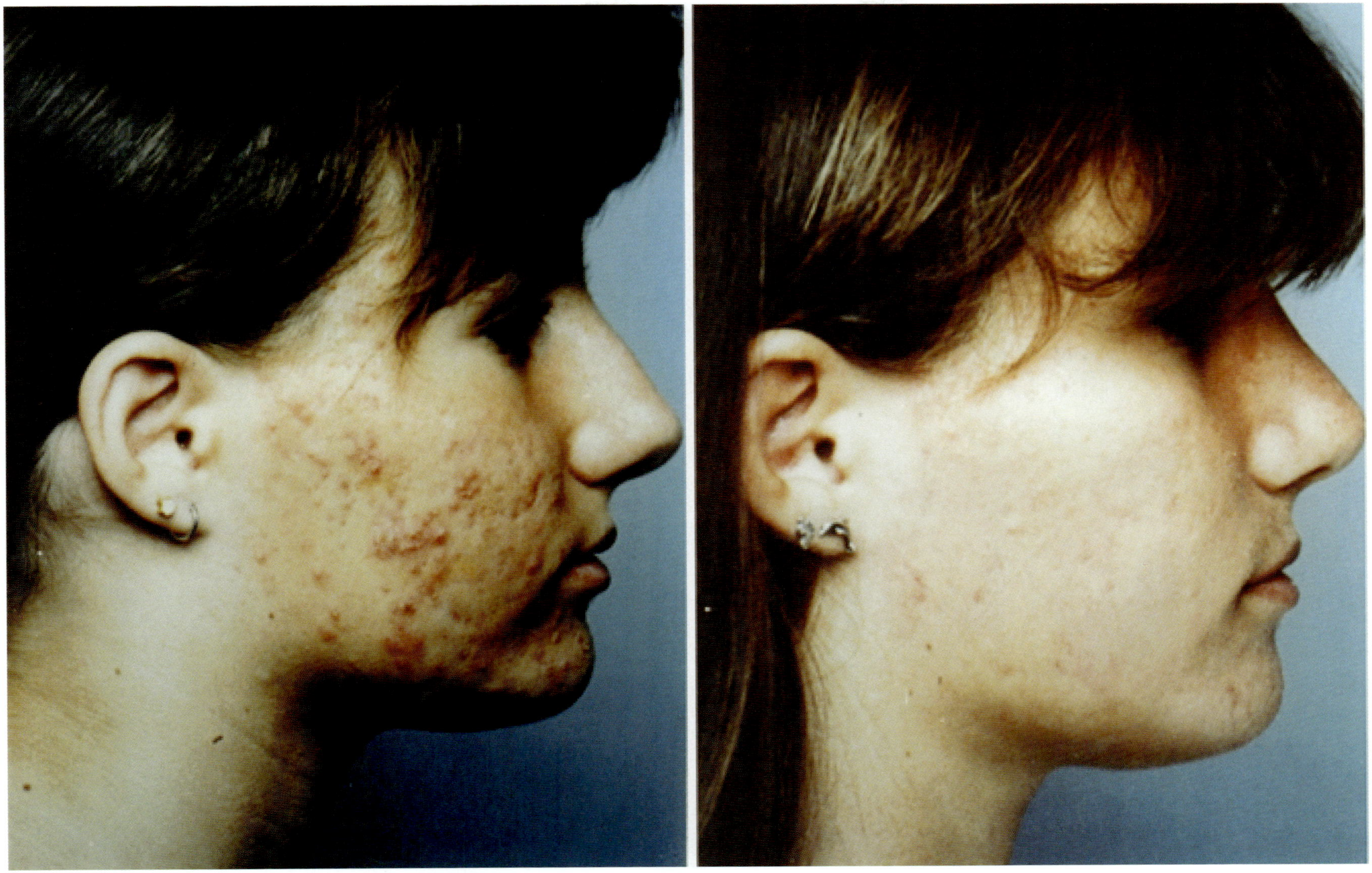

The skin care system is also very effective in preventing and reversing acne.

ADULT ACNE

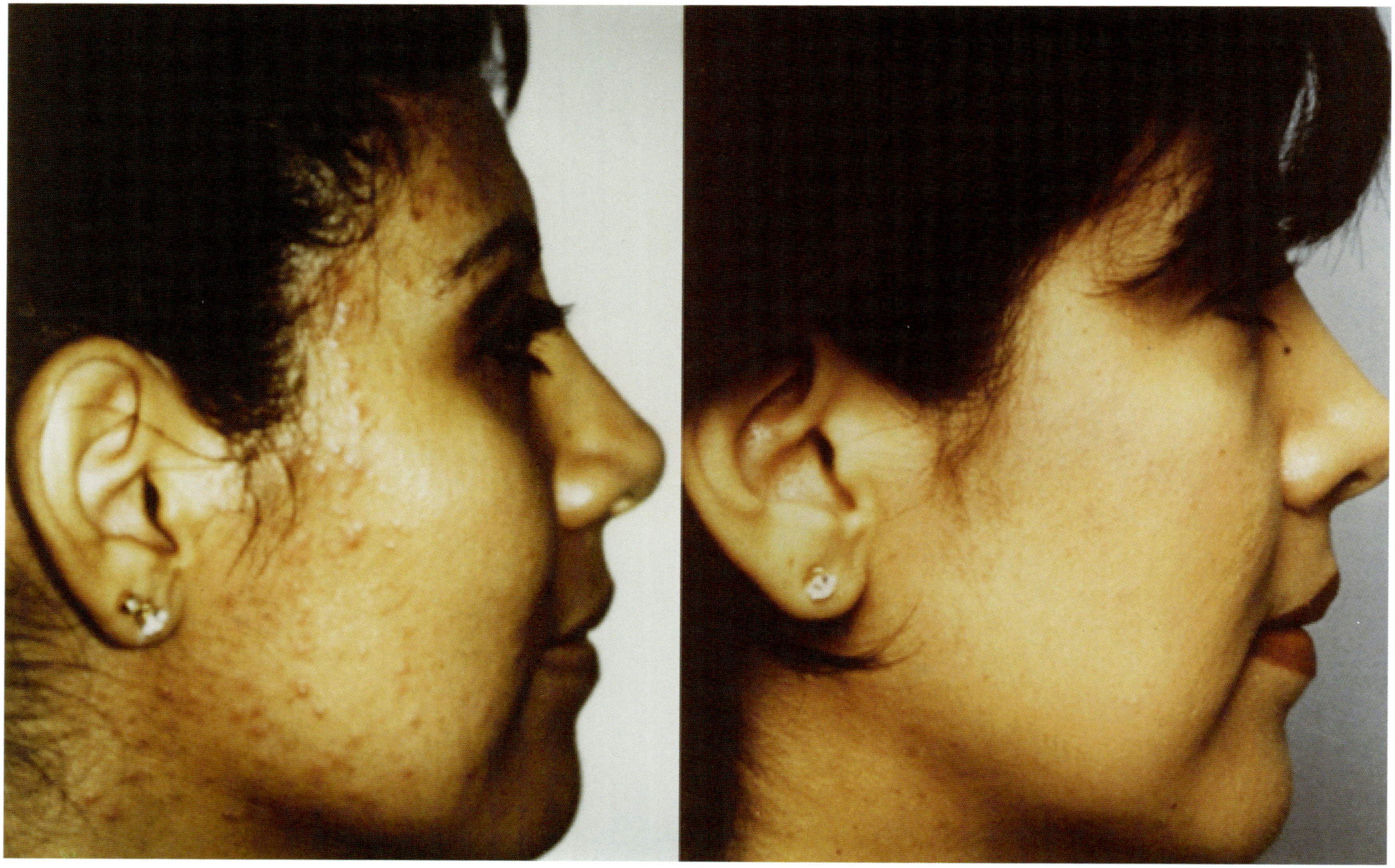

BREAST SURGERY

Both males and females can benefit from breast surgery.

Males can either reduce large breasts which may be due to heredity (gynecomastia) or from obesity.

Males may also enlarge the chest muscle with chest implants.

Females may have;

- ***Breast Enlargements***
- ***Correction of Asymmetry - A difference in the size, shape and position***
- ***Breast Reduction***
- ***Breast Lifts***

MALE BREAST REDUCTION FOR GYNECOMASTIA (HEREDITARY CONDITION)

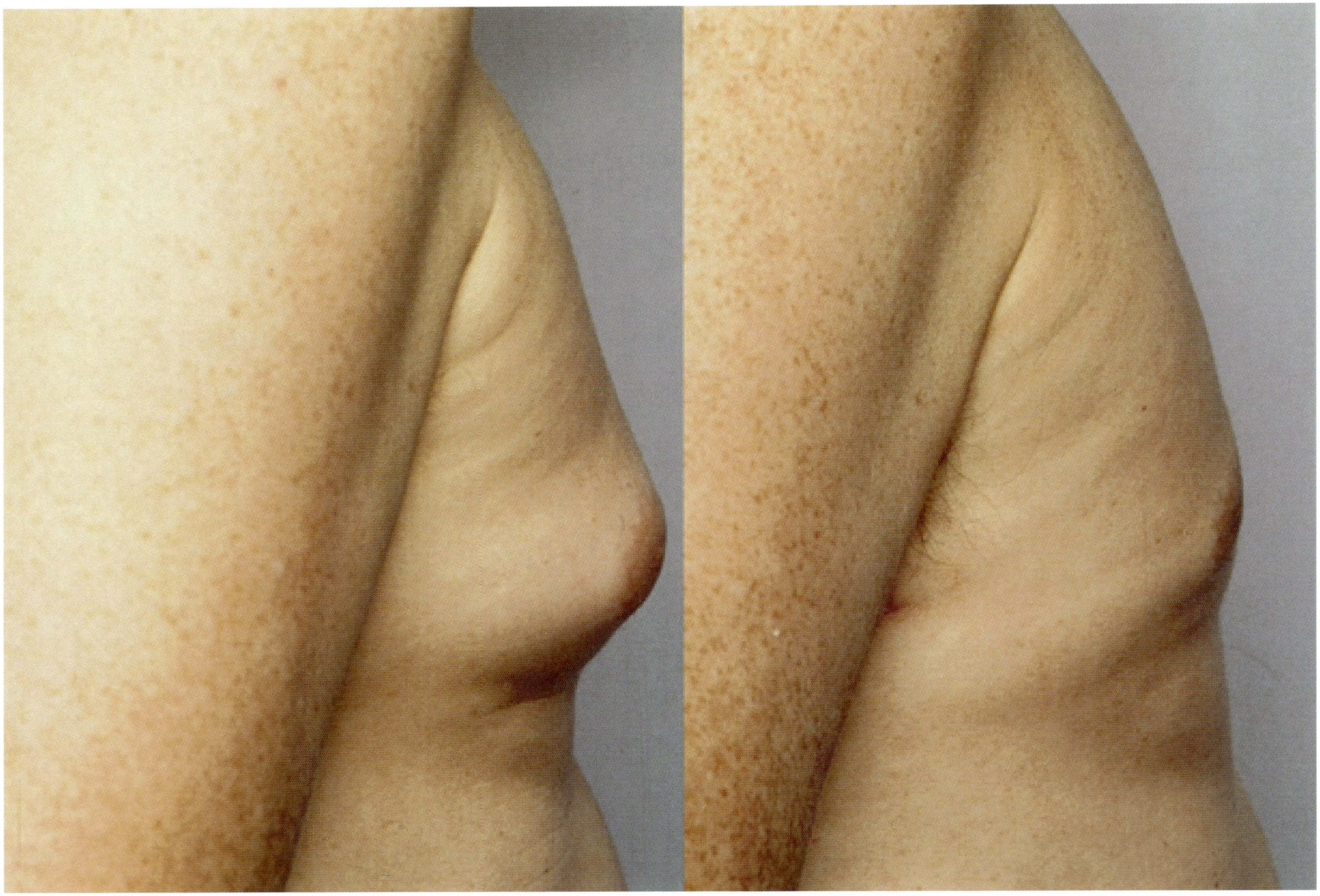

MALE BREAST REDUCTION FOR HEREDITARY CONDITION

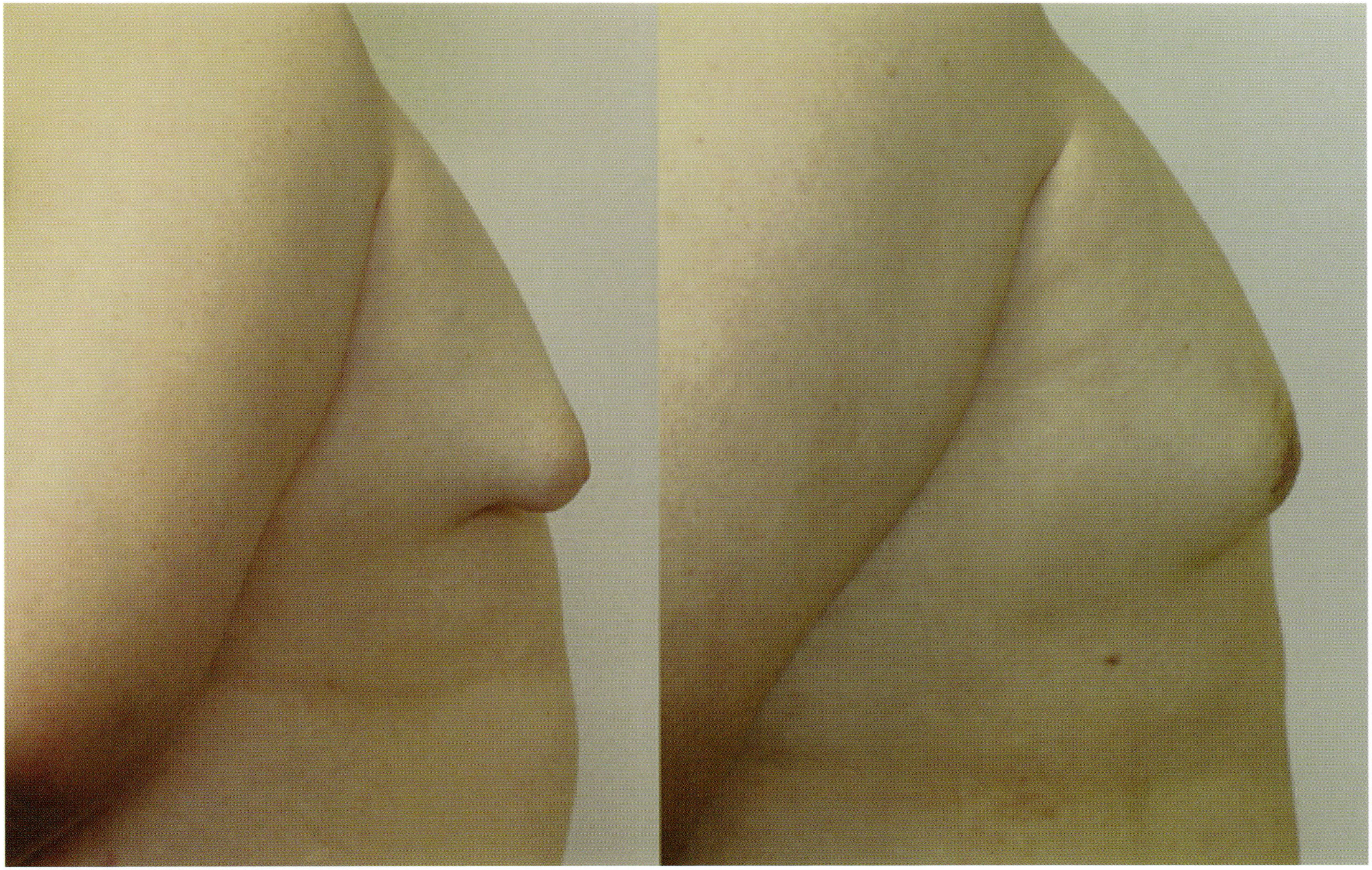

MALE BREAST REDUCTION FOR OBESITY

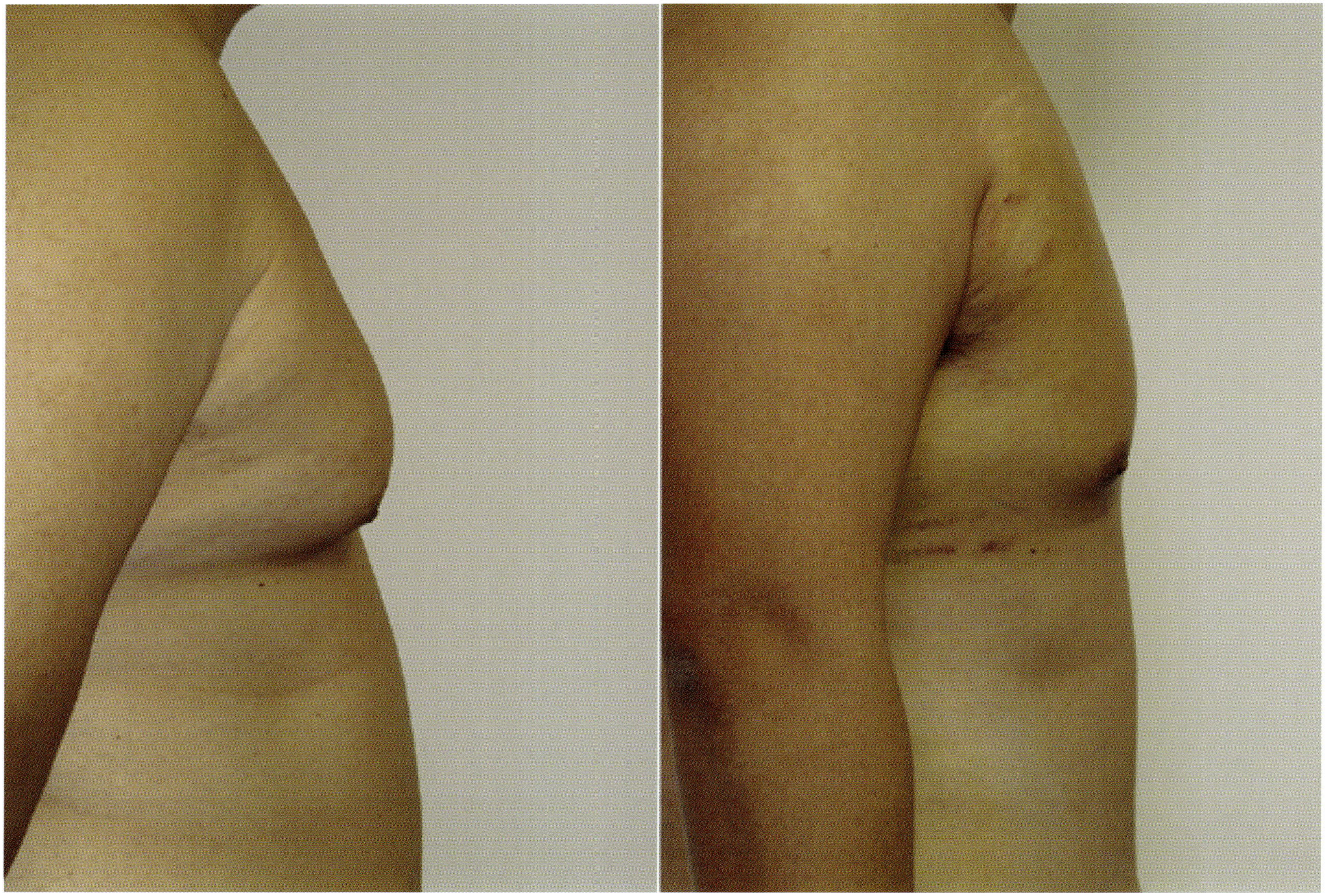

ENLARGING THE CHEST MUSCLE WITH IMPLANTS

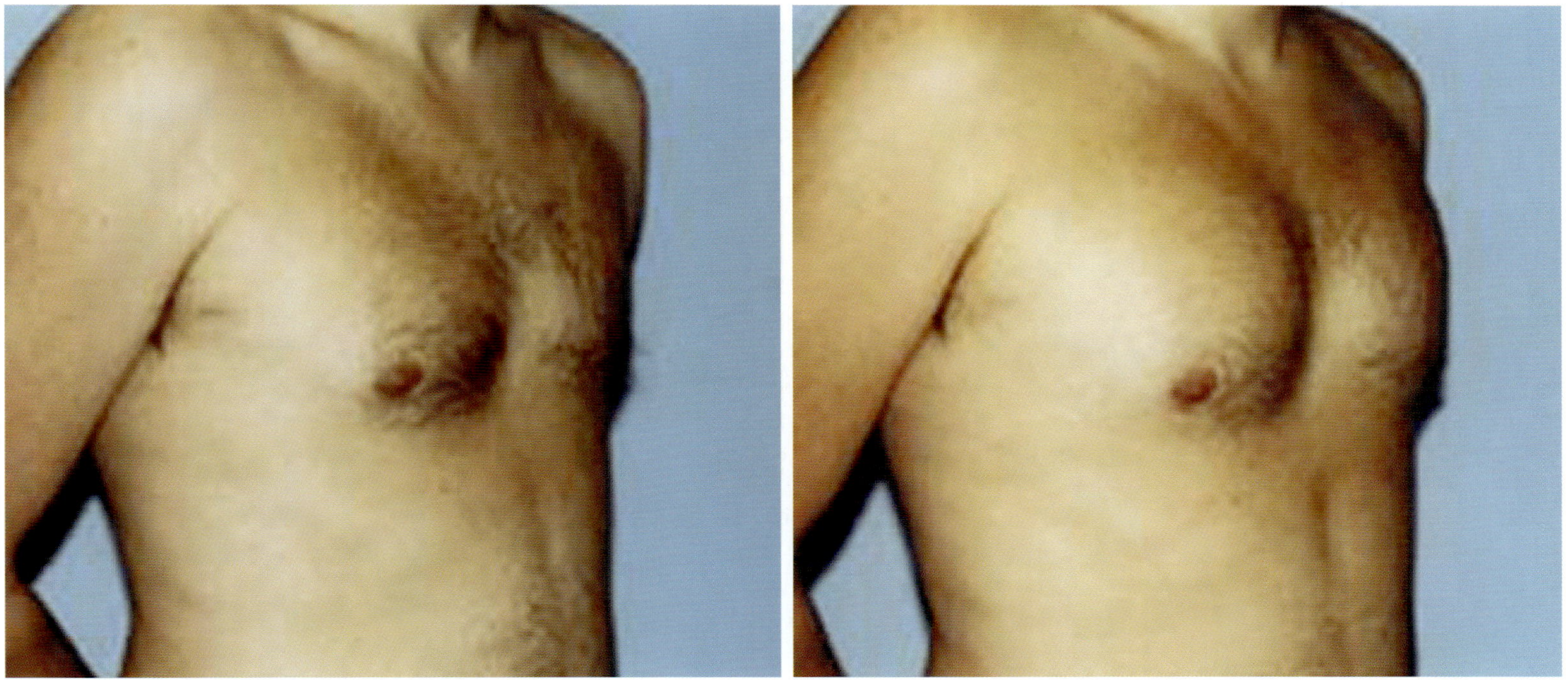

BREAST IMPLANT SURGERY

Breast implants are safe. Breast implants will not cause disease or interfere with the diagnosis of breast disease nor affect nursing.

There are two types of FDA approved implants. Both are silicone shells. One is inflatable with salt water (saline implants) the other is prefilled with silicone gel (silicone implants).

Breast implant patients must make four (4) decisions prior to surgery.

1. ***Incision Site***
    - ***A. Arm Pit***
    - ***B. Nipple (areola)***
    - ***C. Breast Crease***
    - ***D. Umbilical (Belly Button)***

    Any incision can result in visible scarring.

2. Saline or Silicone Implants
    See page 128
3. Size of Implant
    See page 129
4. Under or Over the Muscle
    See pages 130-138

Breast surgery is relatively simple, very safe and is performed under light anesthesia as an out patient surgery. The day after surgery the patient can resume normal activity, personal hygiene, diet and lifestyle.

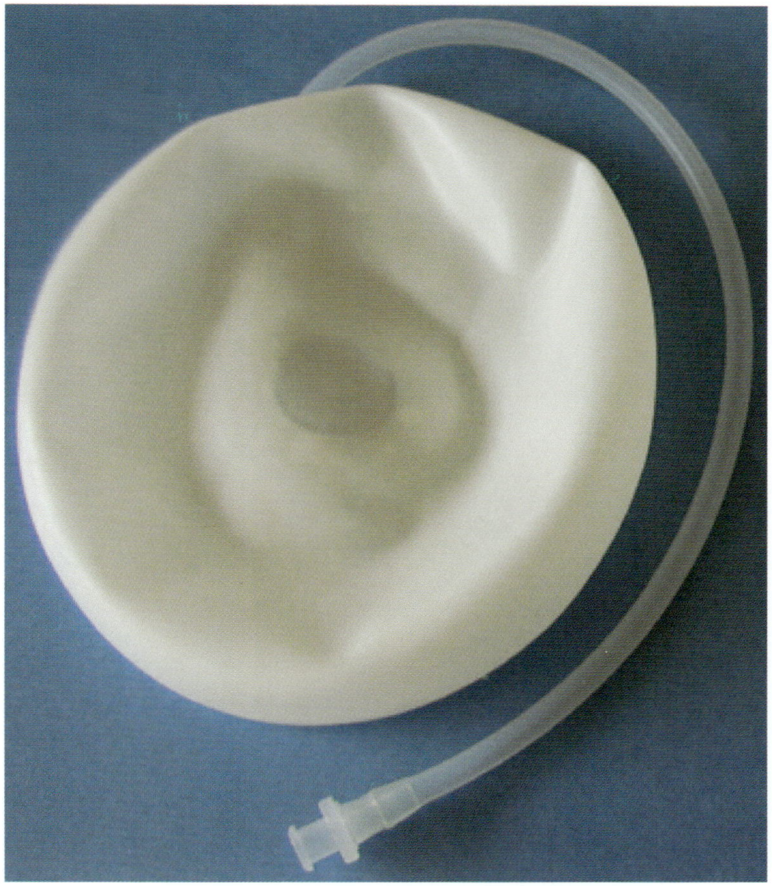

Saline Implant (inflatable implant)

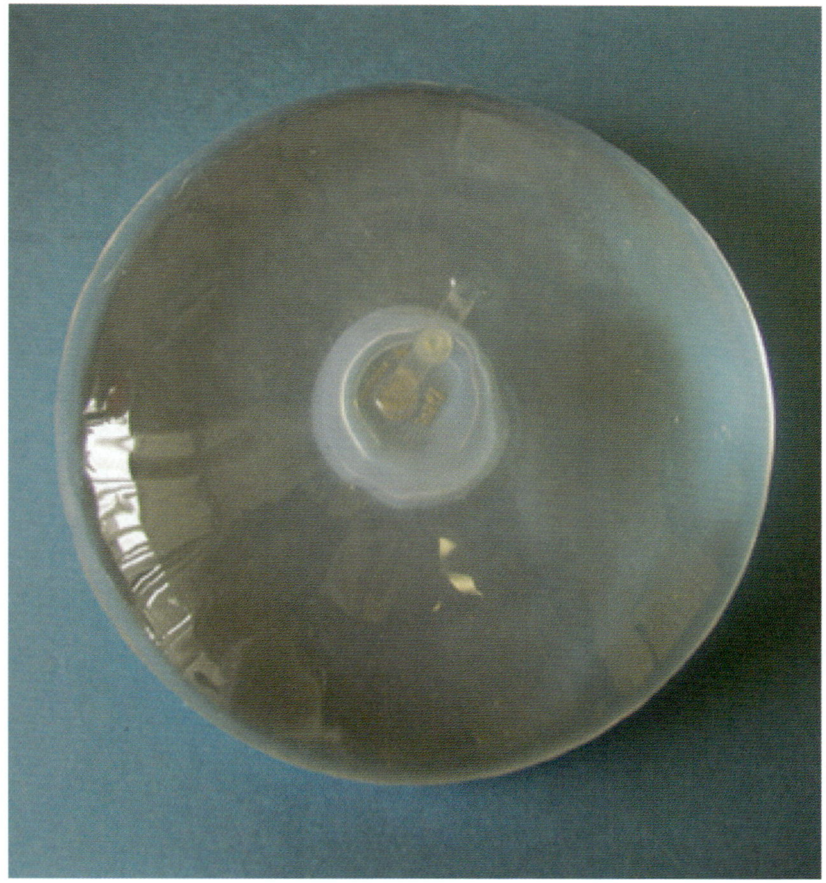

Silicone Implant (prefilled)

PATIENT USING SIZERS TO DETERMINE SIZE OF BREAST

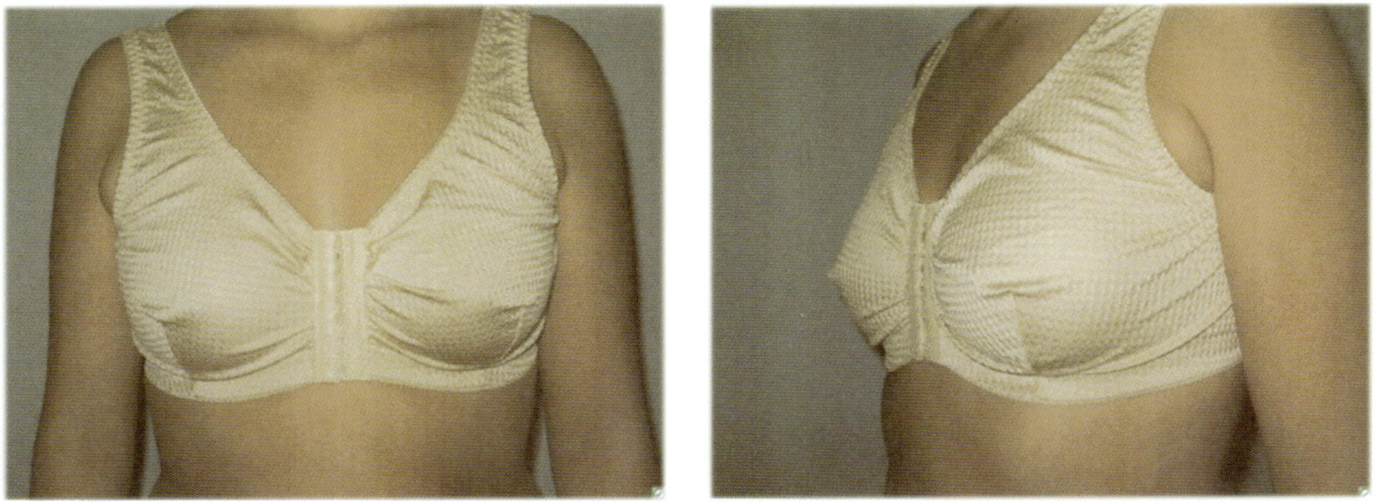

Patient wearing standard bra

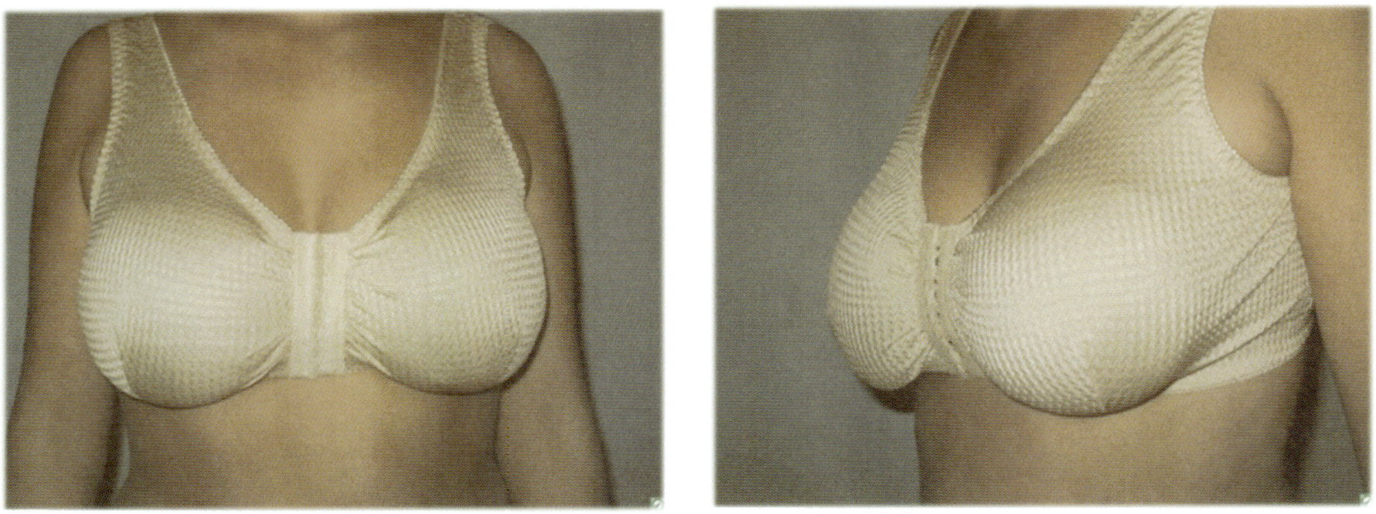

Patient trying on sizers to determine breast size

BREAST IMPLANTS UNDER THE MUSCLE

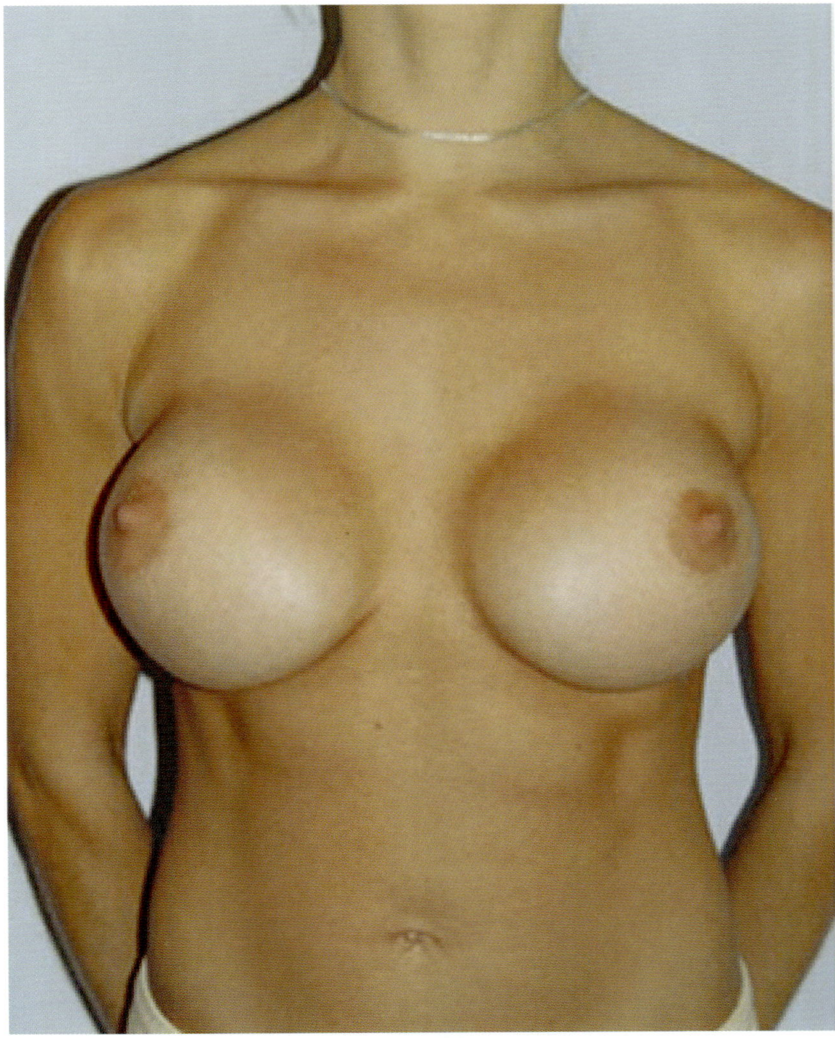

Wide cleavage and nipple malposition

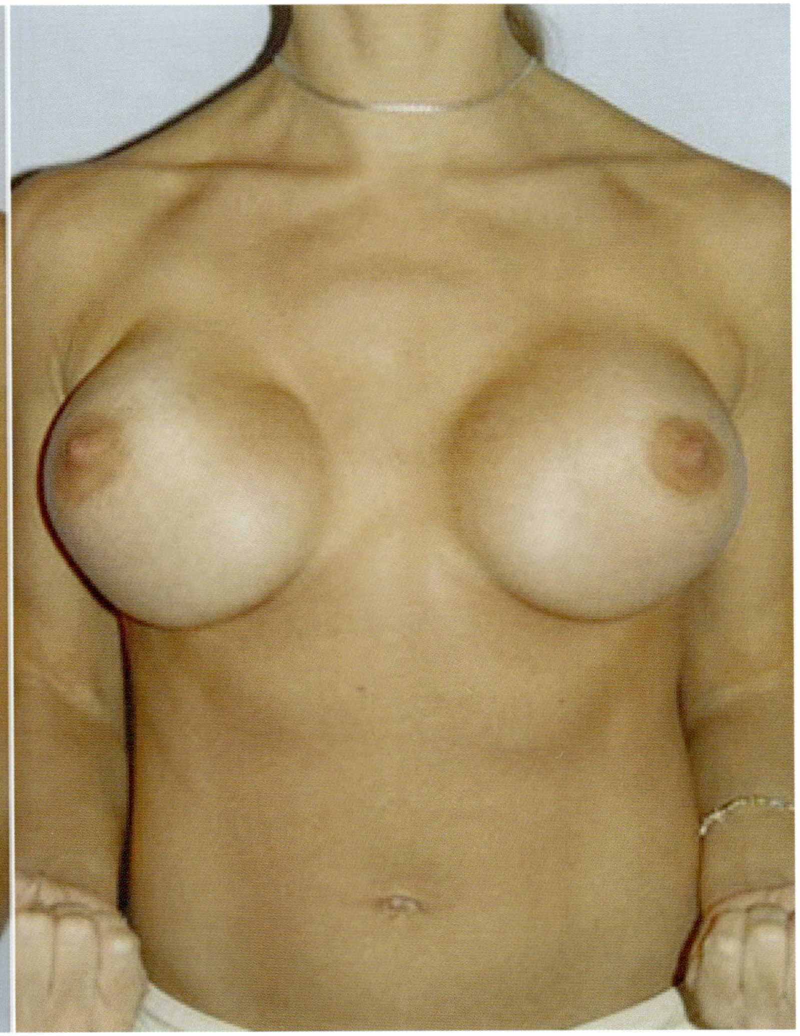

With Muscle contraction – wider cleavage and muscle deformity

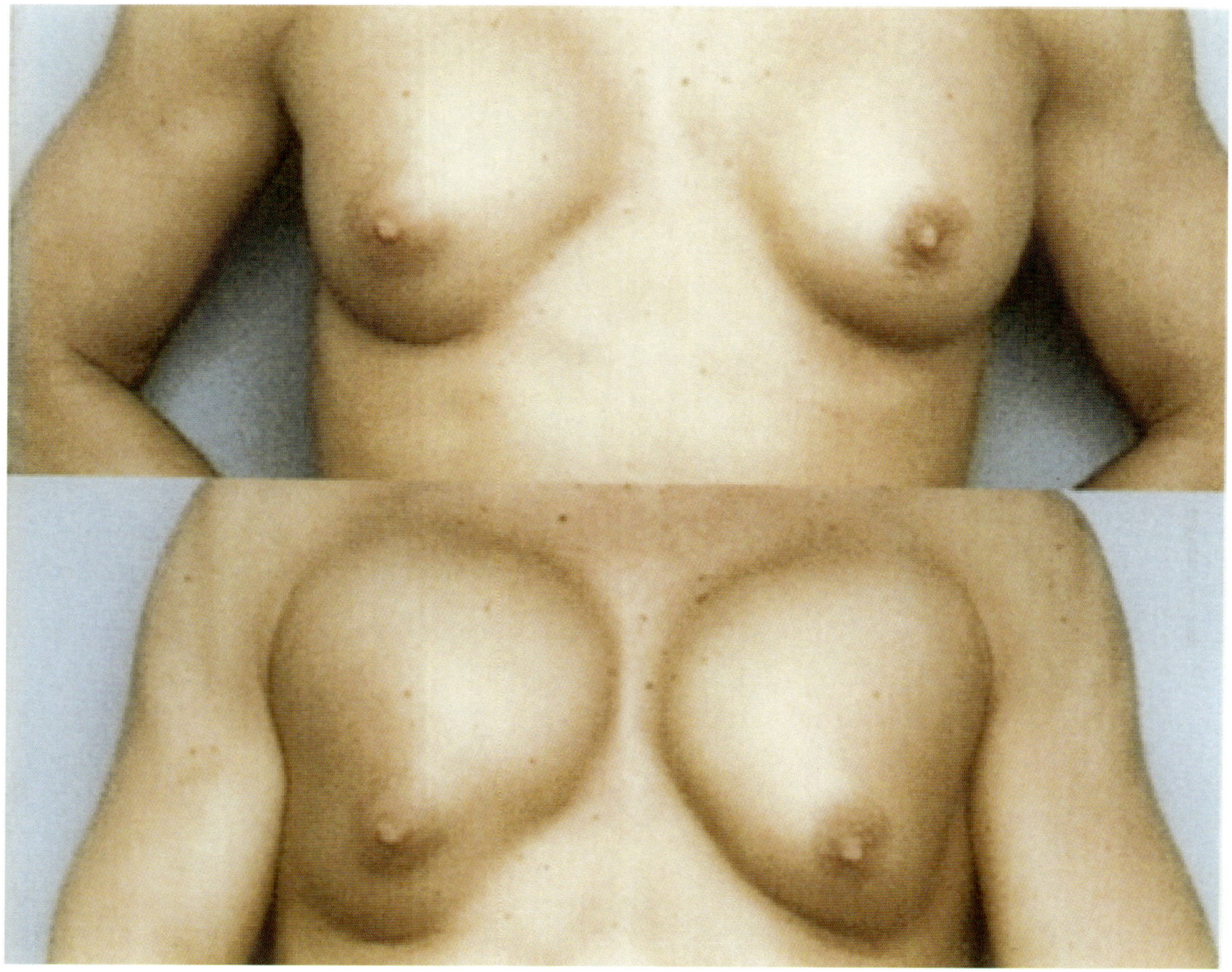

Deformity with muscle contraction

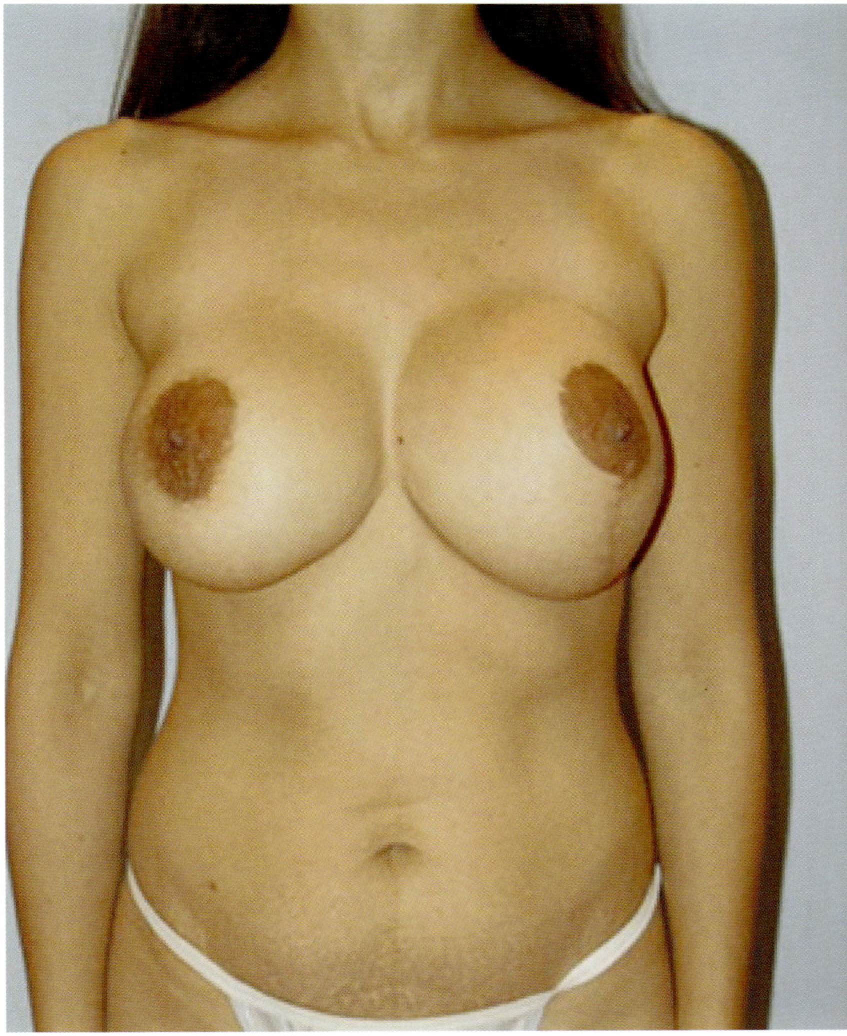

Implants under muscle

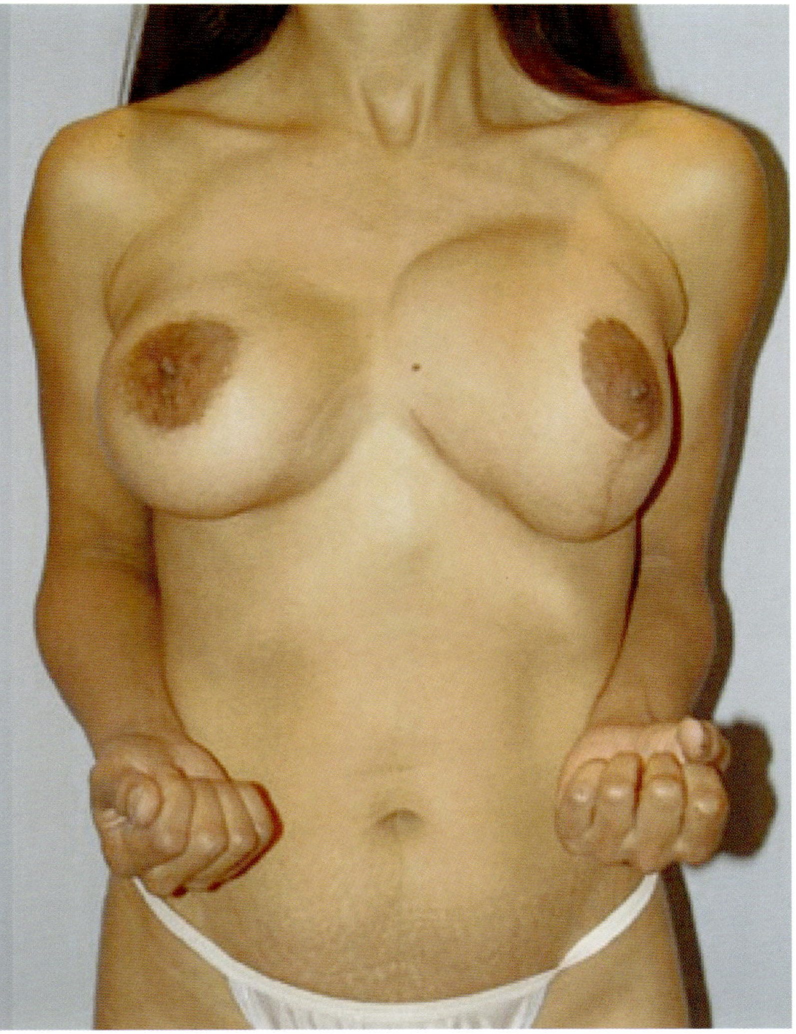

Under muscle deformity

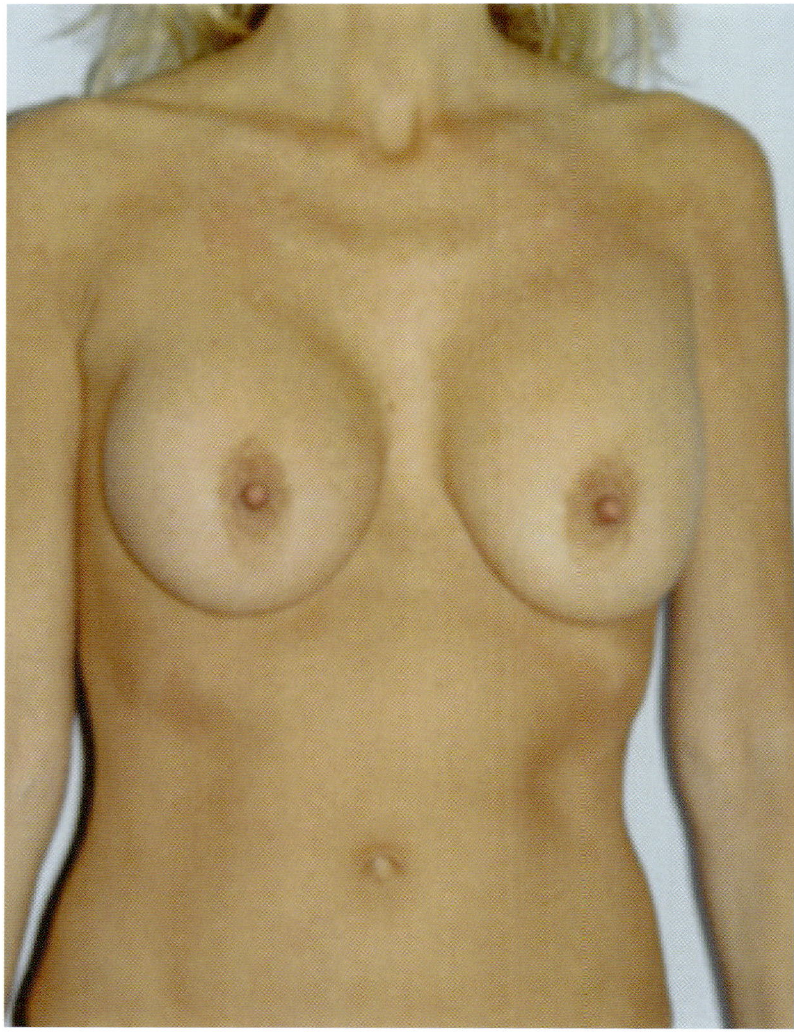

Implants under muscle

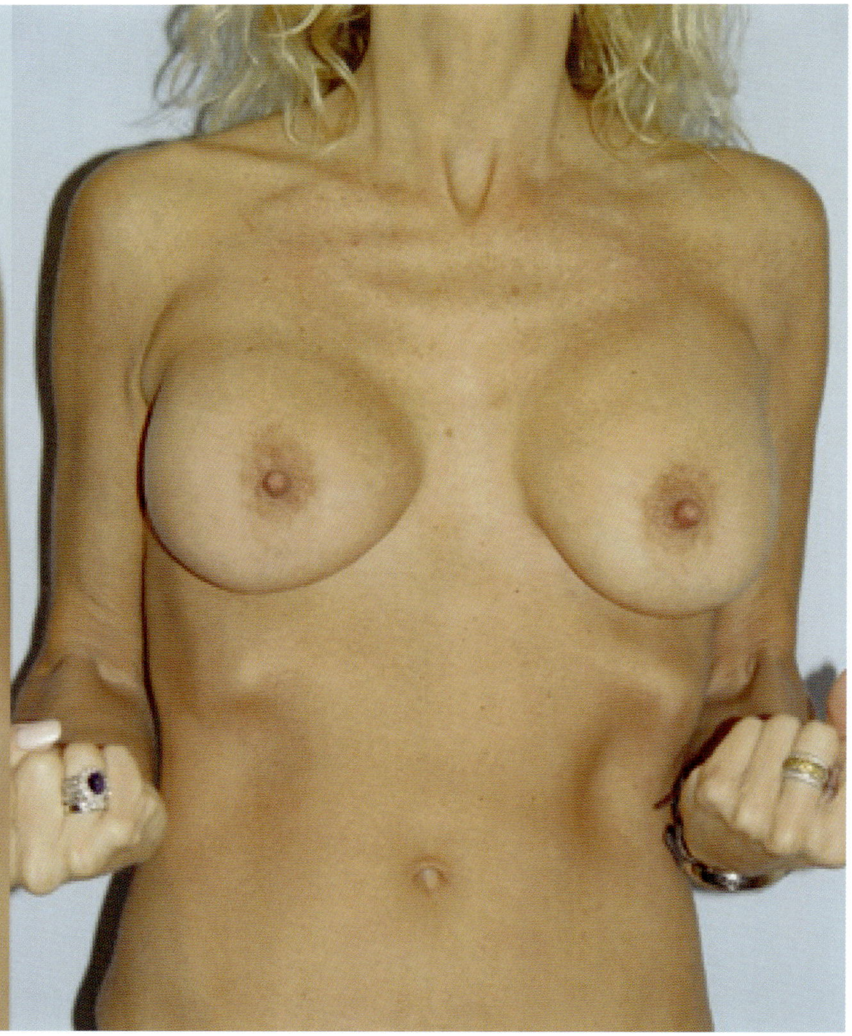

Under muscle deformity

Implants were removed from under the muscle and replaced over the muscle for a much more natural look.

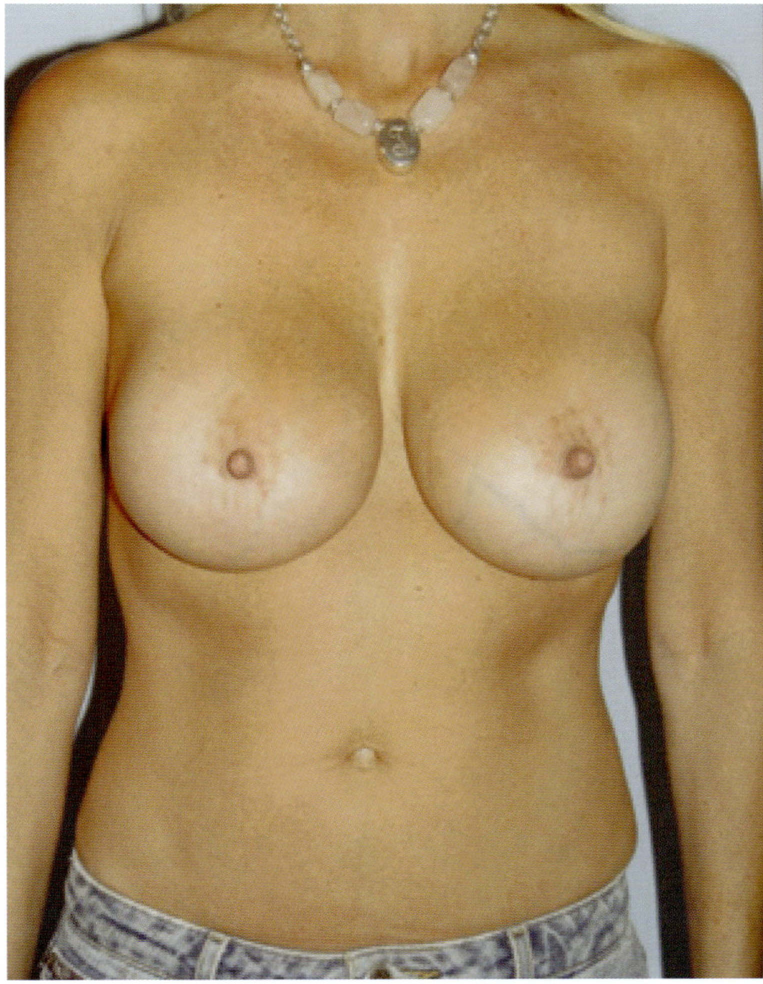

Implants Over The Muscle-Relaxed

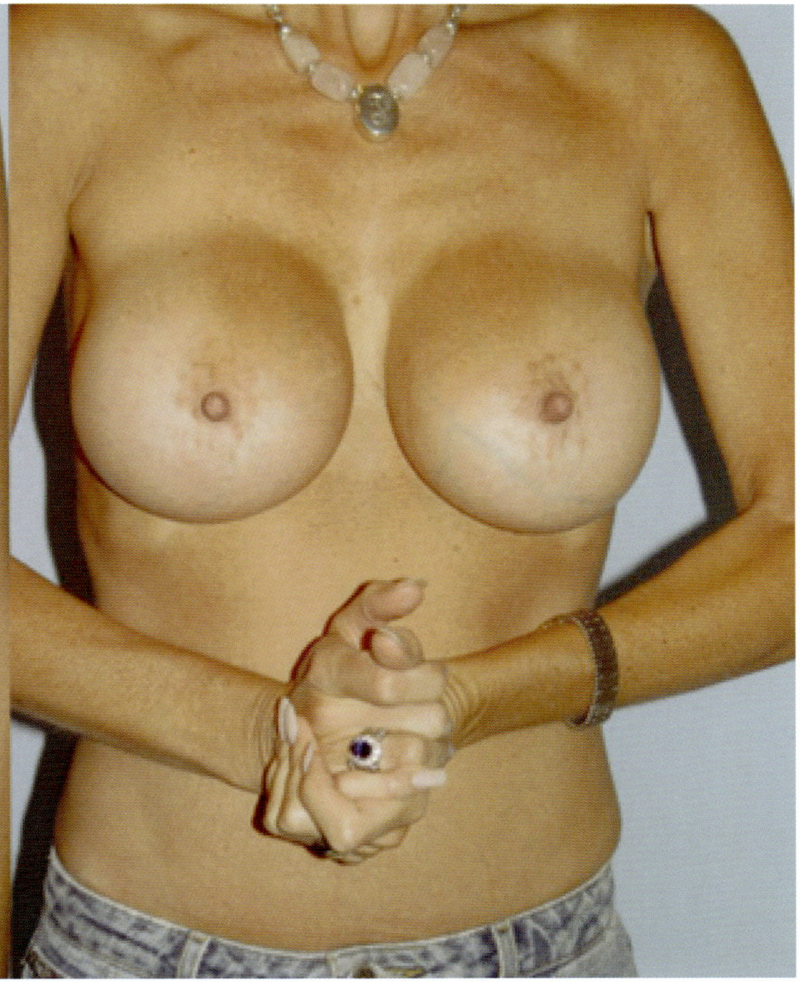

Implants Over The Muscle-Muscle Contraction

IMPLANTS USING SALINE IMPLANTS PLACED OVER THE MUSCLE

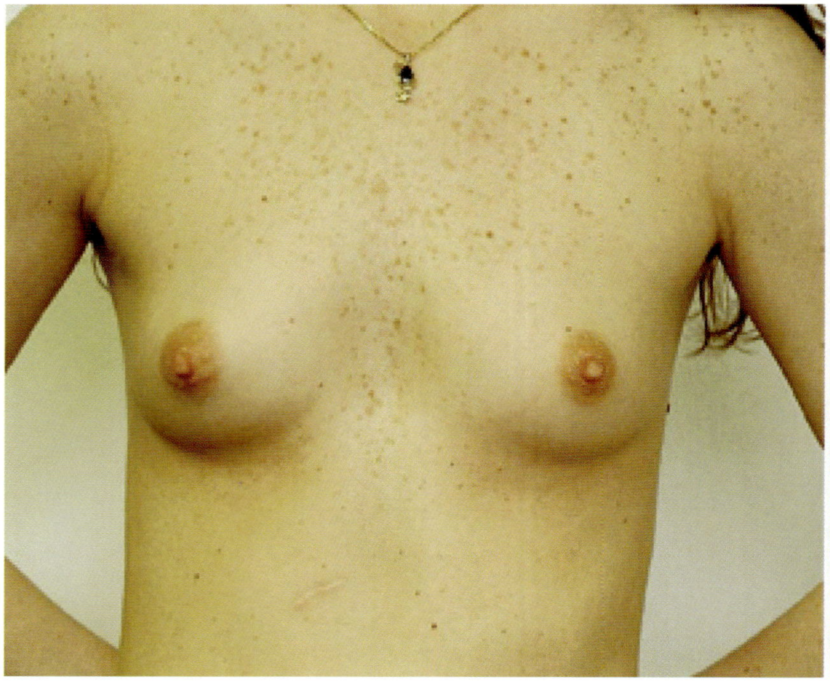

Hereditary

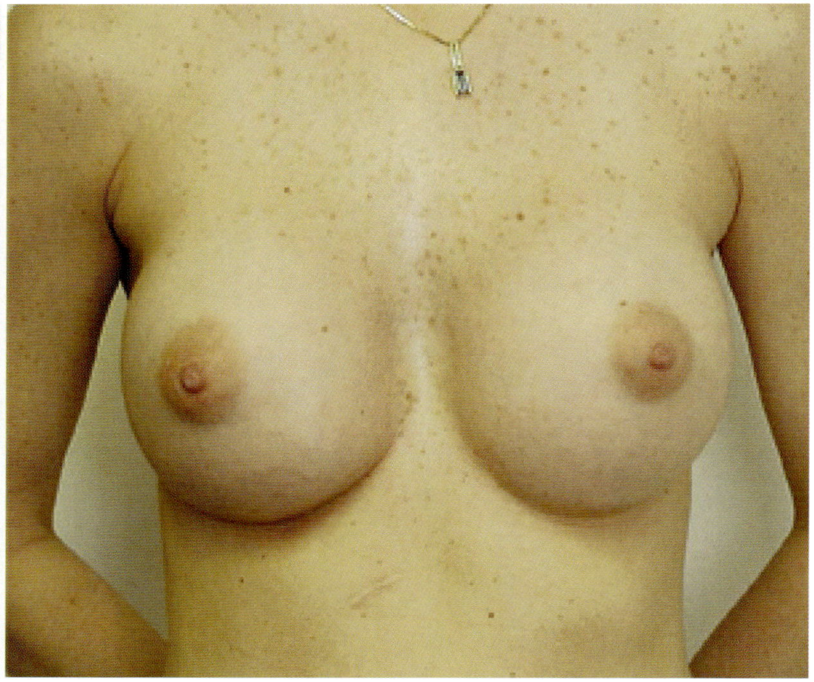

Saline implants placed over the muscle

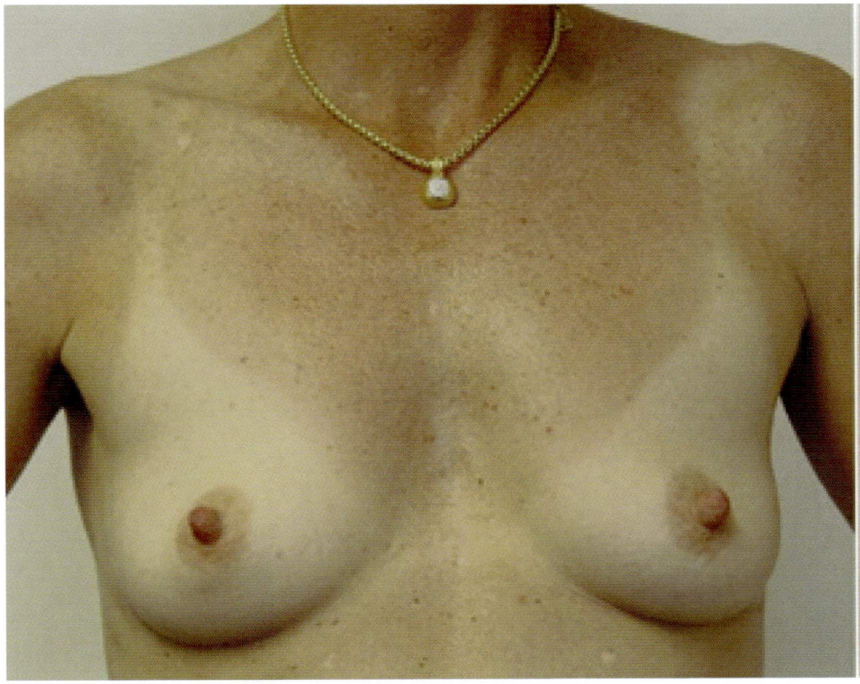

Hereditary

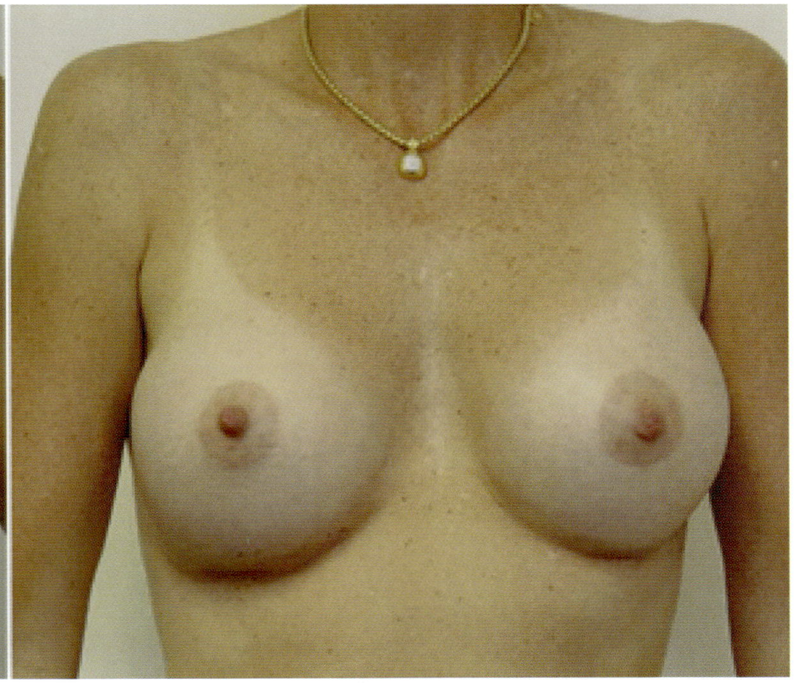

Saline implants placed over the muscle

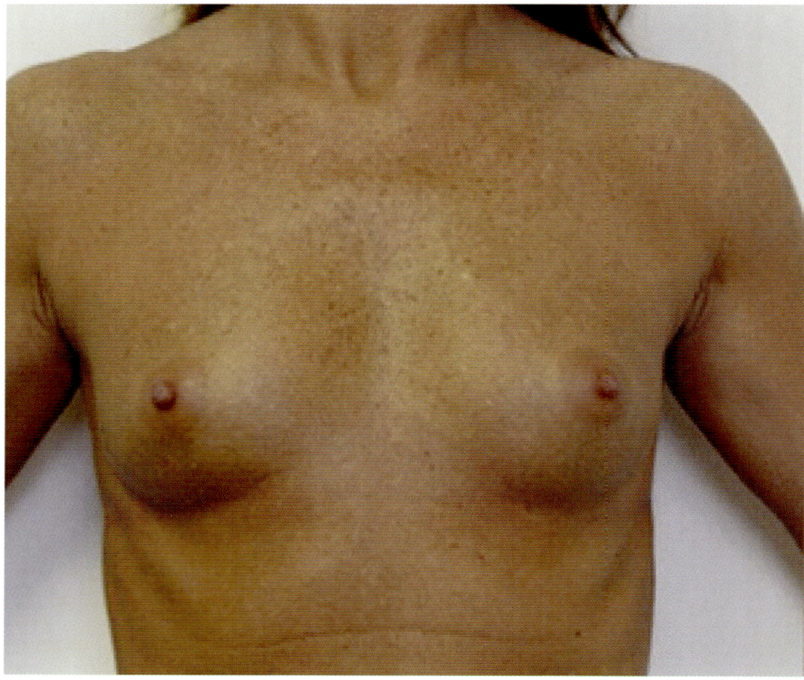

Hereditary

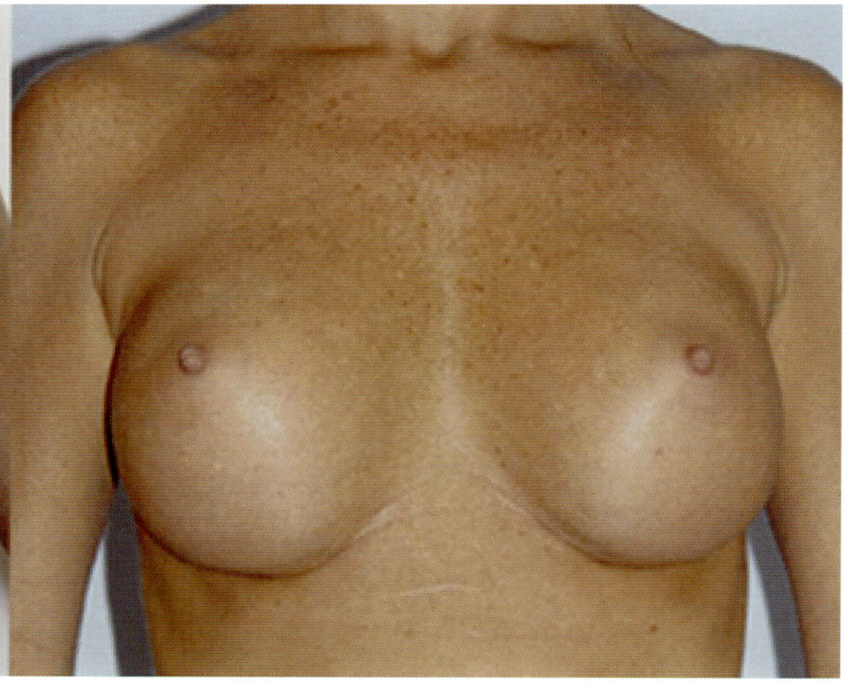

Breast implants placed over the muscle

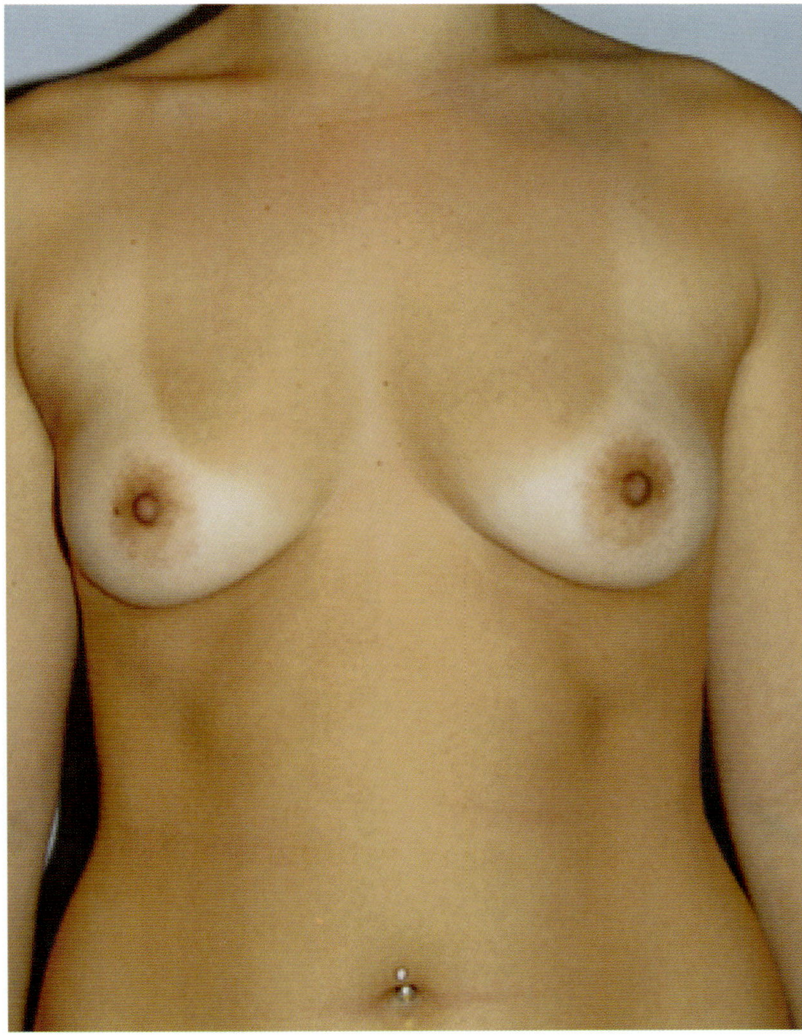

Hereditary

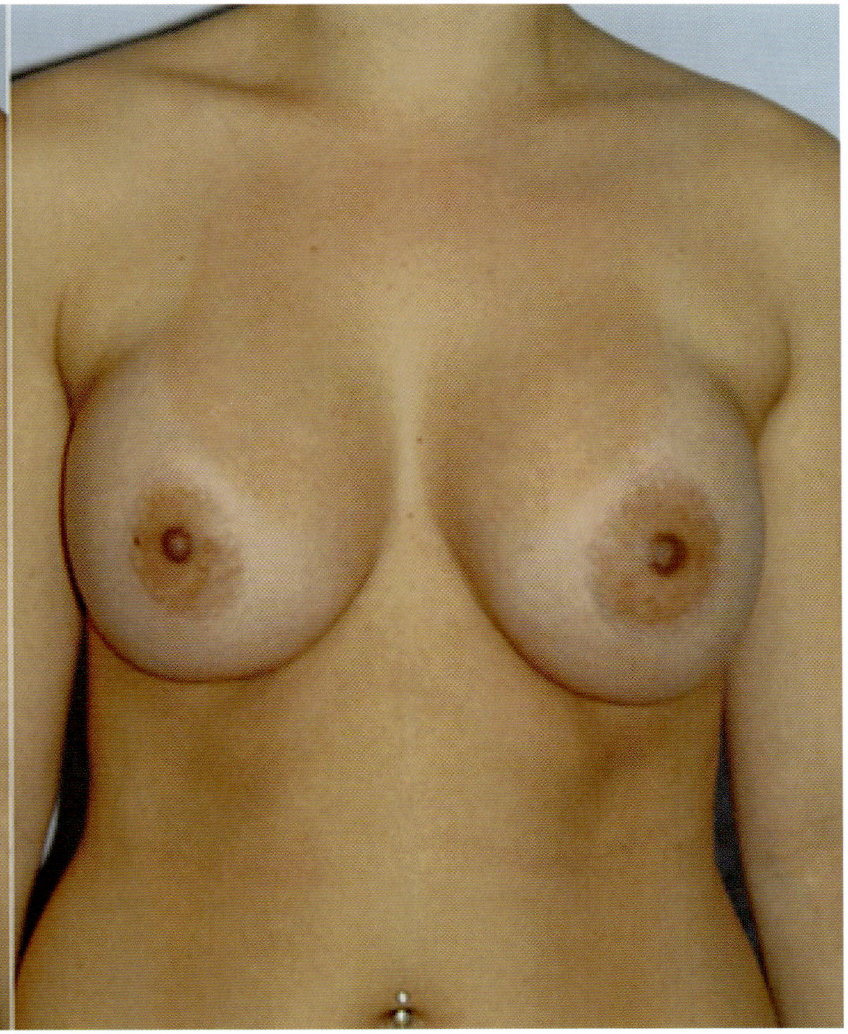

Breast implants placed over the muscle

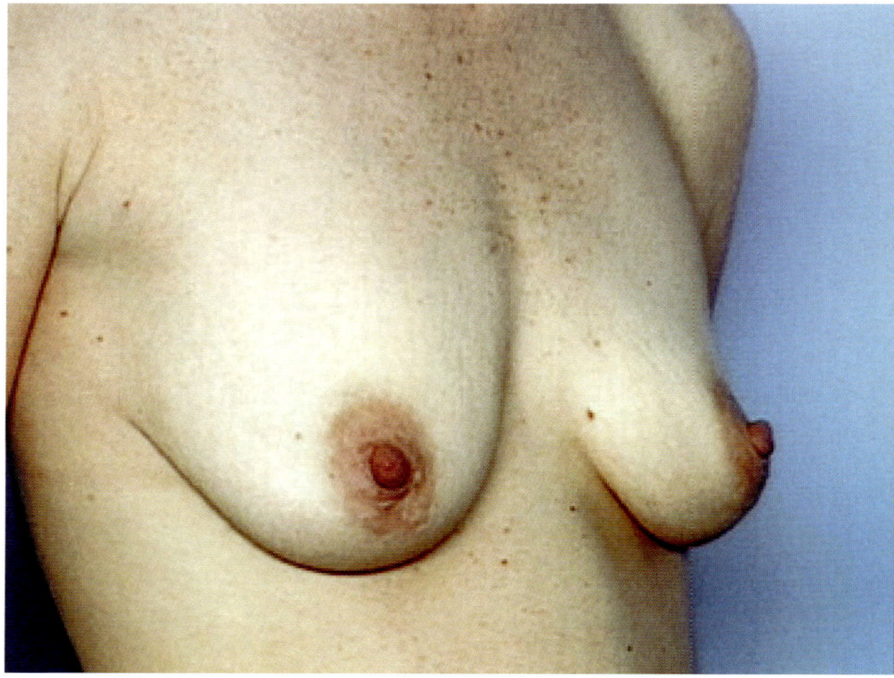

Loss of volume after nursing

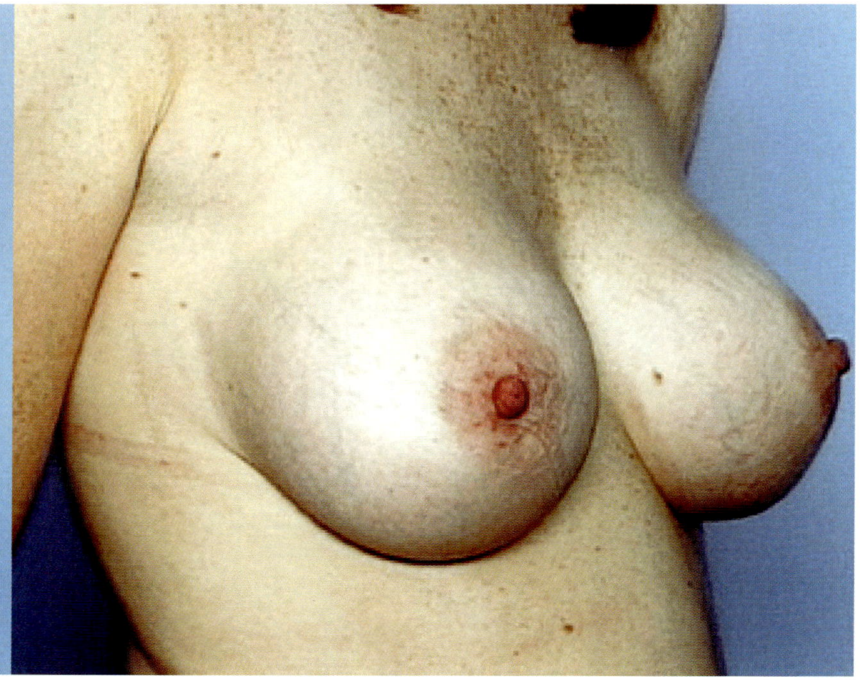

Improvement with breast implants

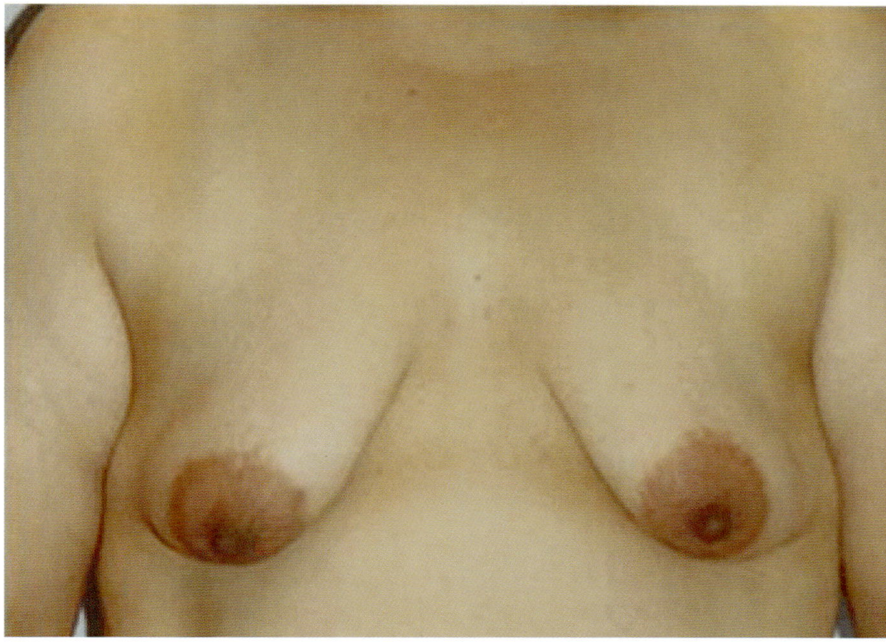

Loss of volume after weight loss

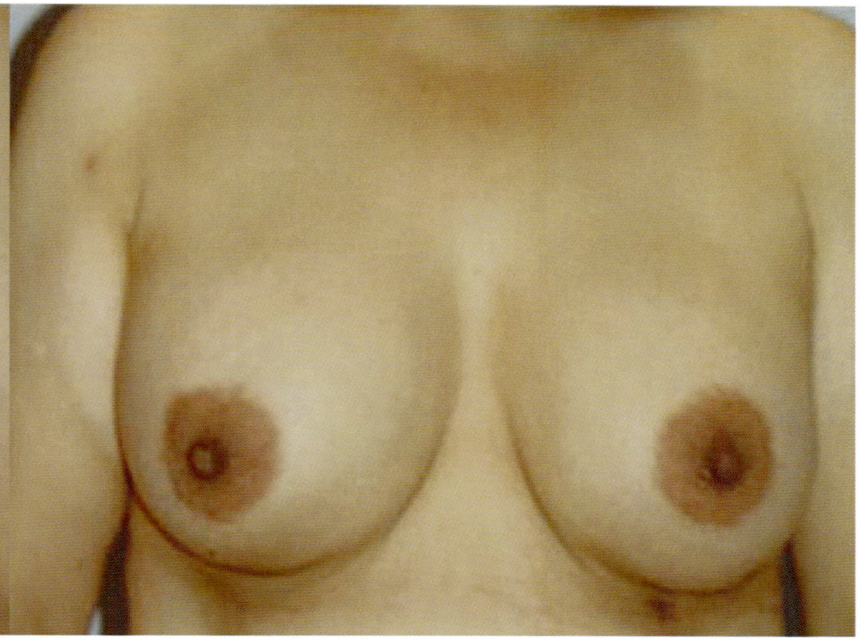

Improvement with breast implants

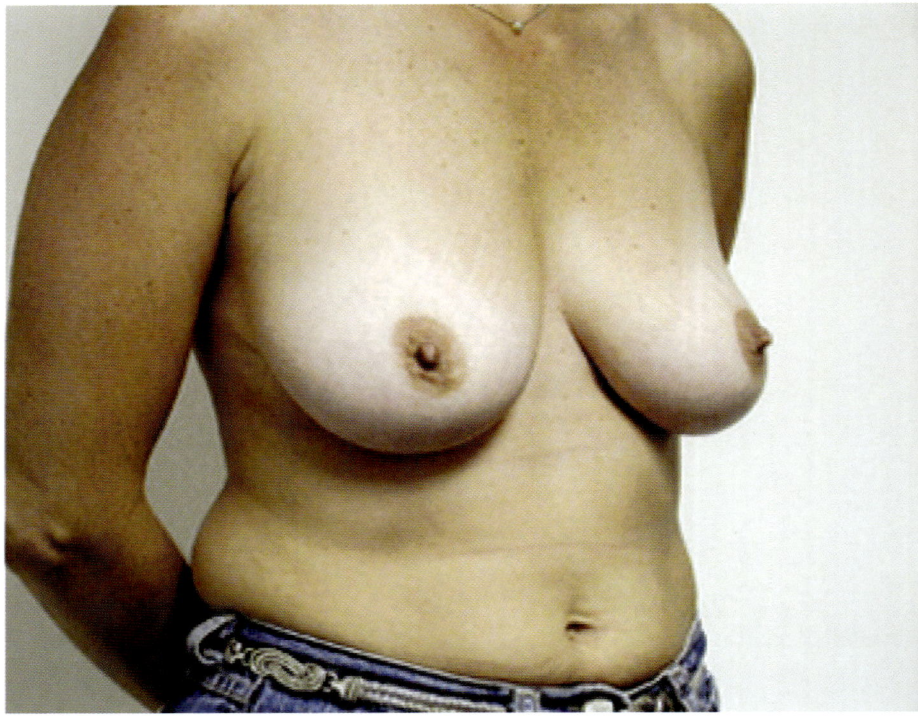

Loss of volume and lowered positioning due to age

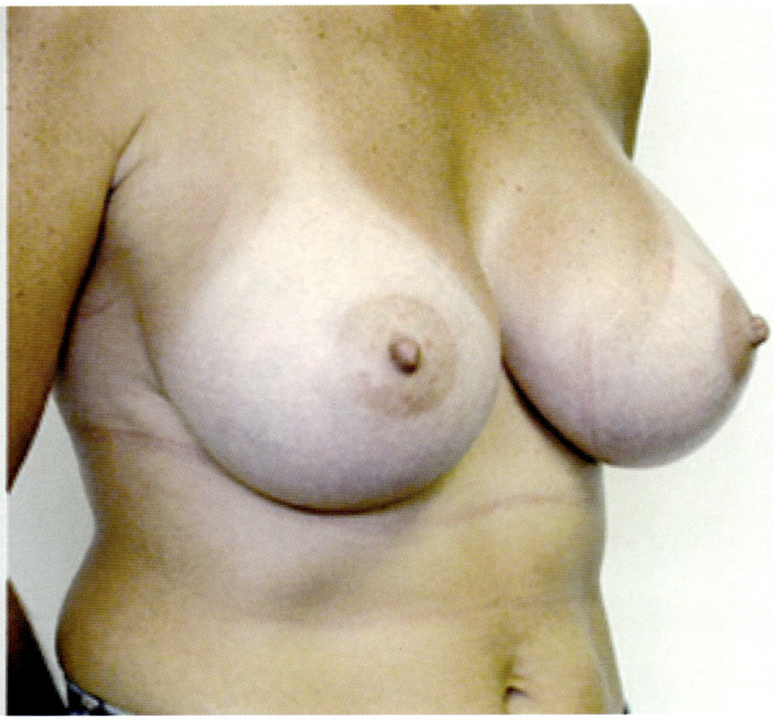

Improvement with breast implants

ASYMMETRICAL BREAST

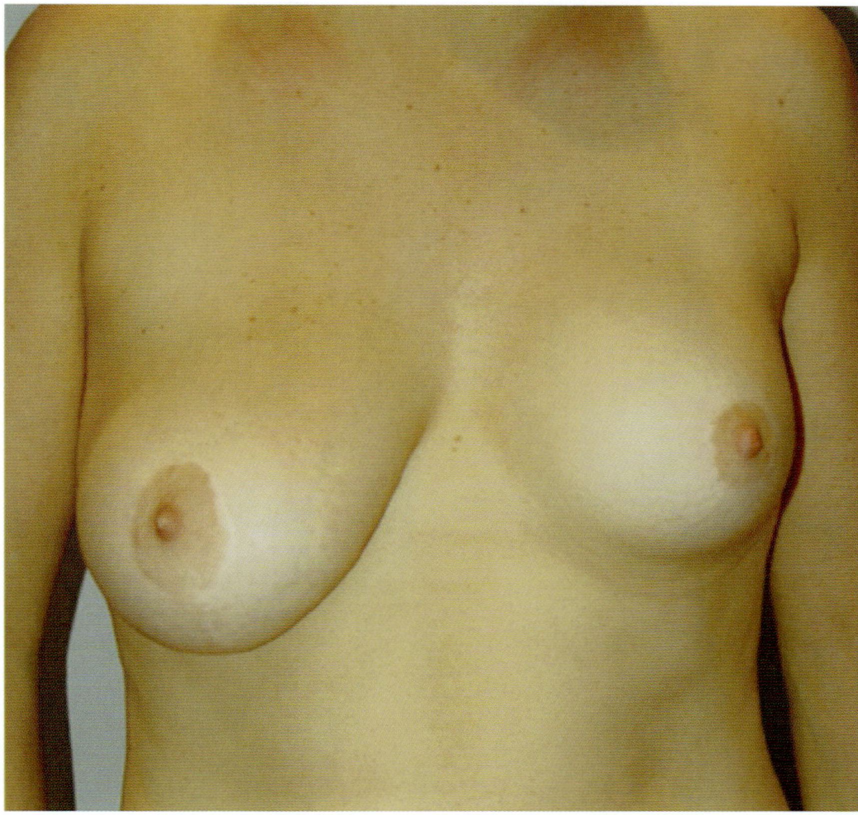

Breast Asymmetry

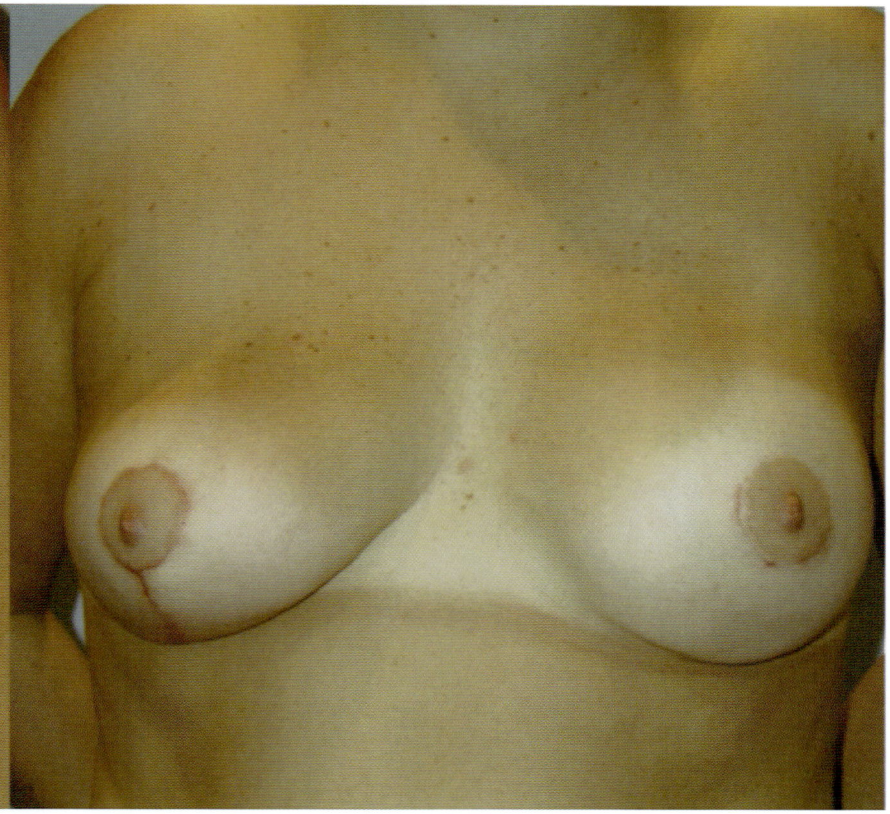

Improvement by breast implant and lift
Early result

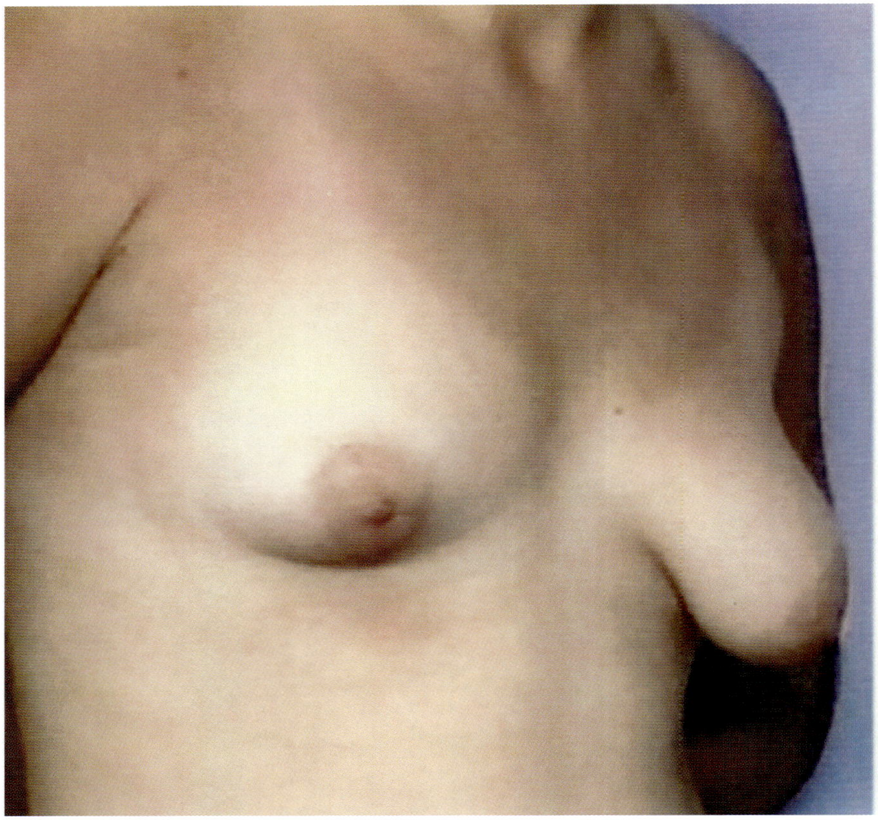

Breast Asymmetry

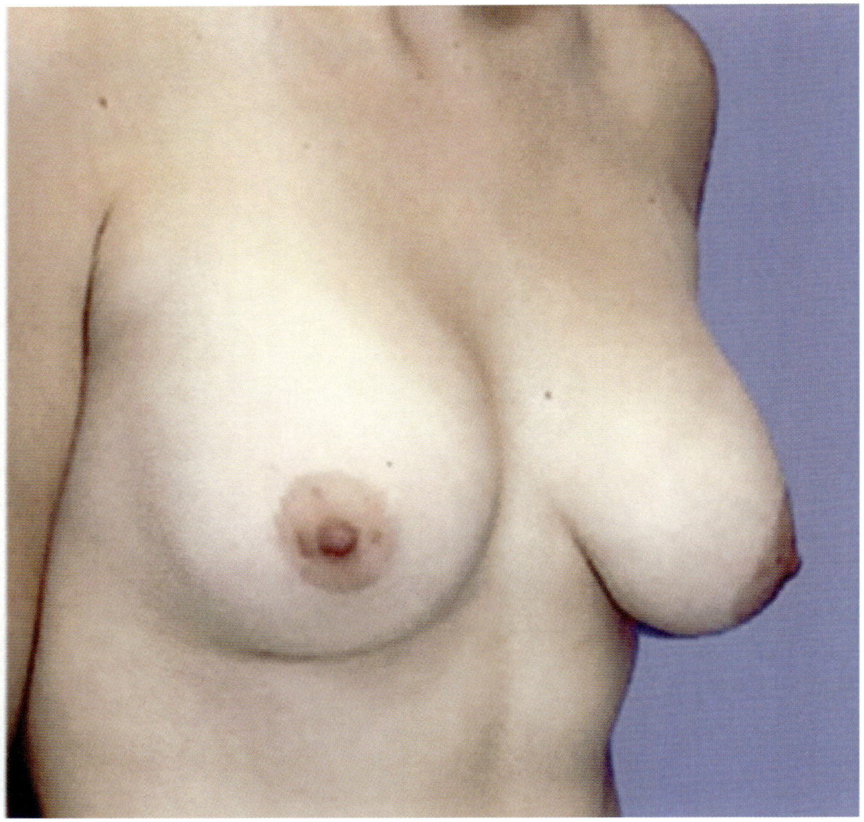

Improvement with breast implants

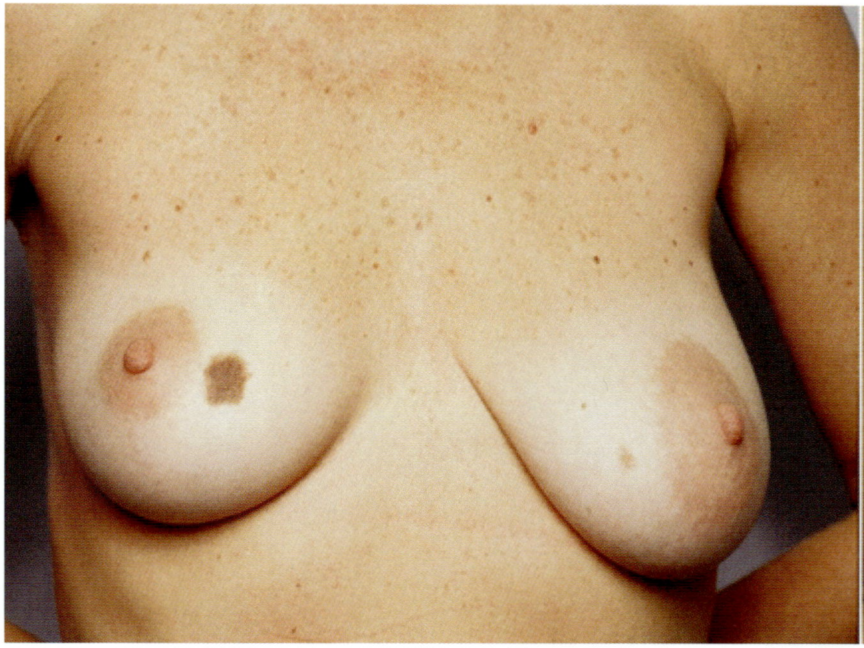

Breast Asymmetry

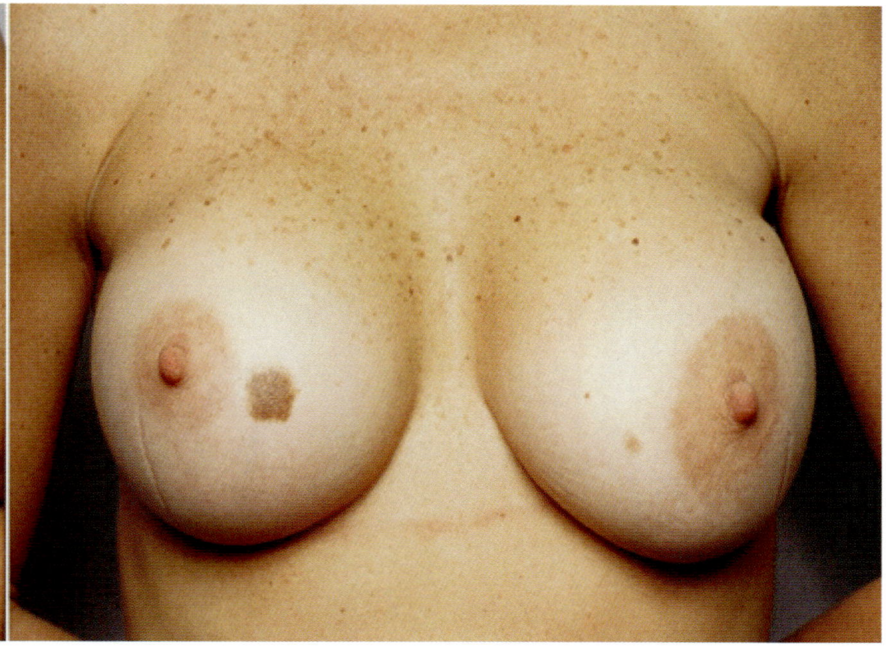

Improvement with breast implants

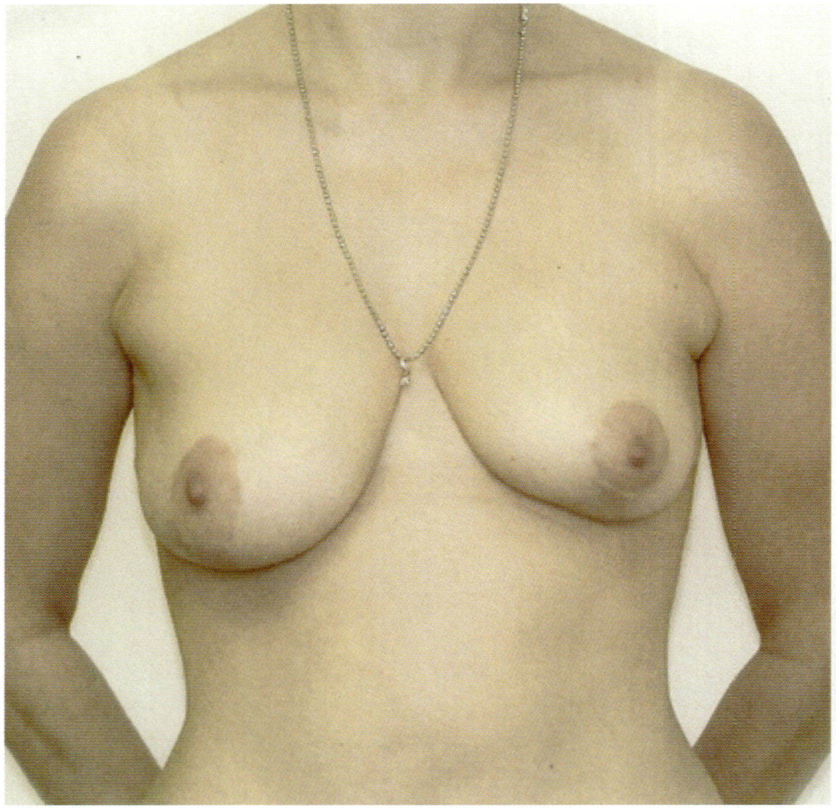

Breast Asymmetry

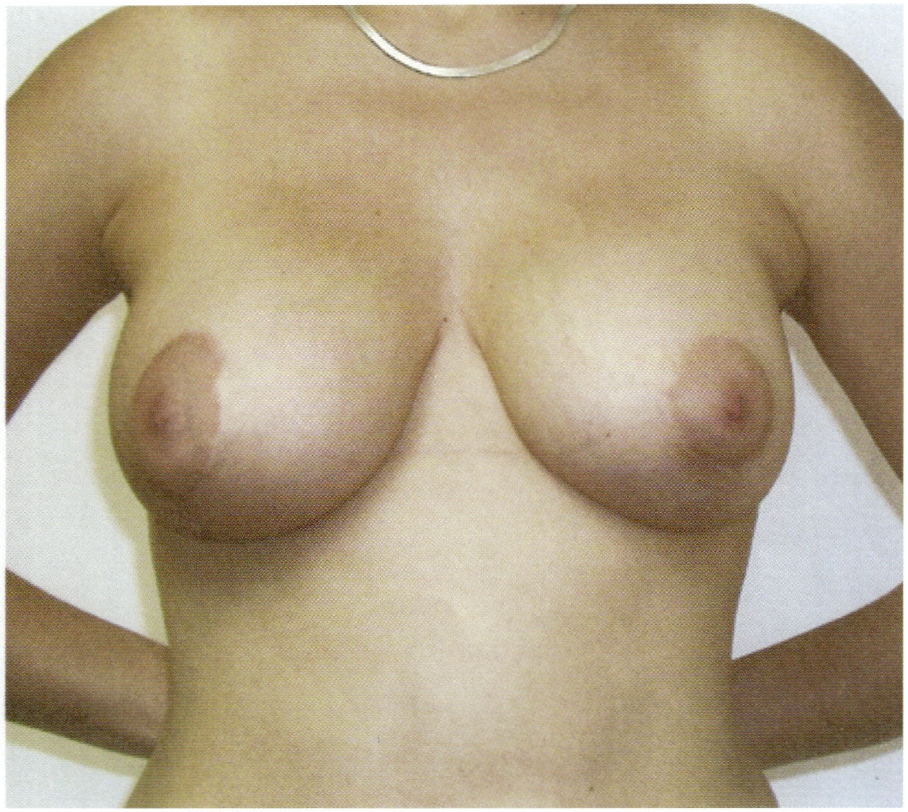

Improvement with breast implants

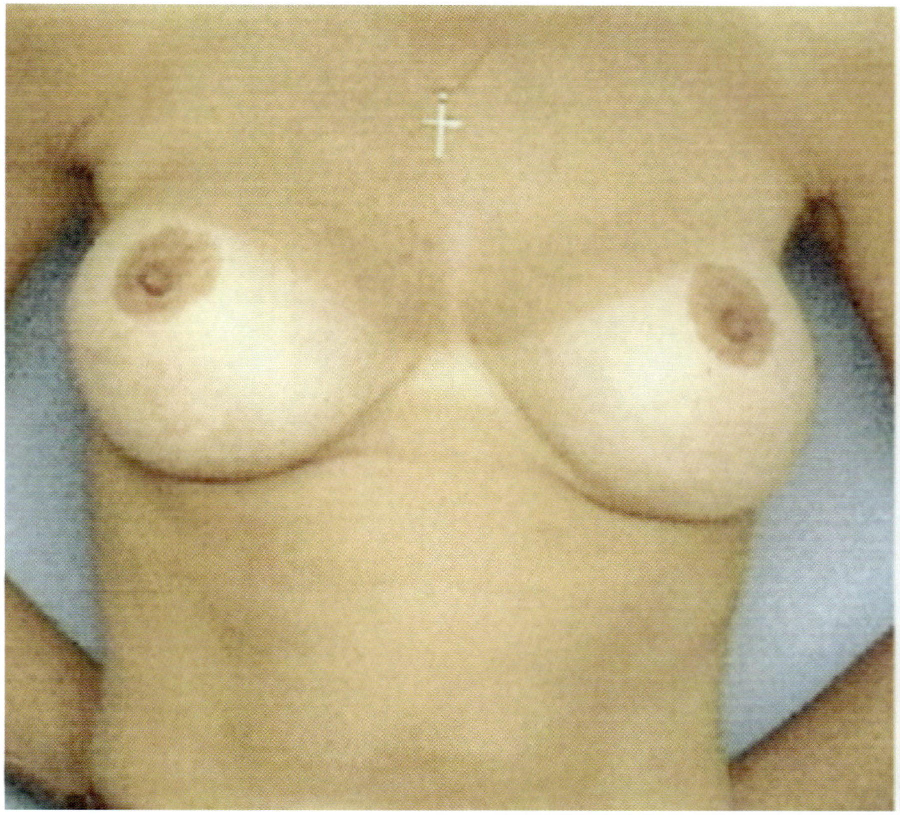

Patient desired smaller breasts

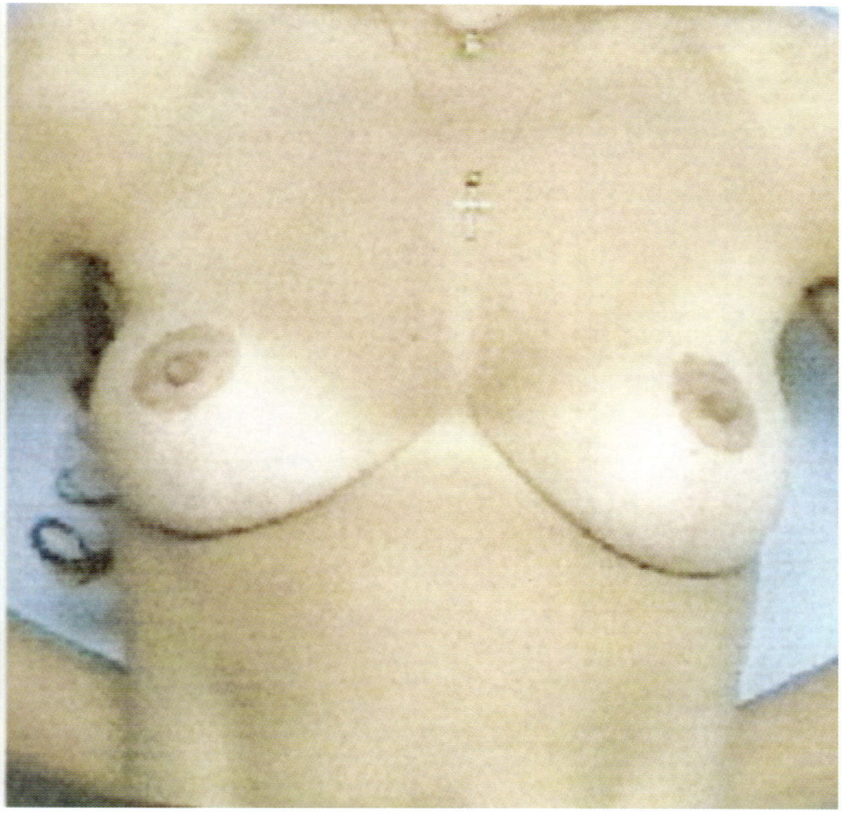

Result using a closed technique (Liposuction)

BREAST REDUCTION AND LIFT

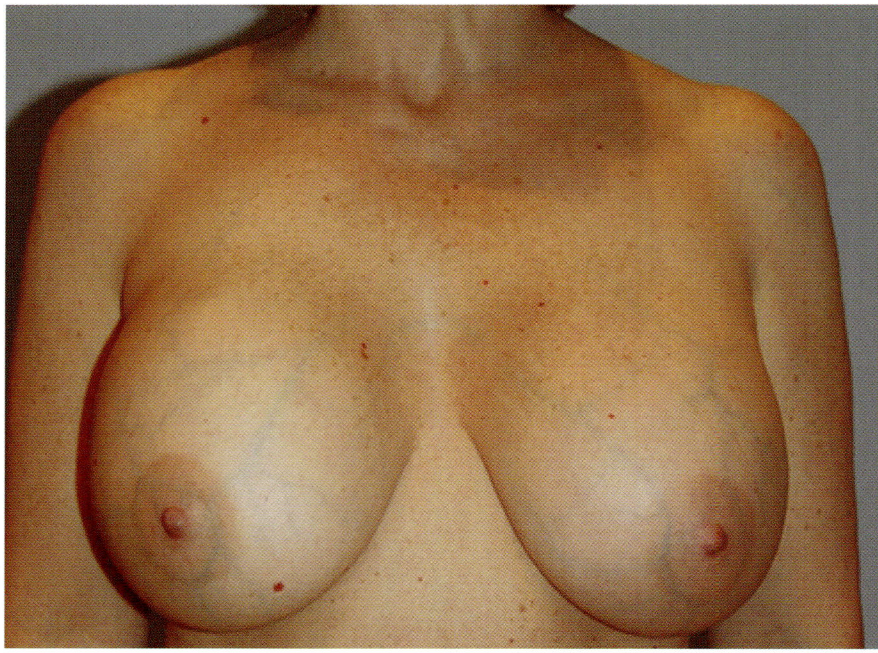

Patient with large, sagging breasts

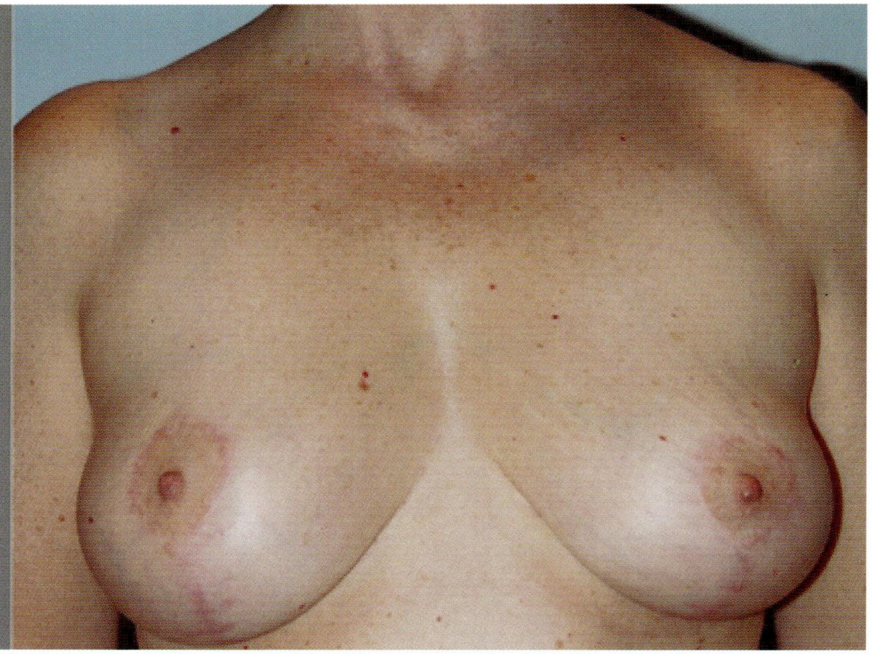

Breast reduction using an open technique (lollypop incision).

BREAST REDUCTION AND LIFT

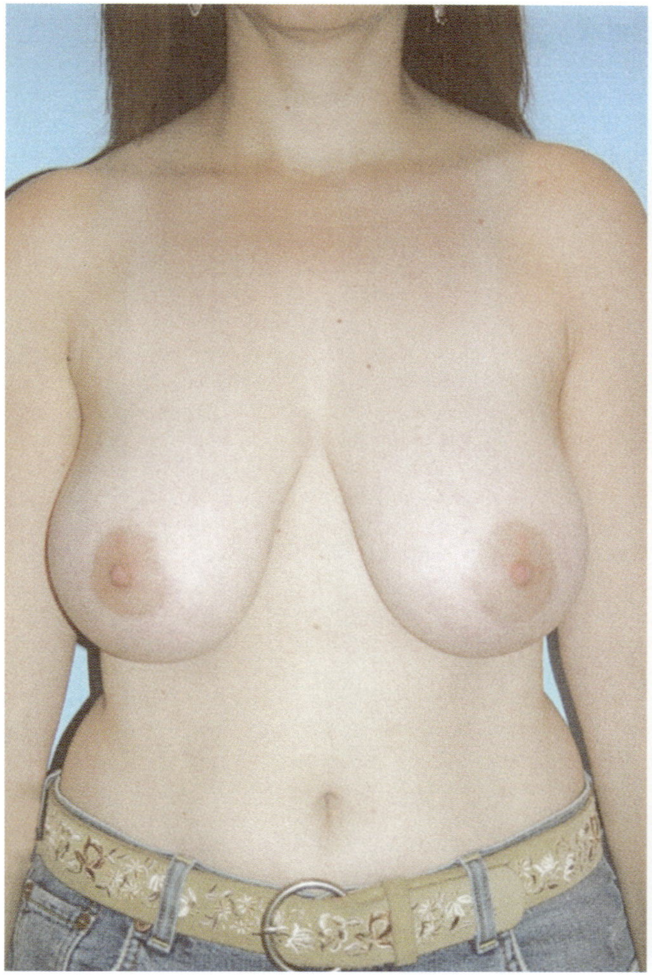

Patient desires smaller and higher breasts

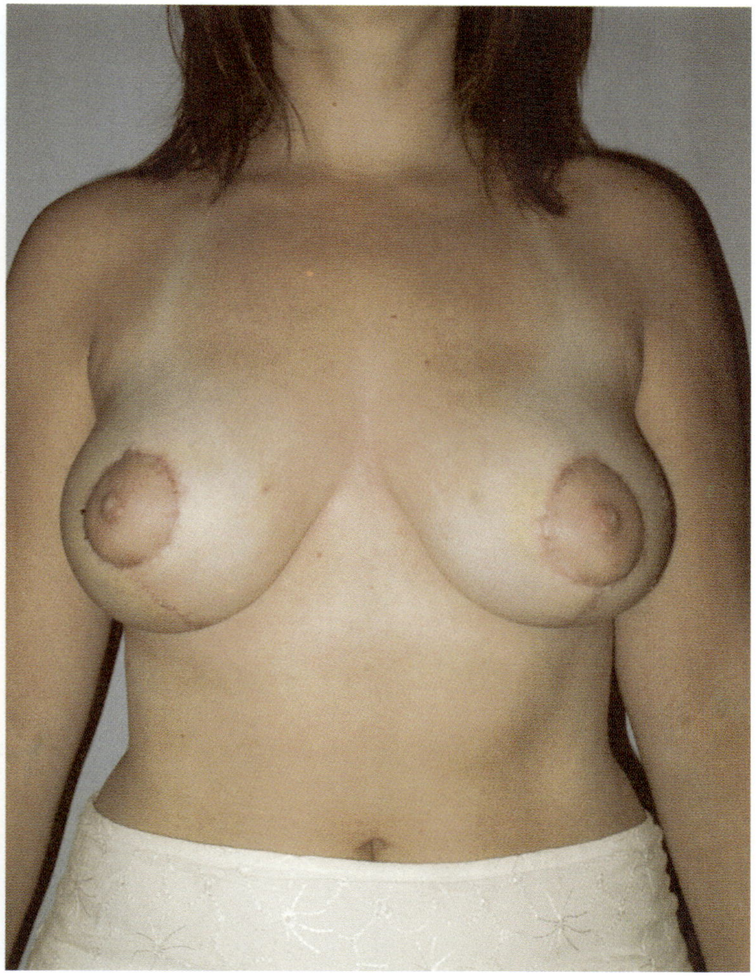

Result of closed reduction and breast lift

BREAST LIFT

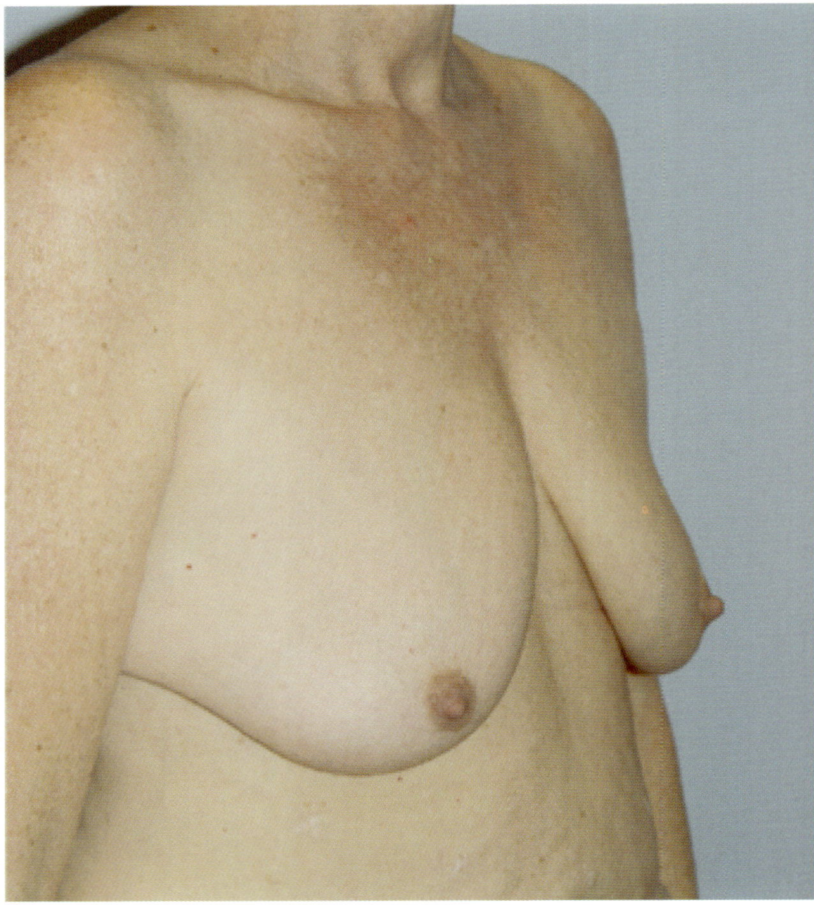

Sagging breasts

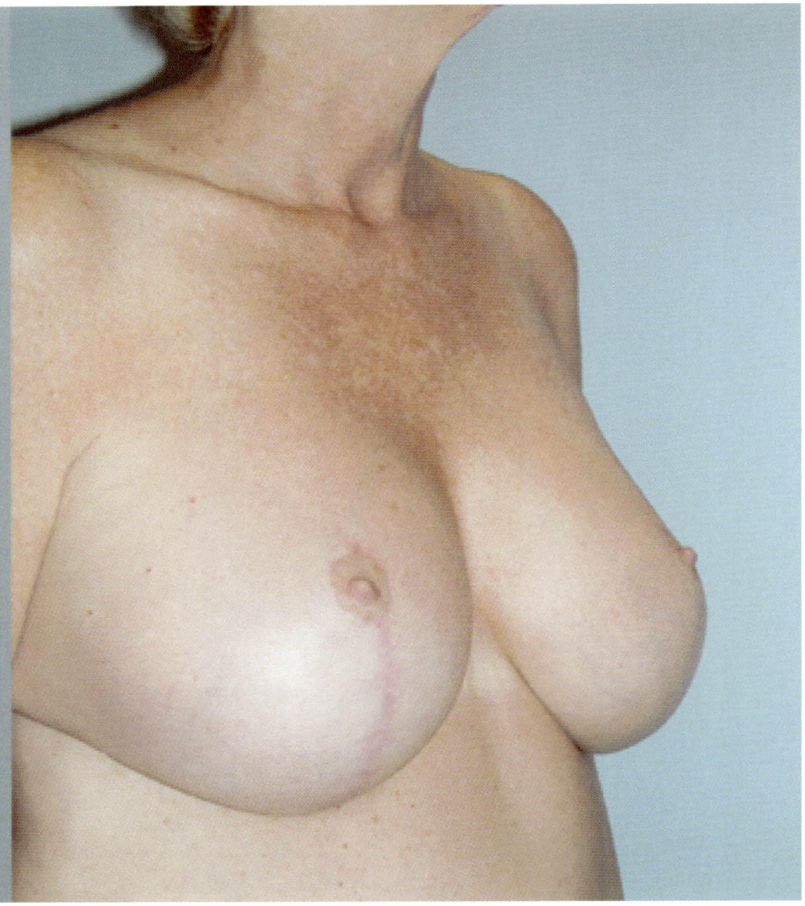

Corrected using an open technique and breast implants - (lollypop incision)

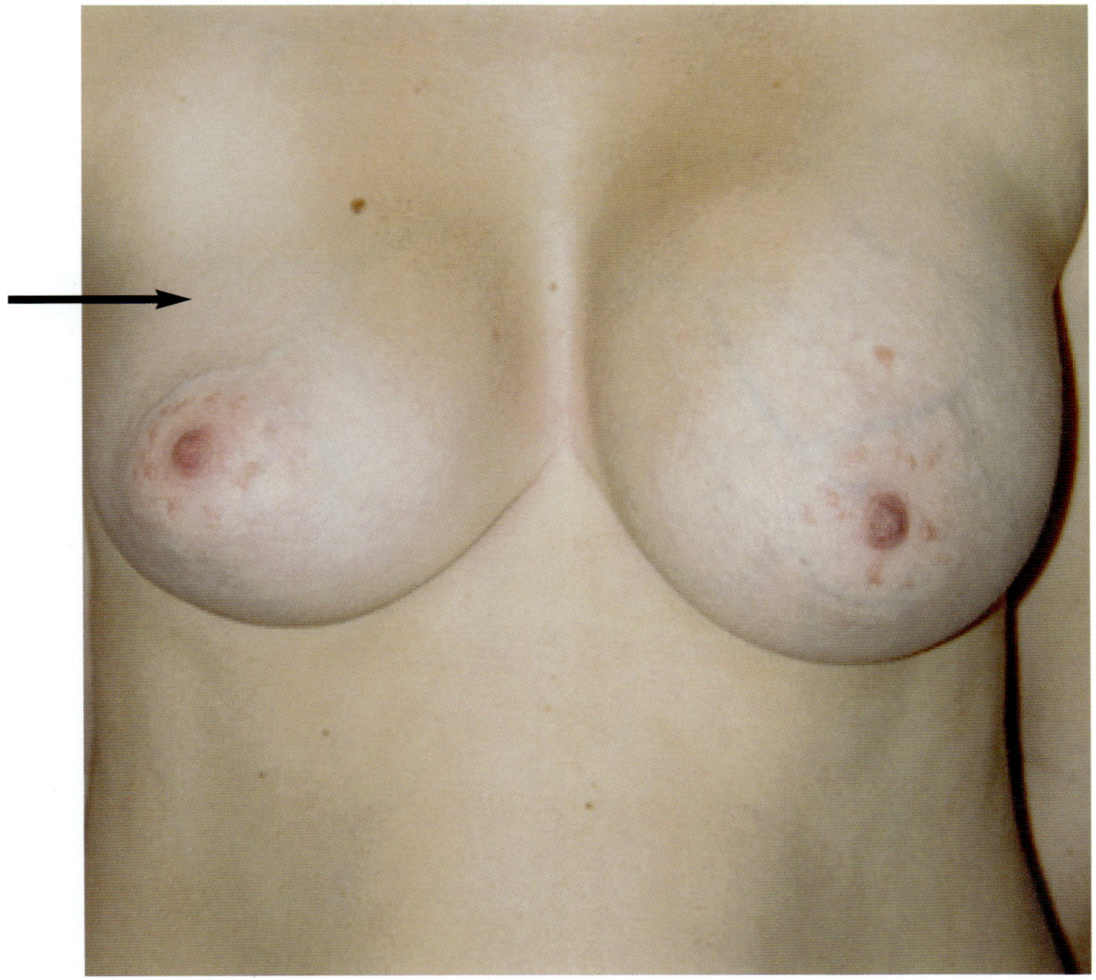

Example of a saline filled implant that leaked and deflated requiring replacement surgery.

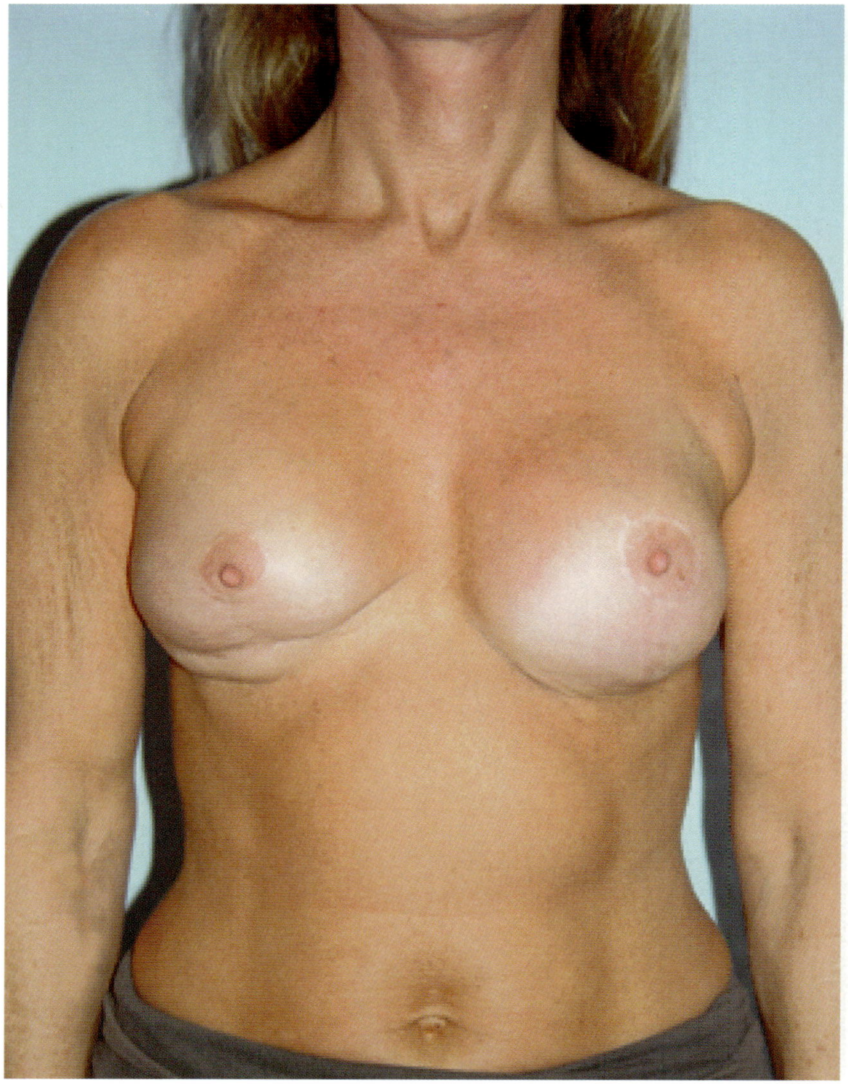

Excessive scar tissue that developed around a breast implant

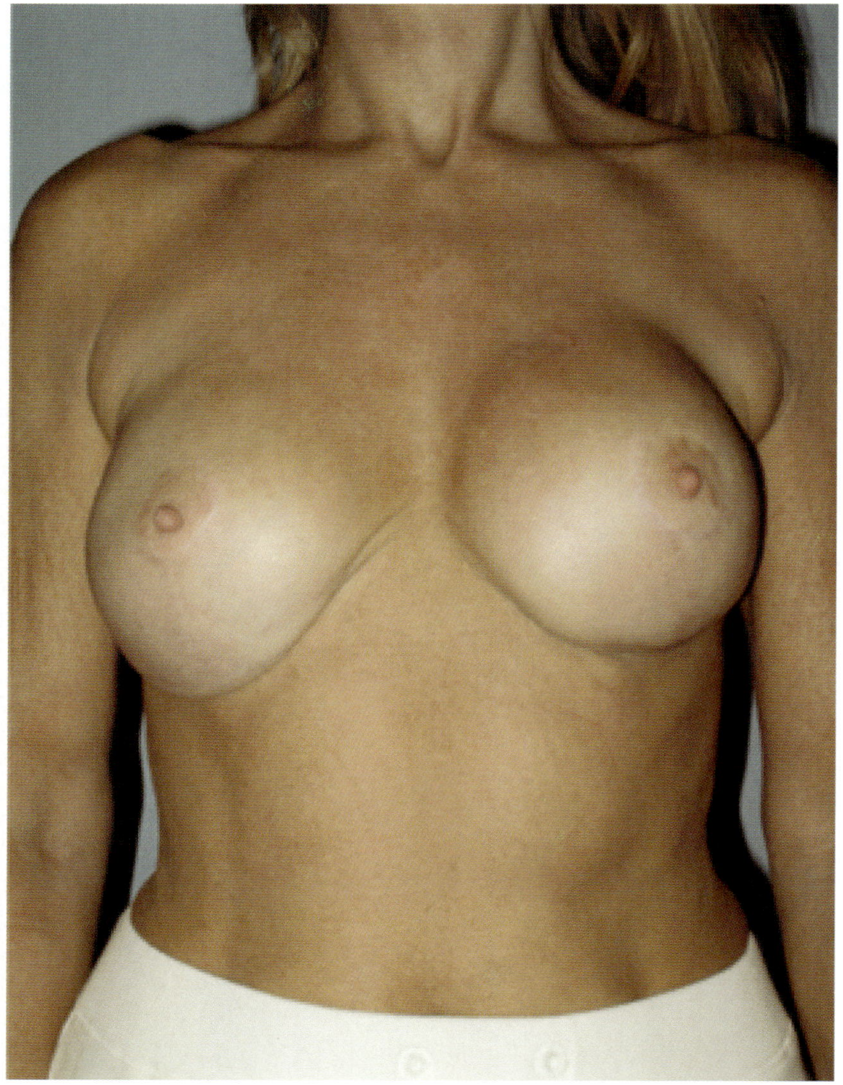

Improvement by breast reconstruction

COSMETIC SURGERY OF THE BODY

The body is a muscle frame work covered by skin. Between the skin and muscle there is a layer of fat. Conditions that respond to body cosmetic surgery may include;

1. *Excess fat which may be hereditary or dietary*
2. *Excess skin - Which may be to post child birth, post weight loss or post liposuction.*
3. *Lack of muscle mass*

Patients who have excess fat are ideally treated with a closed liposuction technique which is designed to remove the excess fat between the skin and muscle, in virtually any area of the body.

The four keys to successful liposuction contouring of the body are:

- *Liposuction Procedure*
- *Patient's Diet*
- *Muscle Tone*
- *Skin Shrinkage*

Patients who have excess skin require open body surgery - which can remove excess skin from any area of the body. Open body surgery requires extensive incisions.

A variety of body implants can be used to simulate muscle mass.

Genital cosmetic surgery continues to increase in popularity. Whether it is female rejuvenation or enlargement in men. Cosmetic foot surgery can correct a variety of unattractive conditions of the feet.

CONTOURING THE BODY BY FAT SCULPTURING USING A CLOSED TECHNIQUE. REDUCTION OF THE UPPER ARMS

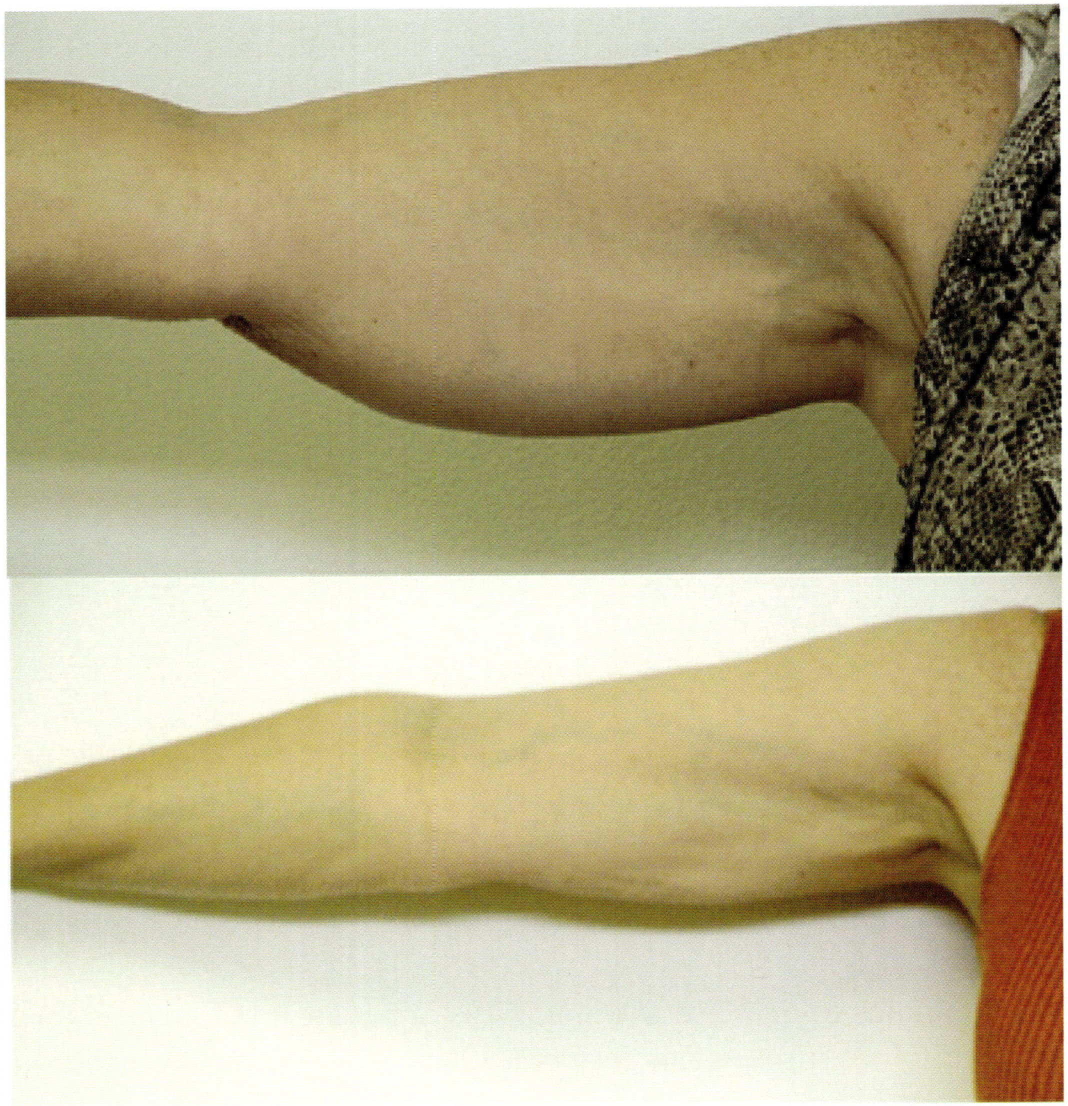

Patient desired tummy tuck - advised to first reduce fat by liposuction alone. This is a result of closed body surgery (liposuction) which eliminated the need for a tummy tuck.

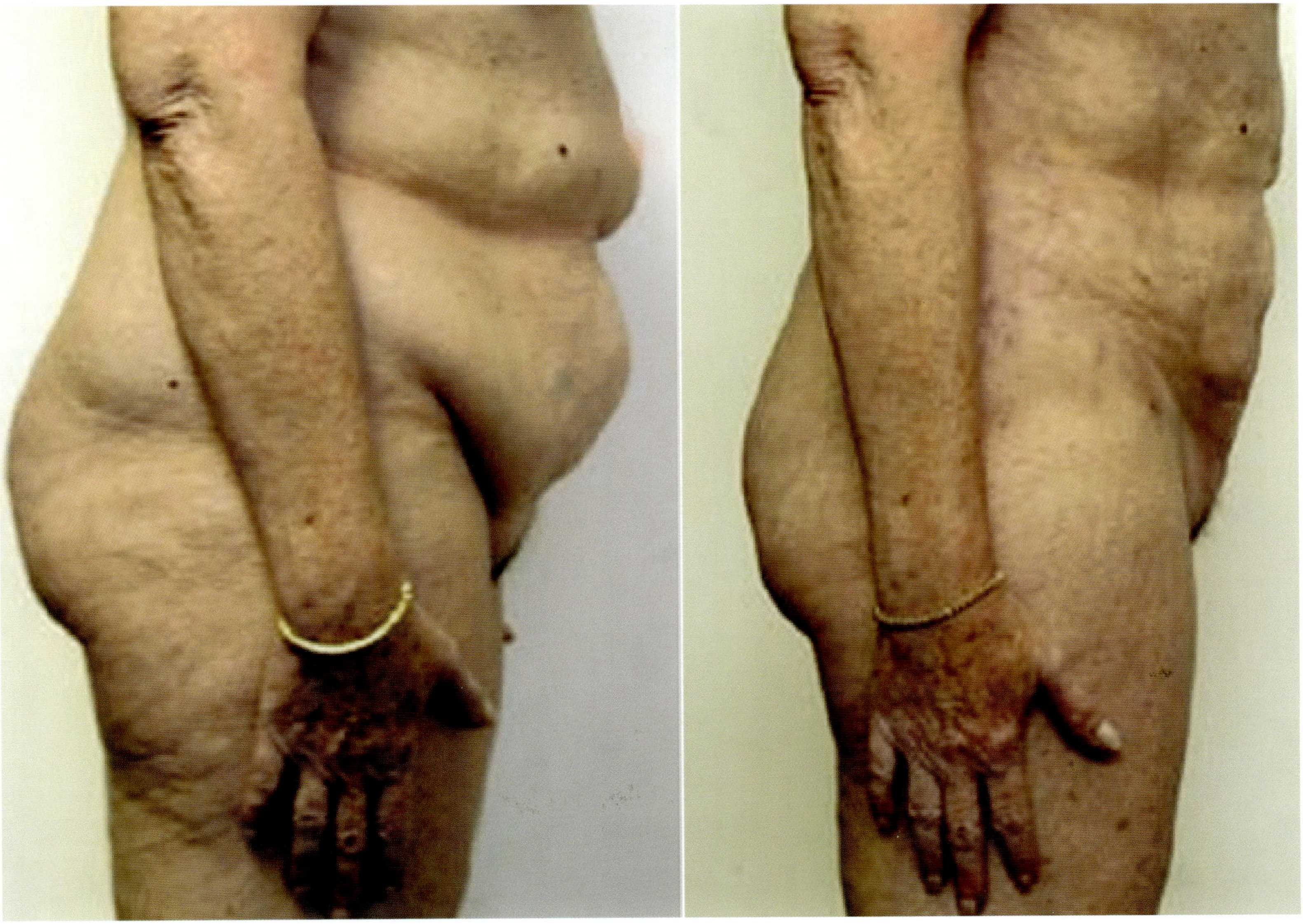

CONTOURING THE BELLY FAT BY LIPOSUCTION

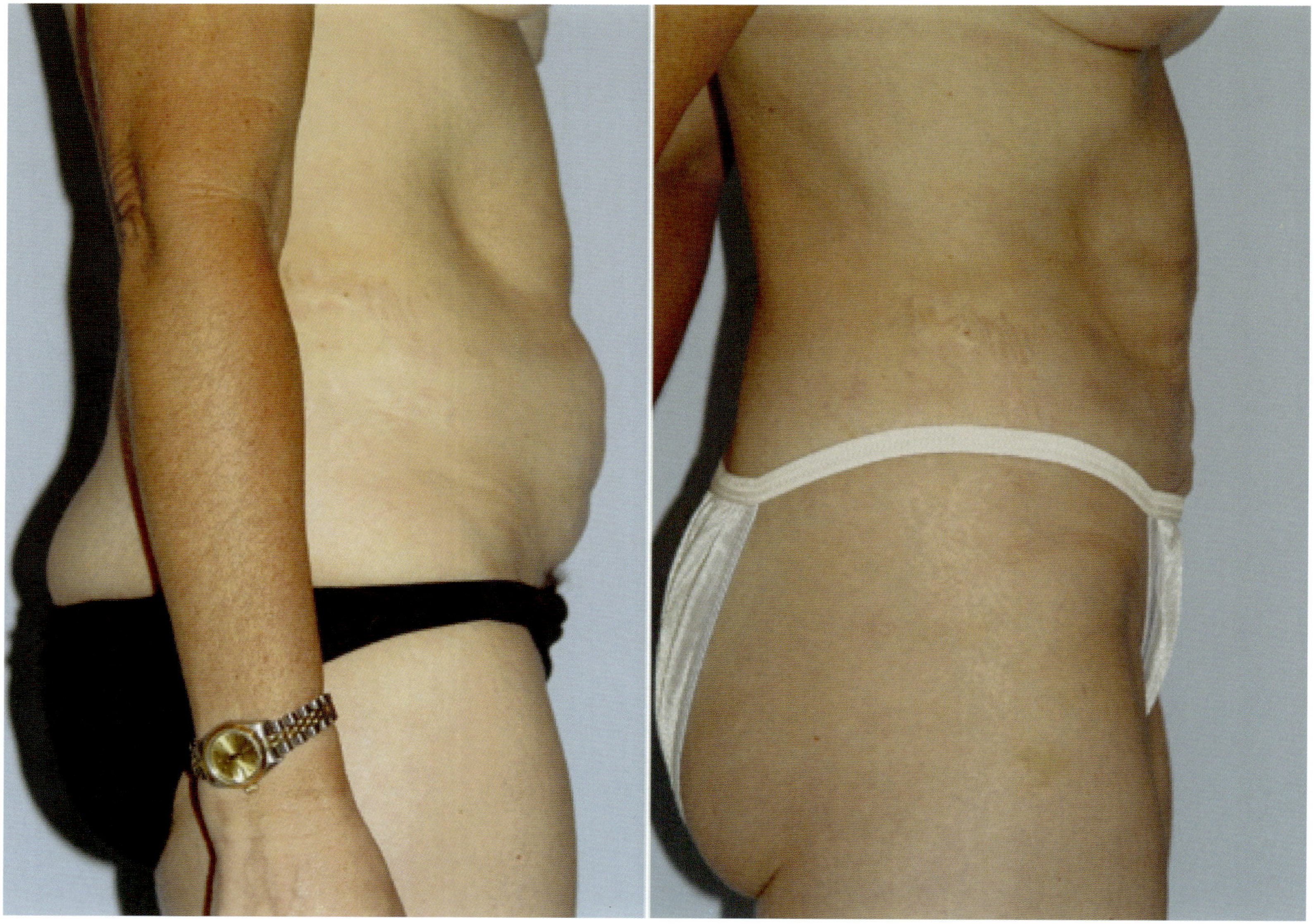

CONTOURING THE WAIST OF A MALE

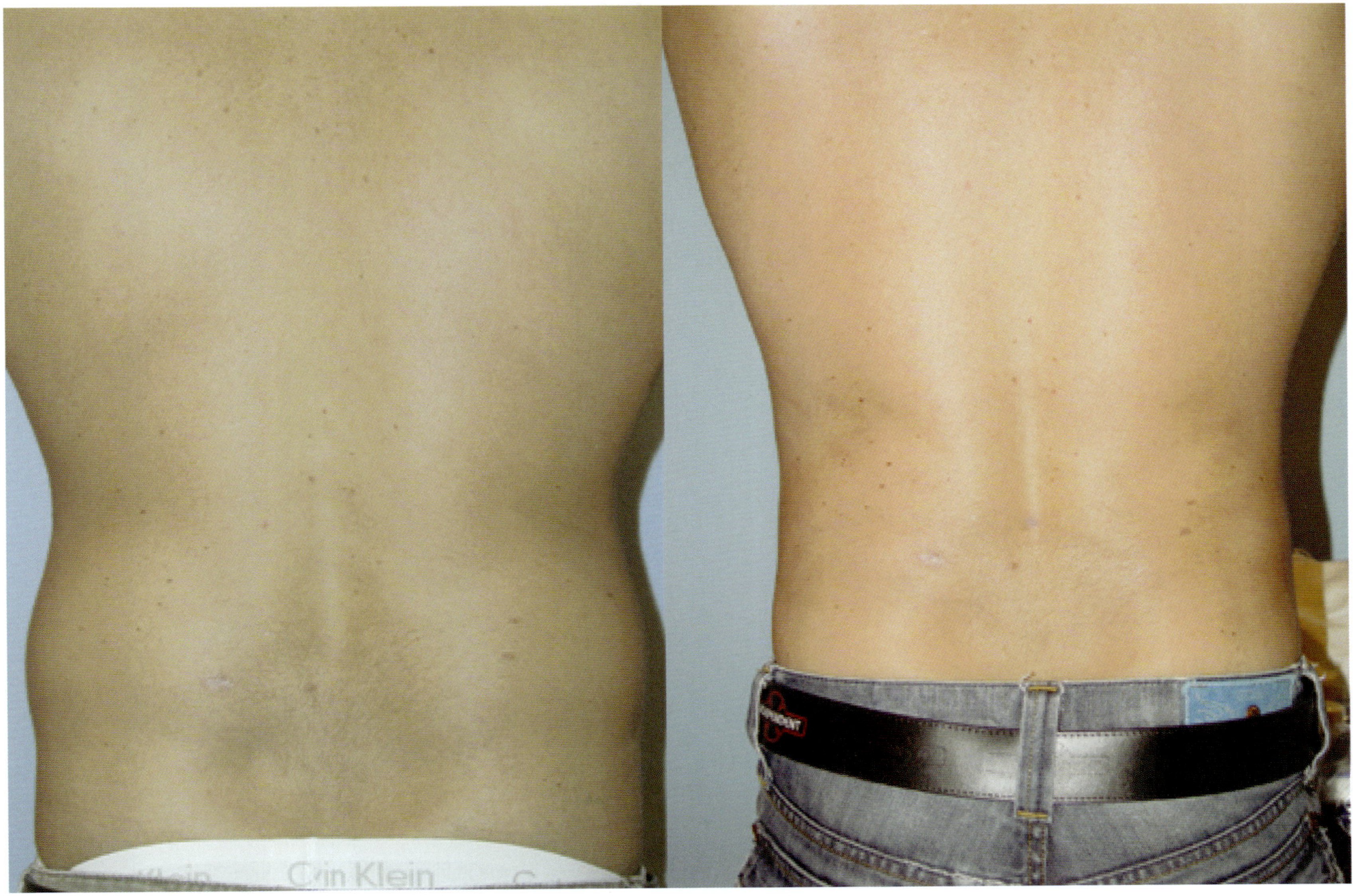

REDUCING THE BUTTOCKS AND THIGH AREA

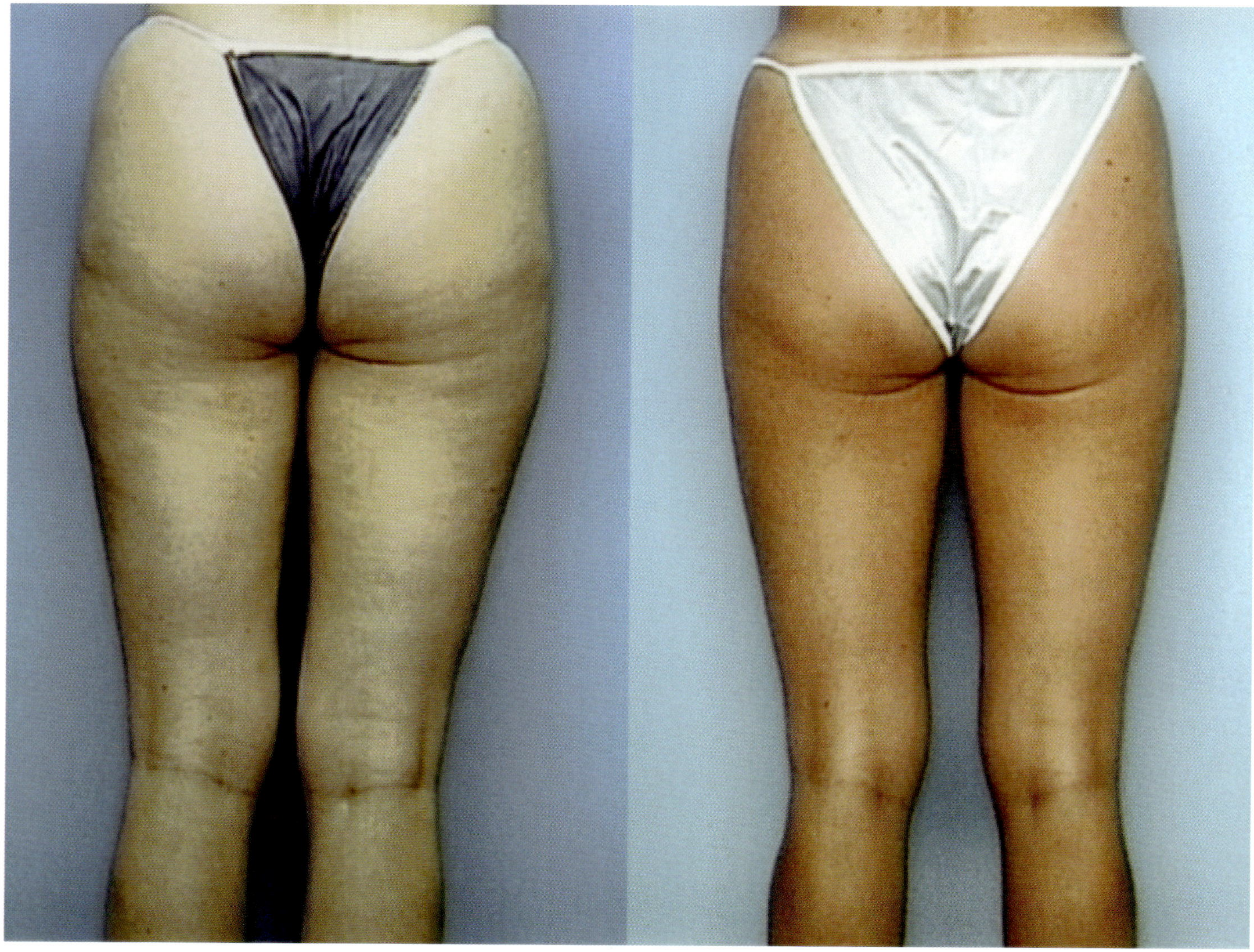

REDUCING SADDLEBAGS

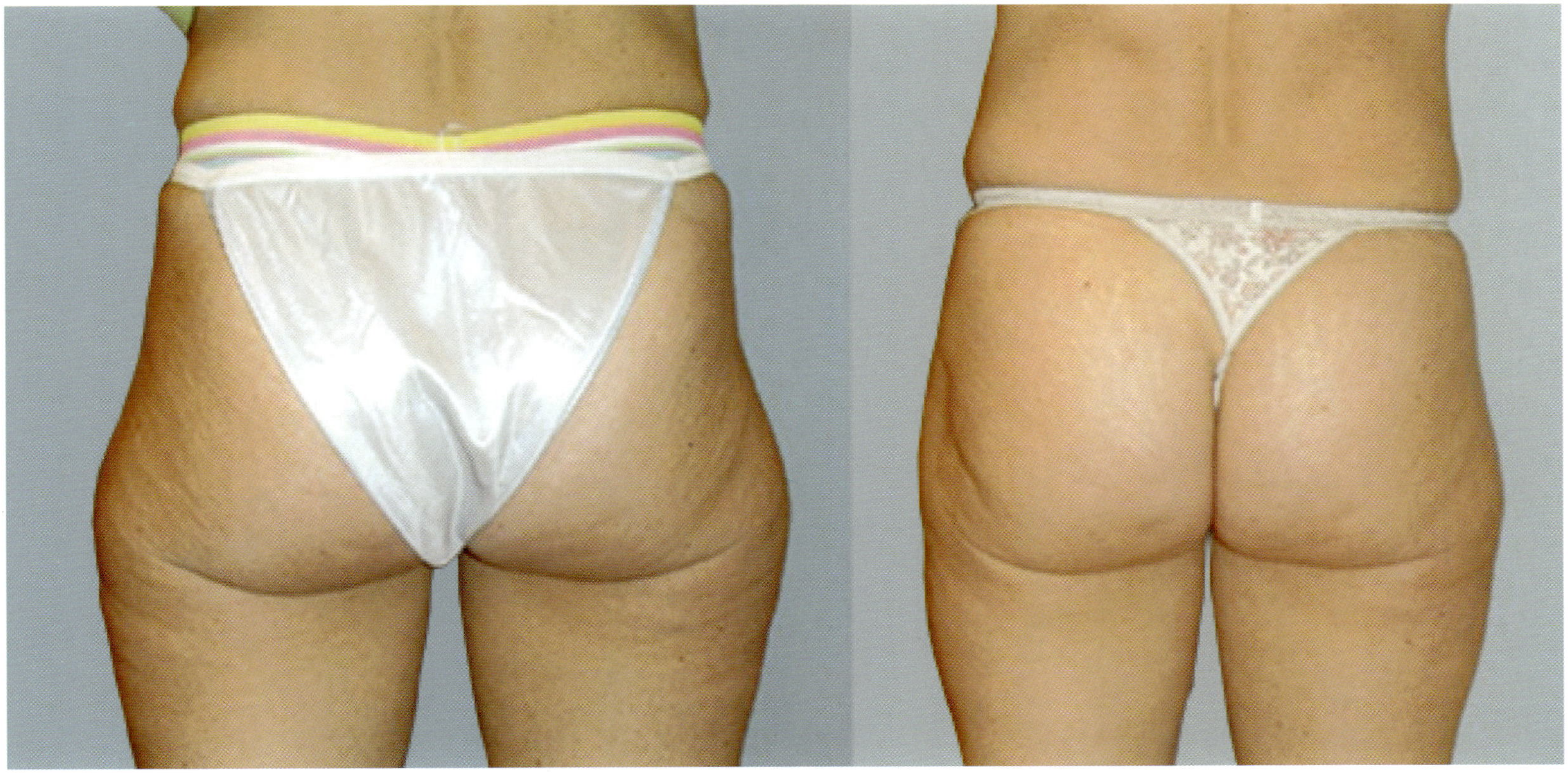

SKIN TIGHTENING OF THE BODY USING AN OPEN TECHNIQUE

There are three types of open body surgery

1. *To tighten excess skin due to age or childbirth.*
2. *To remove excess fat and tighten skin - hereditary.*
3. *To remove excess skin due to loss of large amounts of weight - post bariatric.*

ARM LIFT

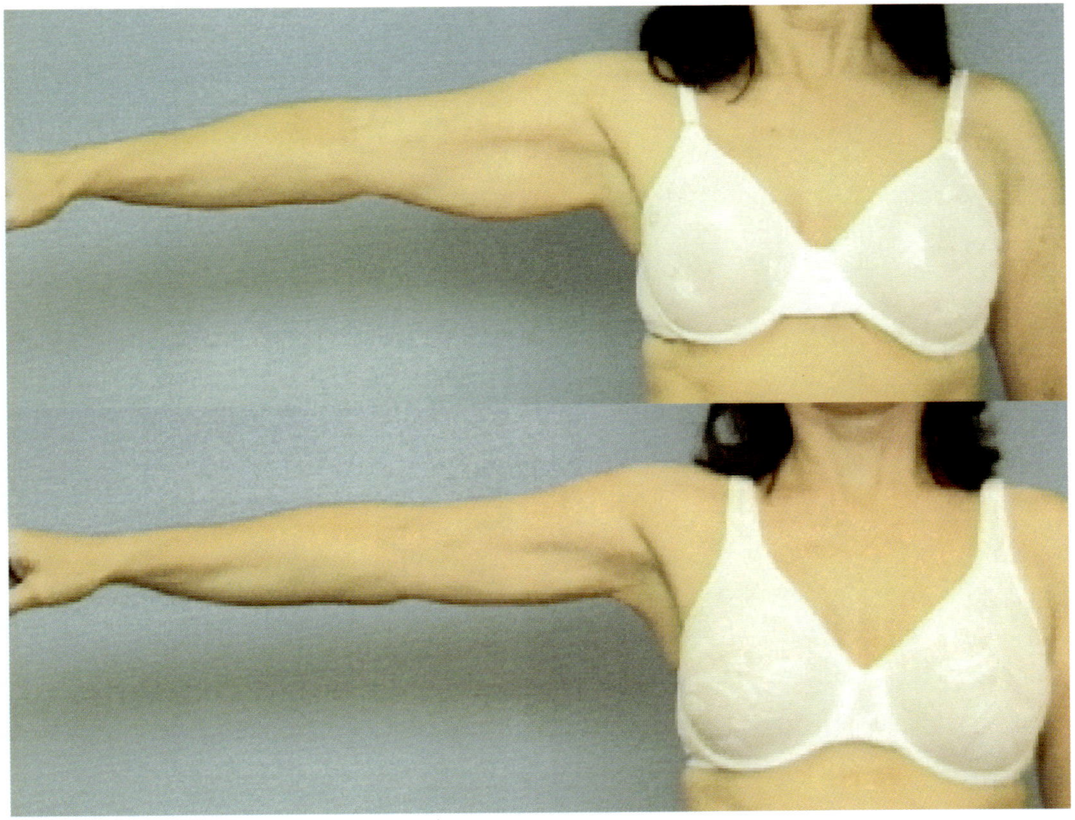

TUMMY TUCK

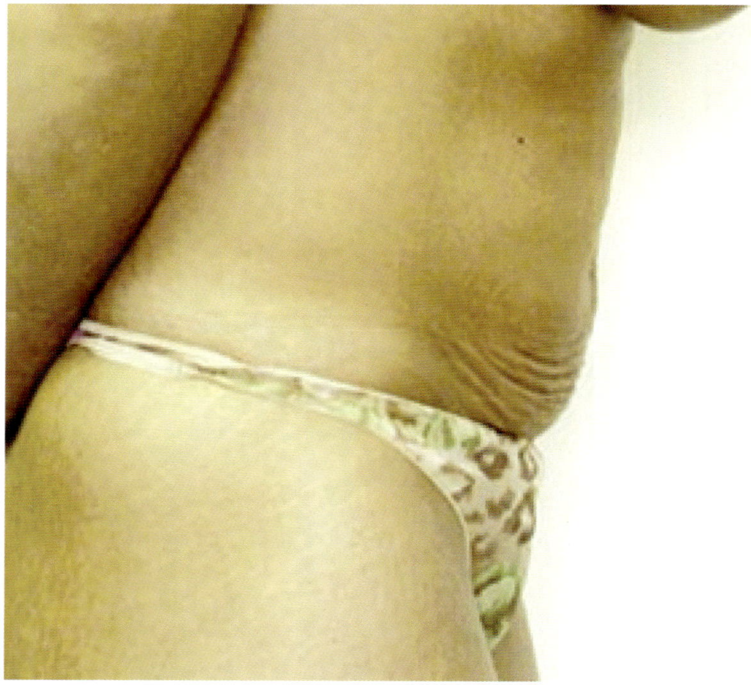

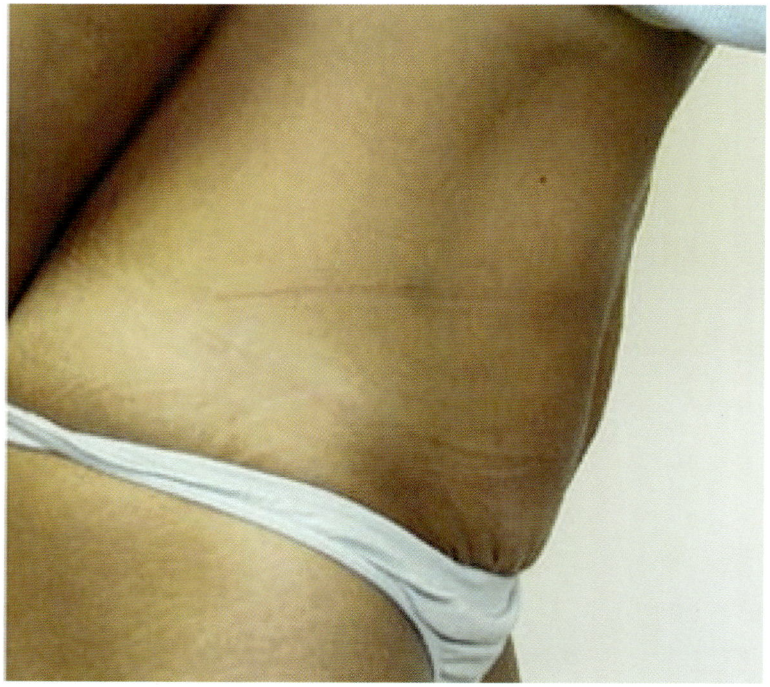

TUMMY TUCK

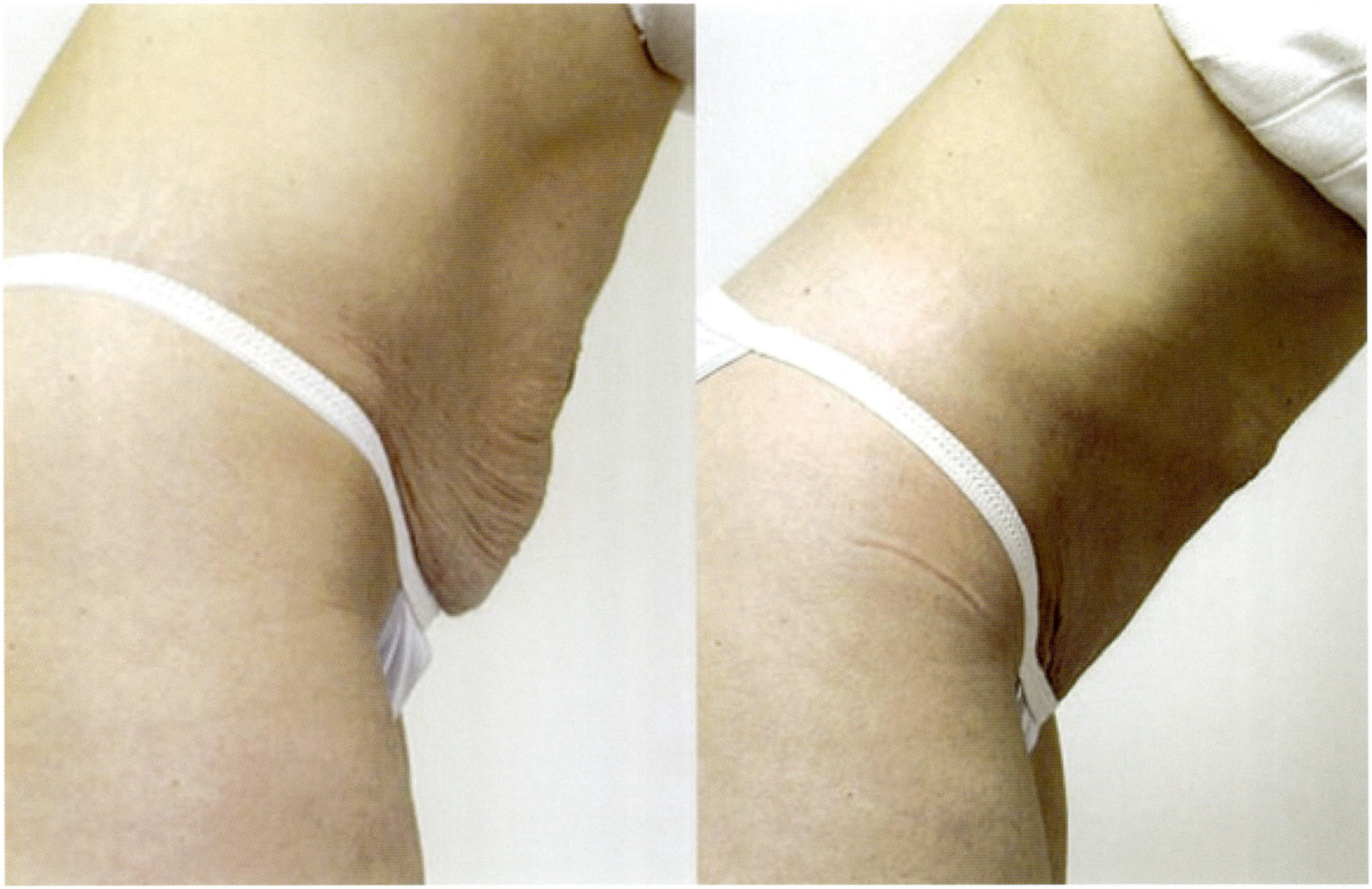

TUMMY TUCK

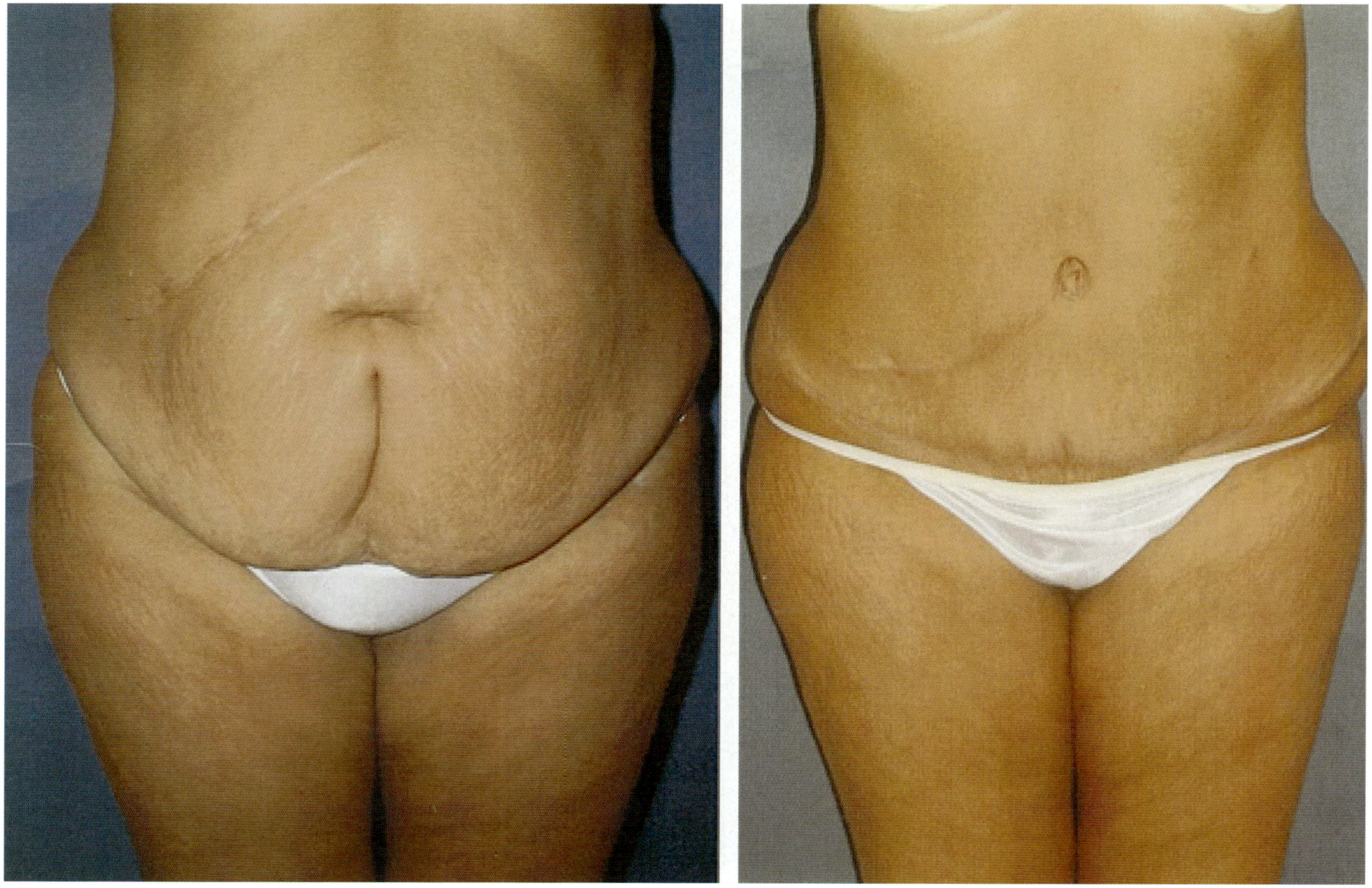

Courtesy of Dr. Robert Cattani, MD
www.drcattani.com

TUMMY TUCK

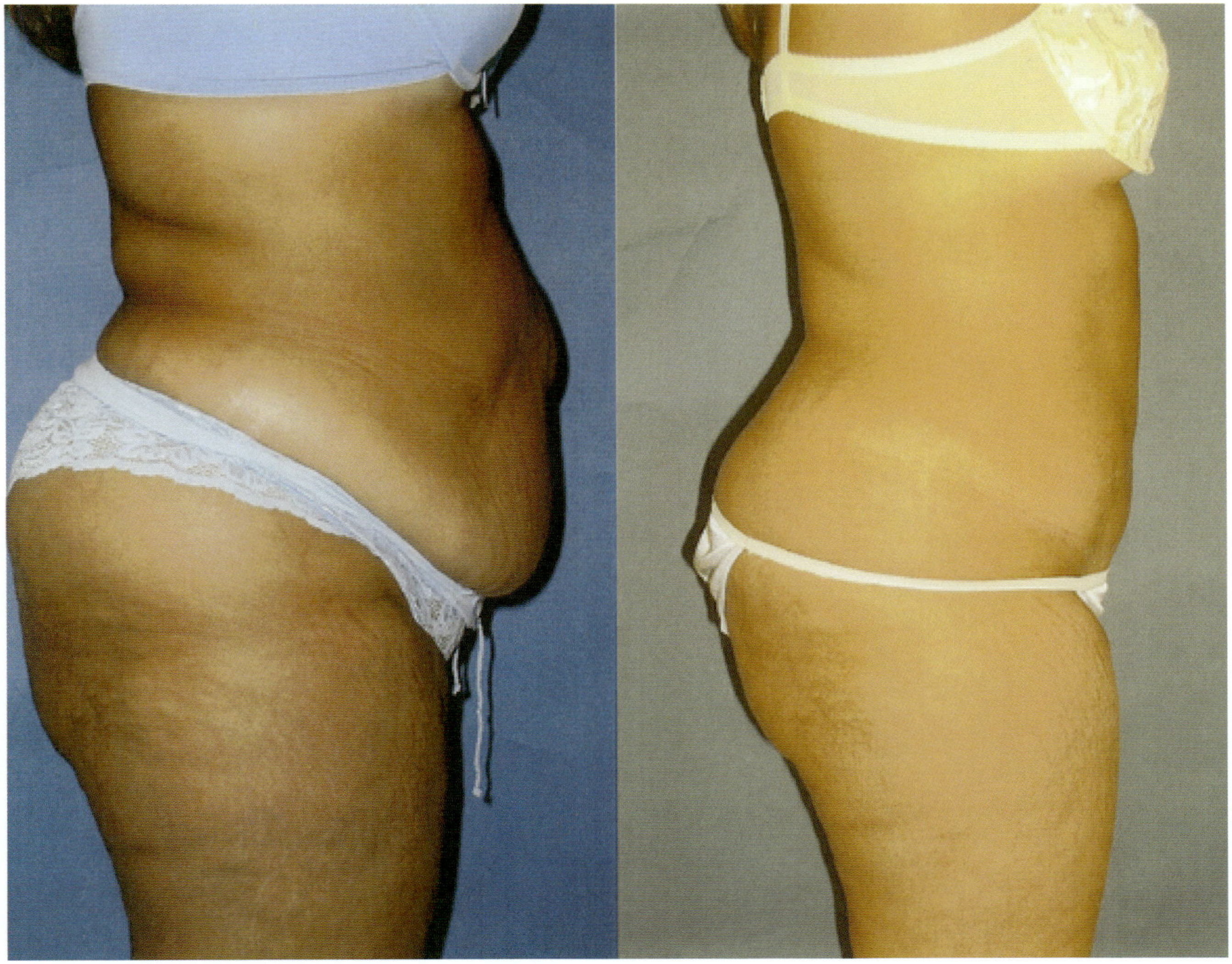

Courtesy of Dr. Robert Cattani, MD
www.drcattani.com

TUMMY TUCK

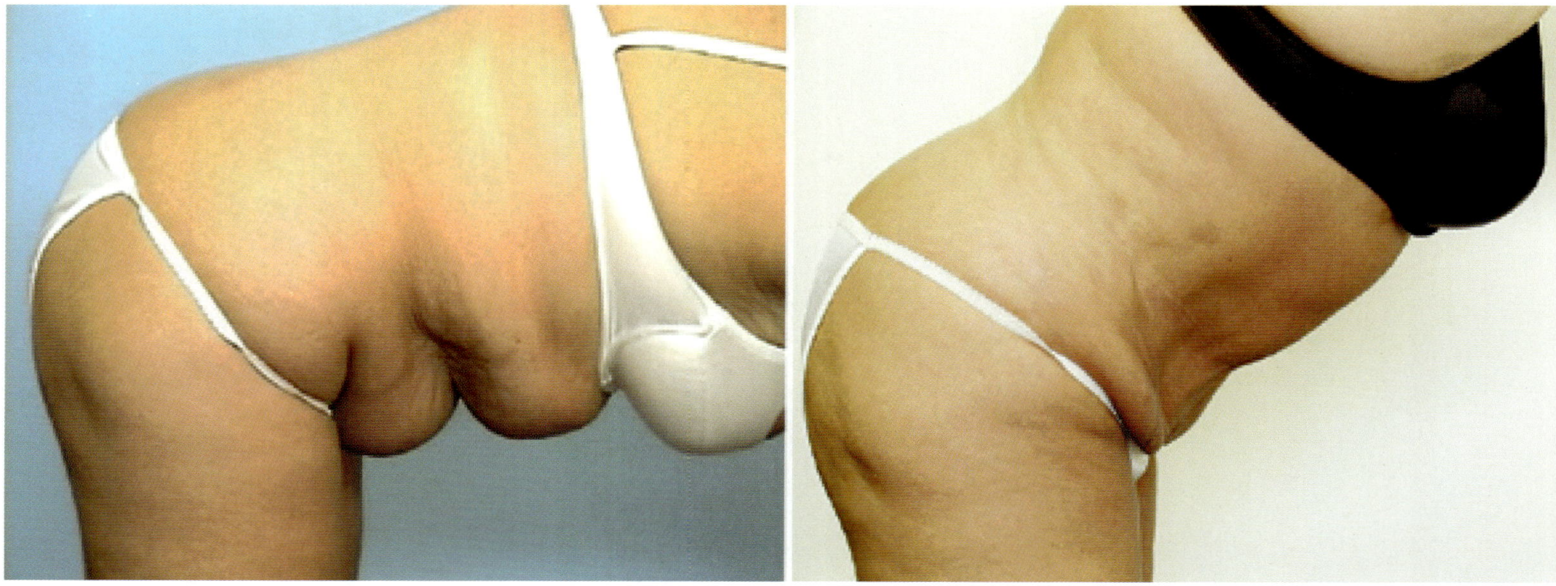

Courtesy of Dr. Robert Cattani, MD
www.drcattani.com

THIGH LIFT

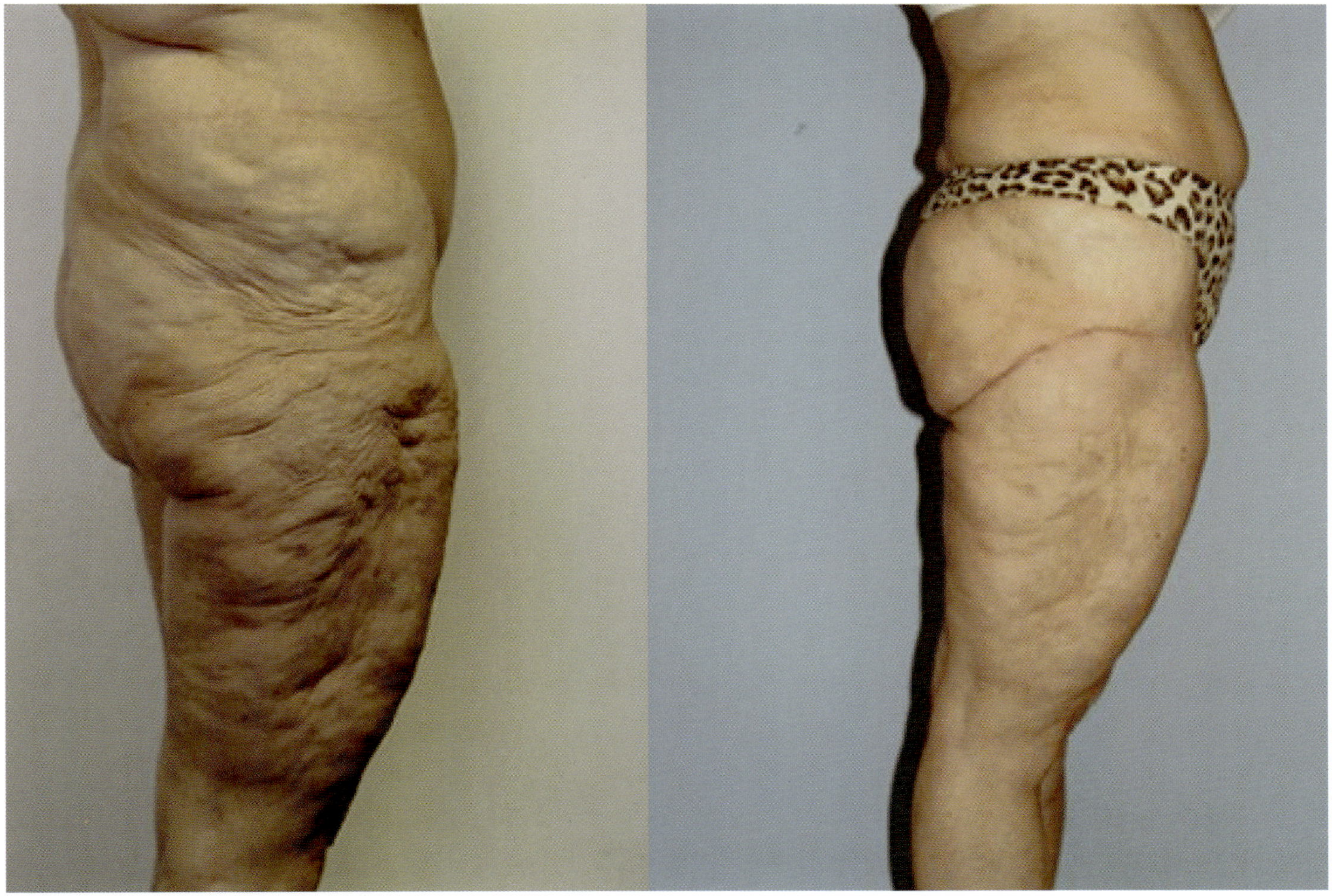

POST BARIATRIC WEIGHT LOSS BODY CONTOURING

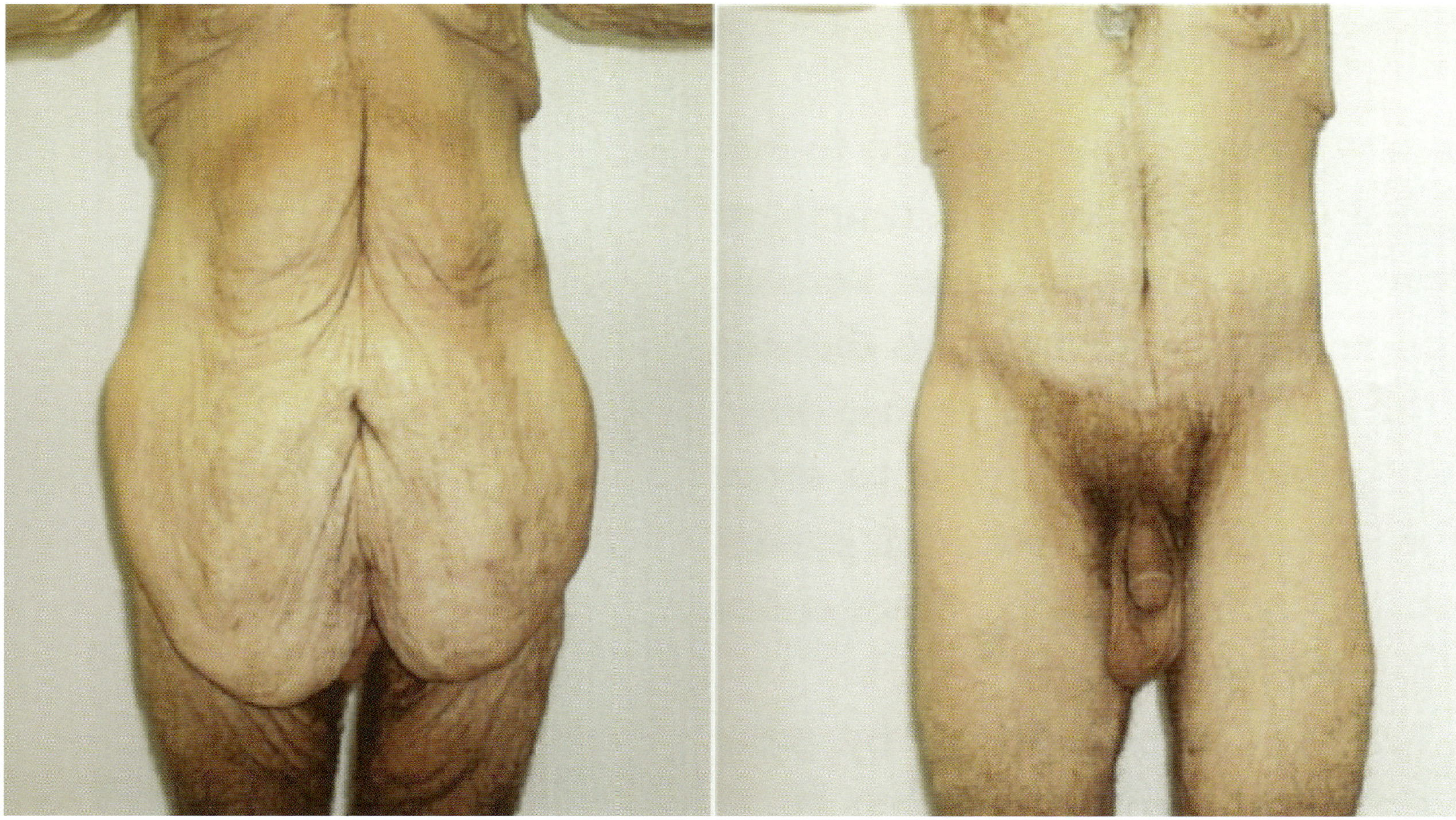

VAGINAL REJUVENATION

Vaginal rejuvenation and cosmetic procedures of the genitals are becoming more popular and can do the following:

1. Tighten the Vagina
2. Enhance the G - Spot
3. Hymen Repair and Revirgination
4. Reduce the Labia

LABIA REDUCTION

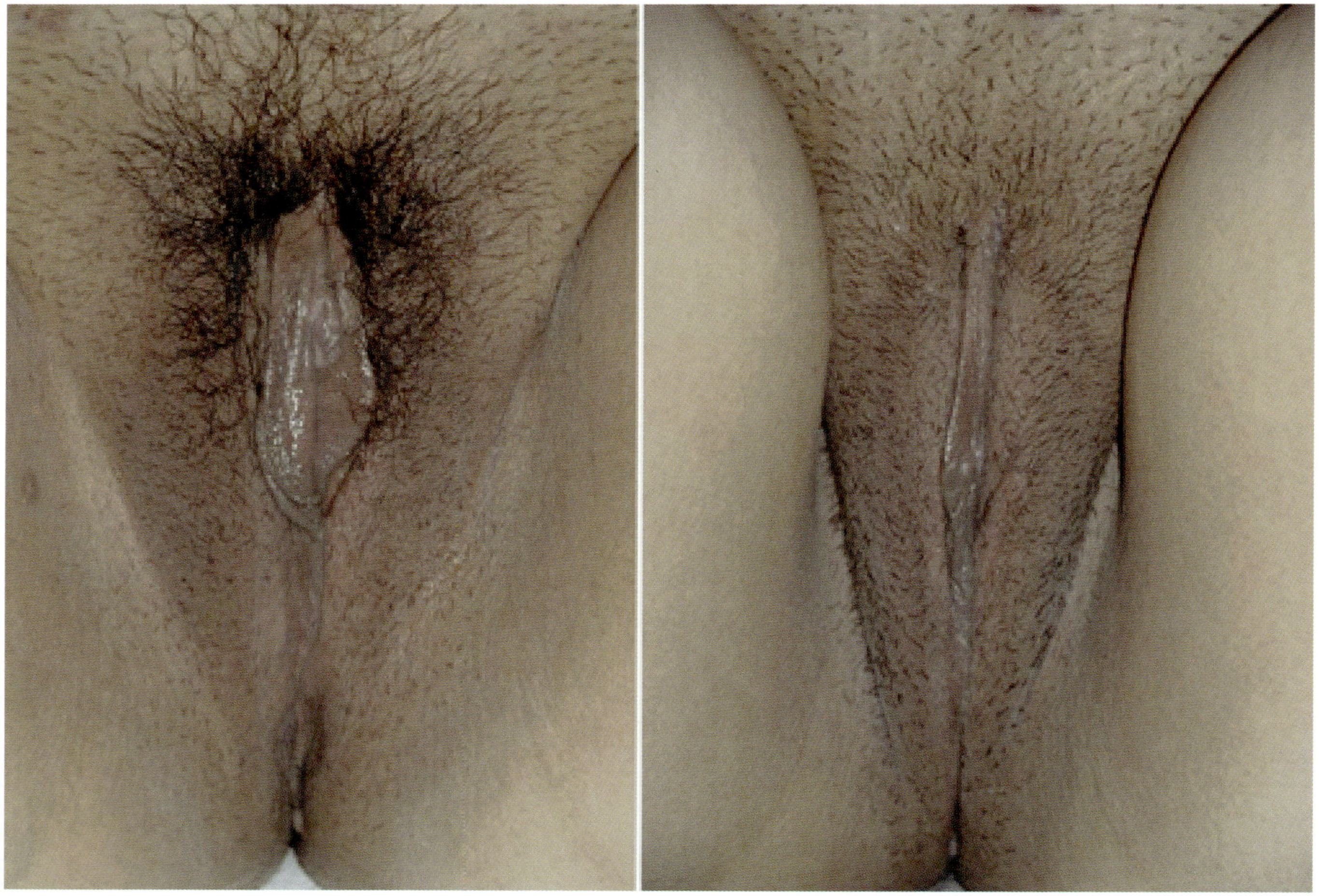

Courtesy of Dr. Aram Bonni, MD
www.beautybybrennan.com

LABIA REDUCTION

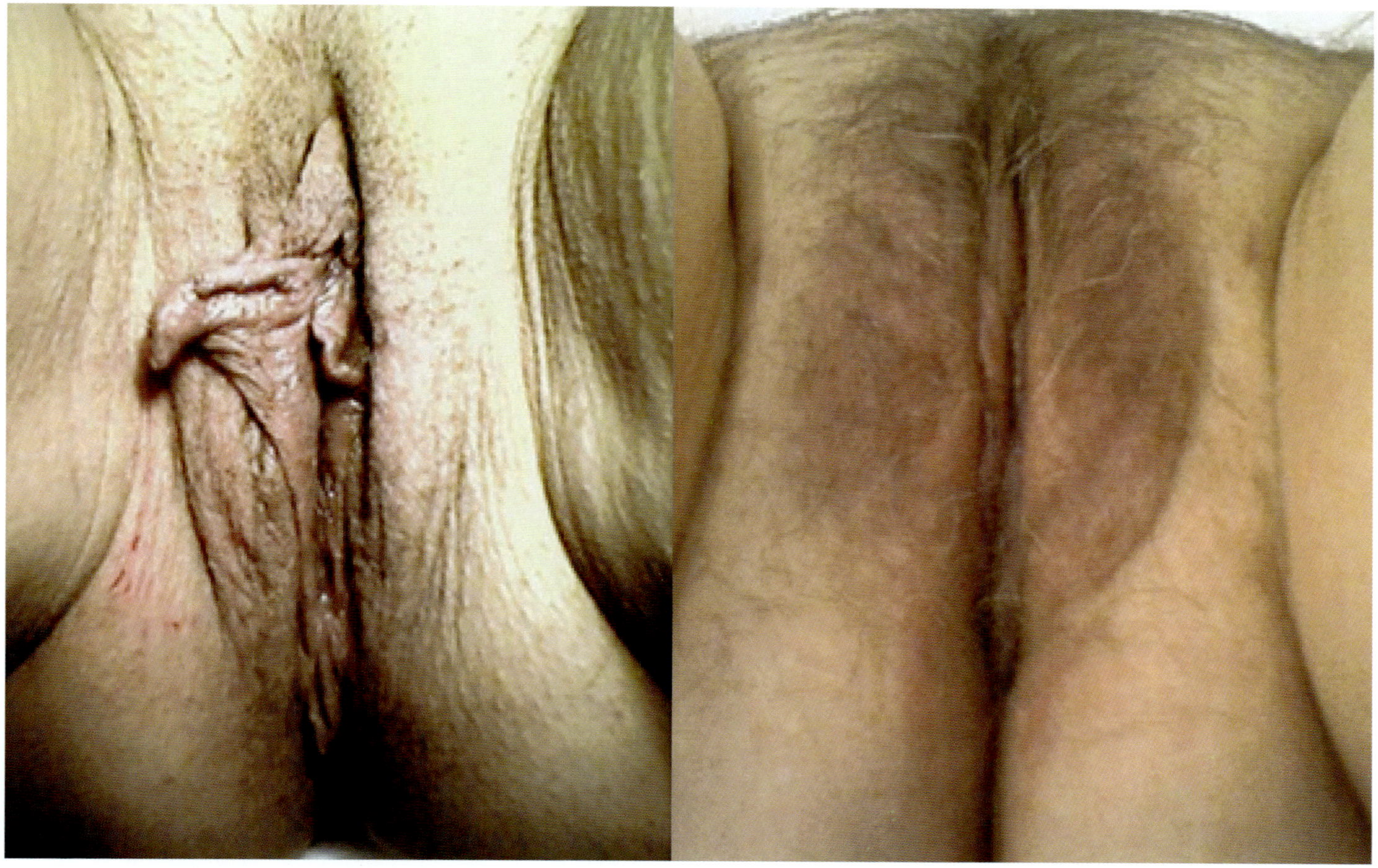

Courtesy of Dr. Aram Bonni, MD
www.beautybybrennan.com

PENILE ENLARGEMENT

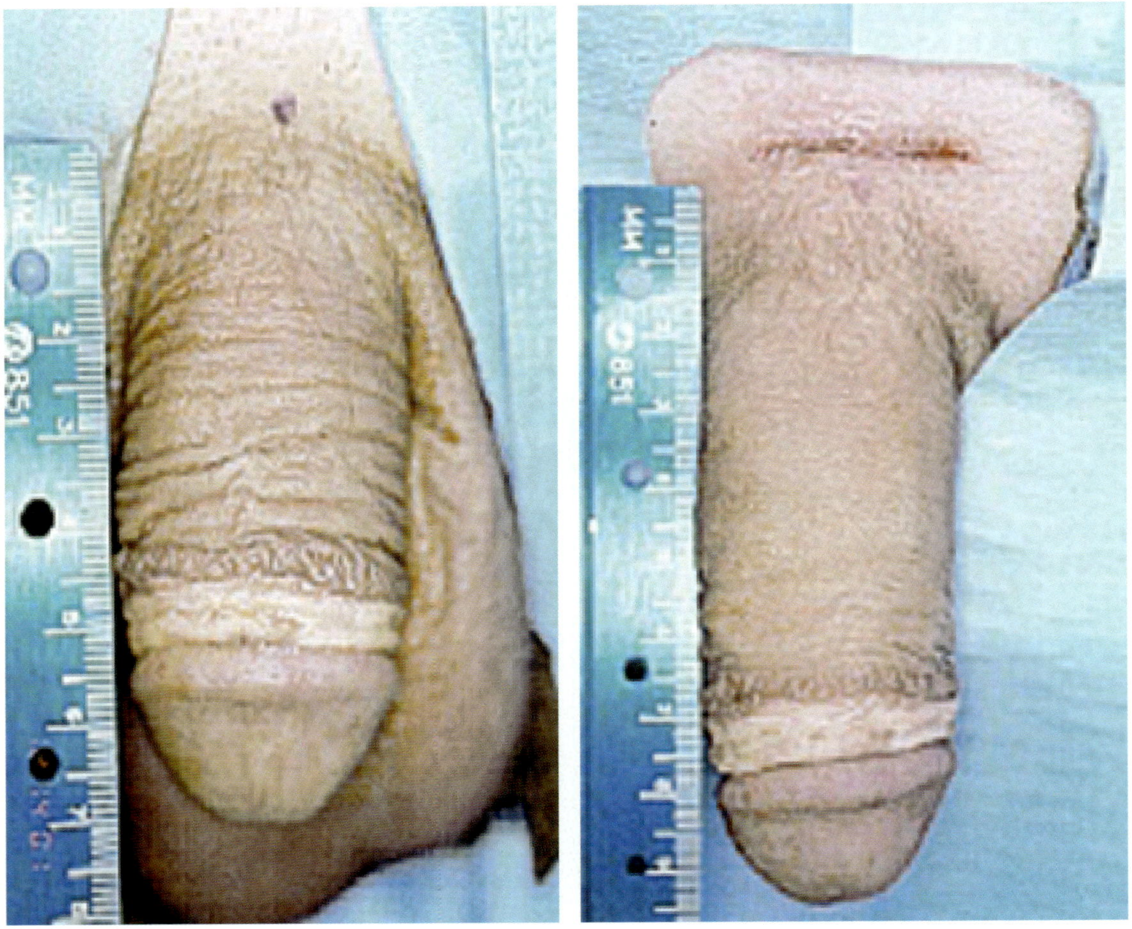

Courtesy of Dr. E. Douglas Whitehead, MD
www.drwhitehead.com

BUTTOCKS IMPLANT

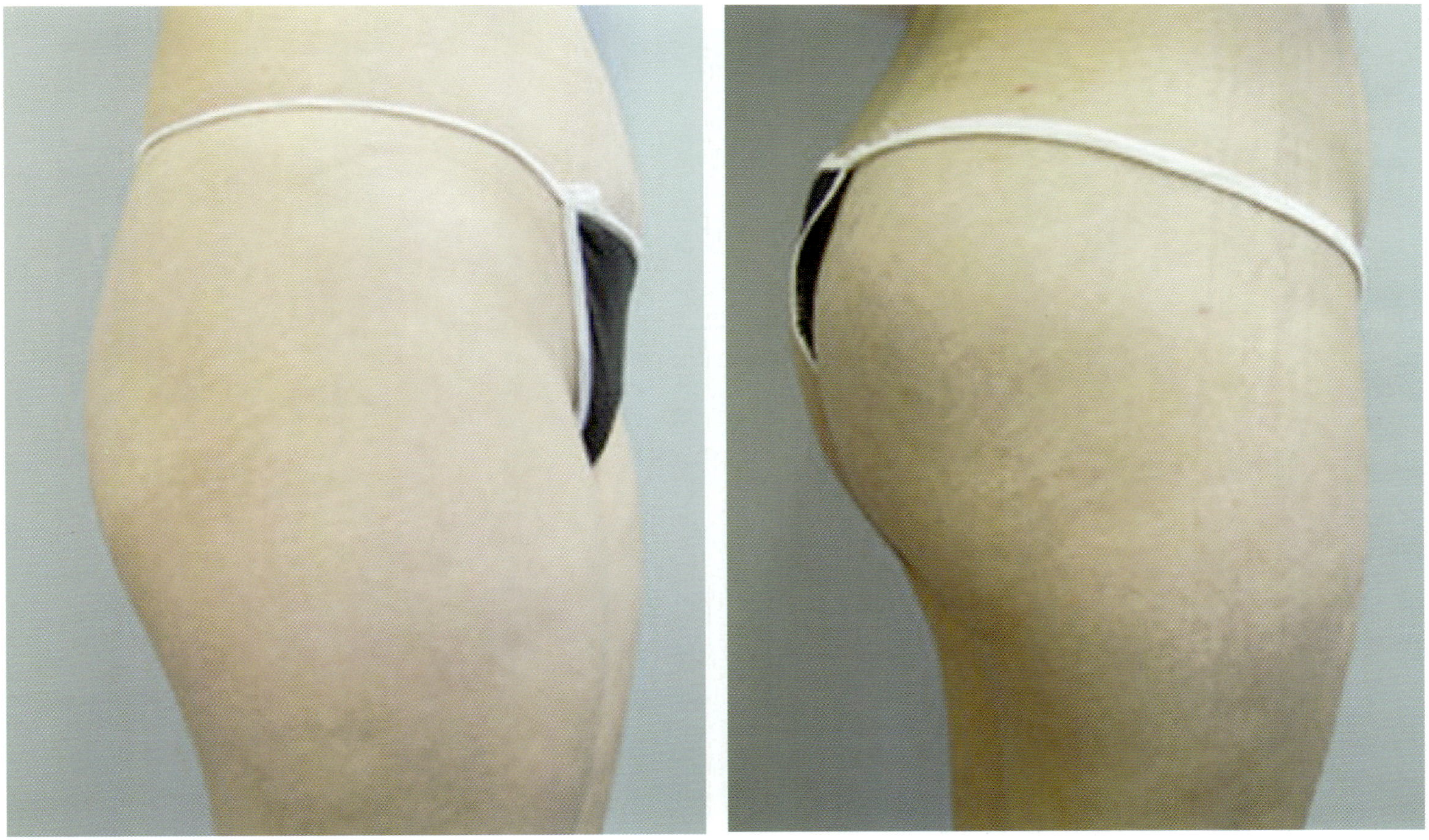

Courtesy of Dr. Nikolas V. Chugay, DO
www.bodyimplants.com

CALF IMPLANT

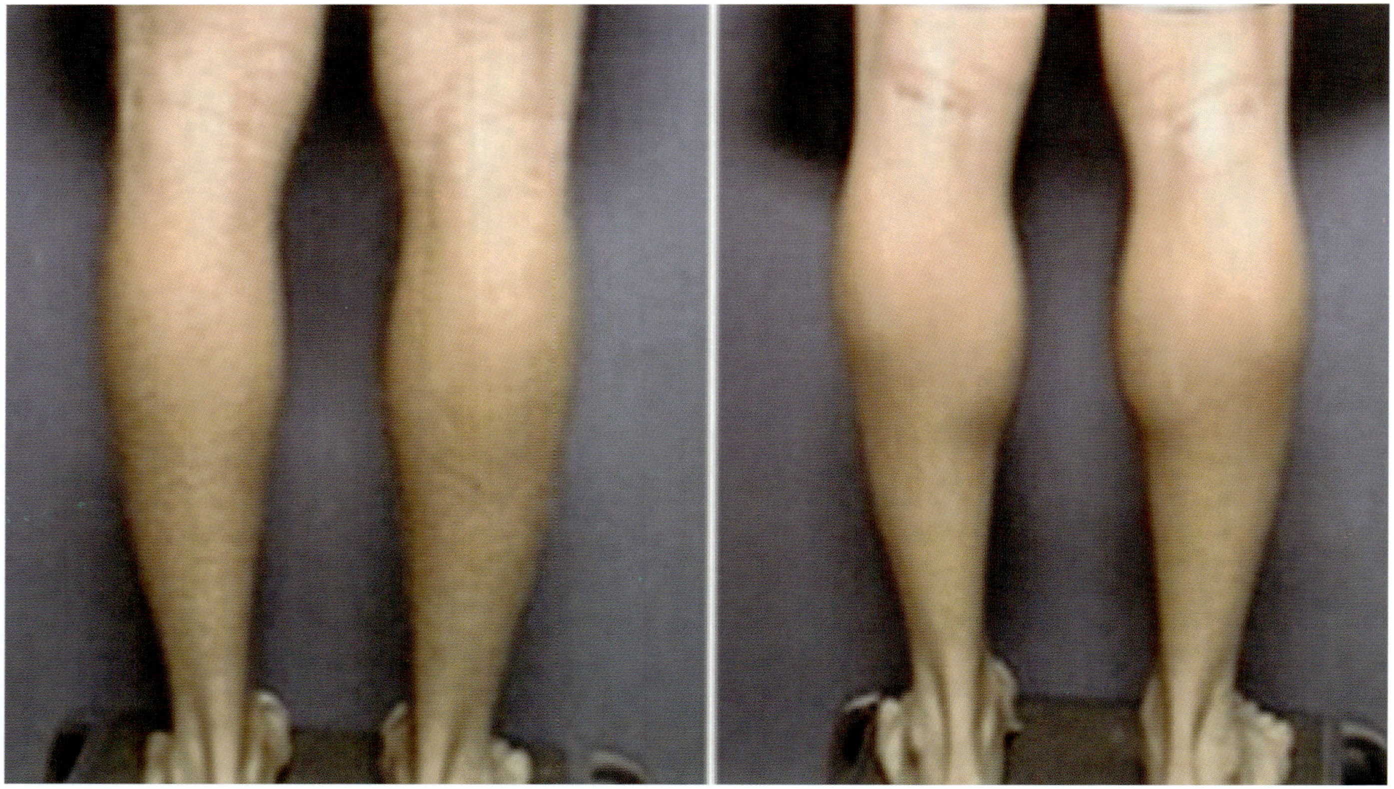

COSMETIC FOOT SURGERY

A variety of conditions are amendable to cosmetic foot surgery.

The most common conditions shown here are;

1. *Short Toe Syndrome*
2. *Bunions*
3. *Hammertoes*

SHORT TOE SYNDROME

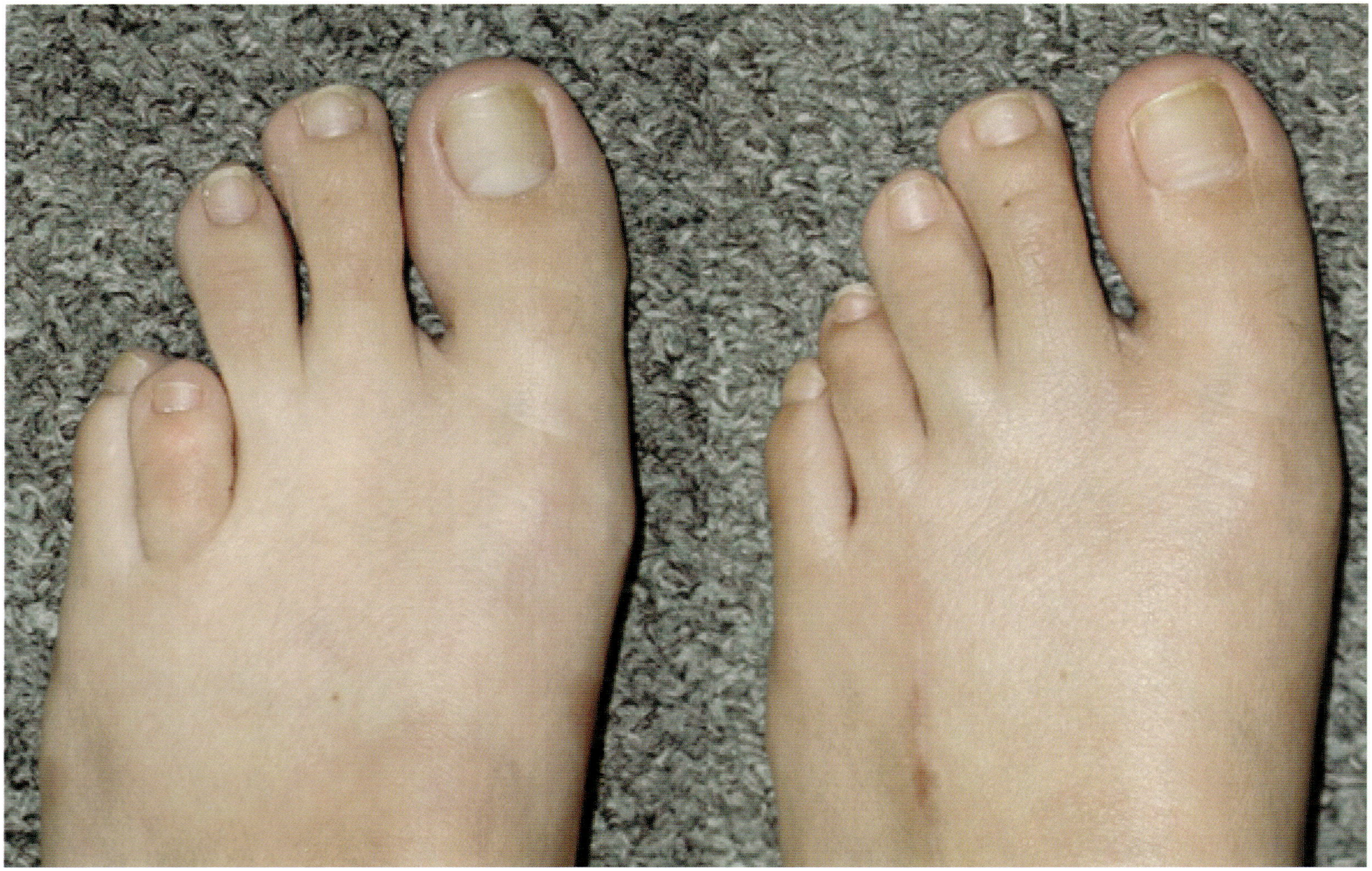

Courtesy of Dr. David Lee, DPM
www.arizonapodiatry.com

SHORT TOE SYNDROME

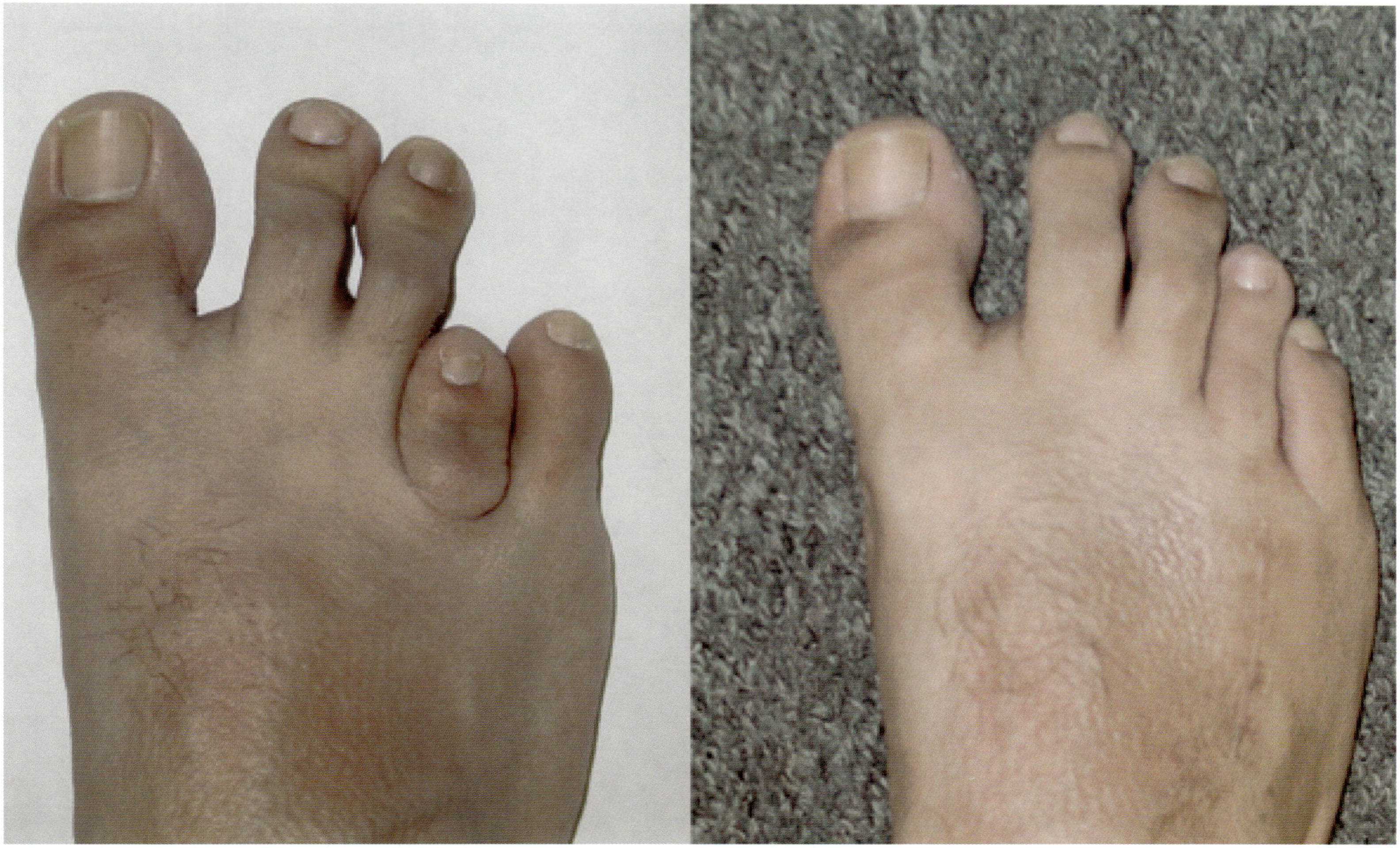

Courtesy of Dr. David Lee, DPM
www.arizonapodiatry.com

BUNION

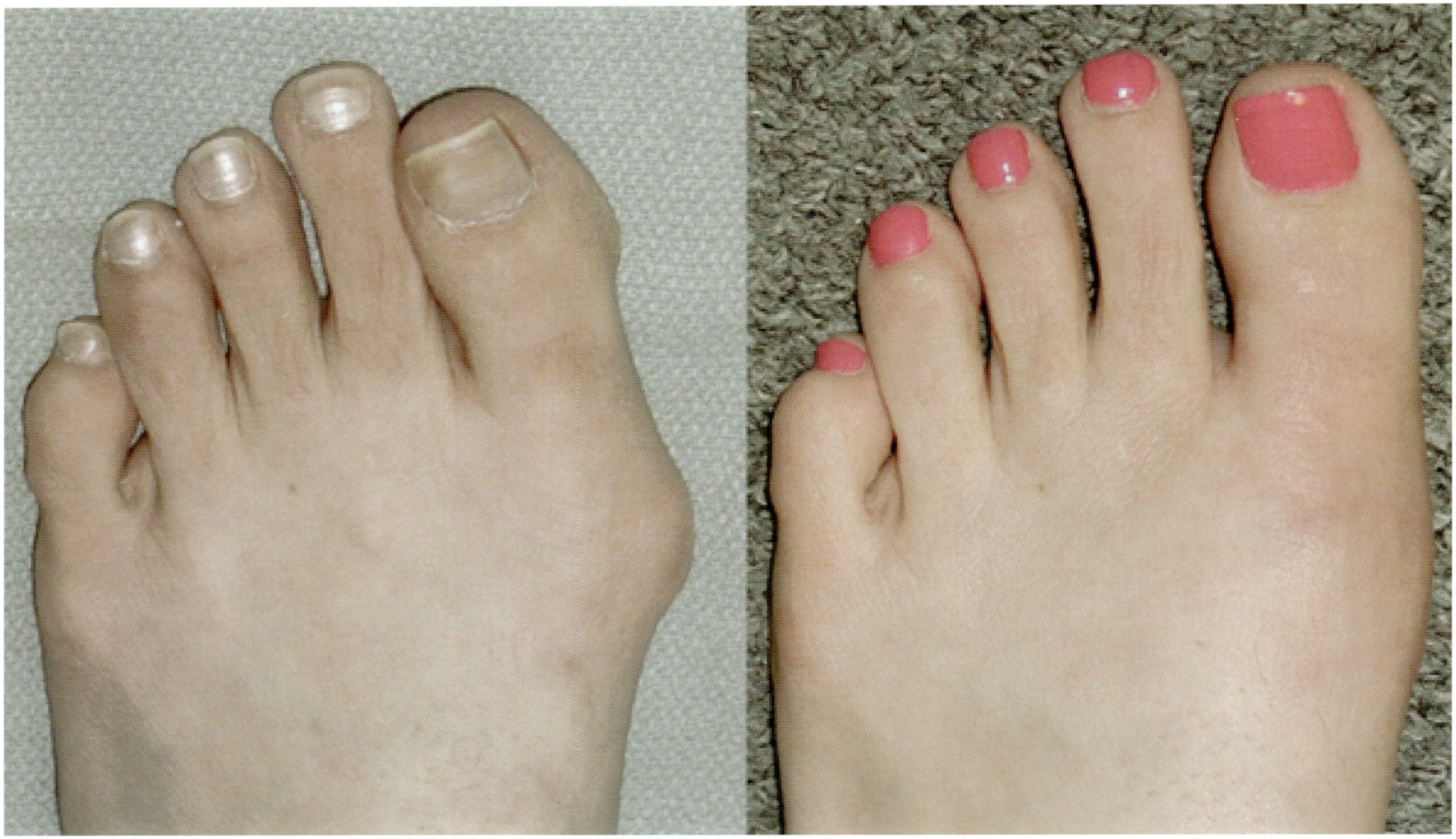

Courtesy of Dr. David Lee, DPM
www.arizonapodiatry.com

BUNION

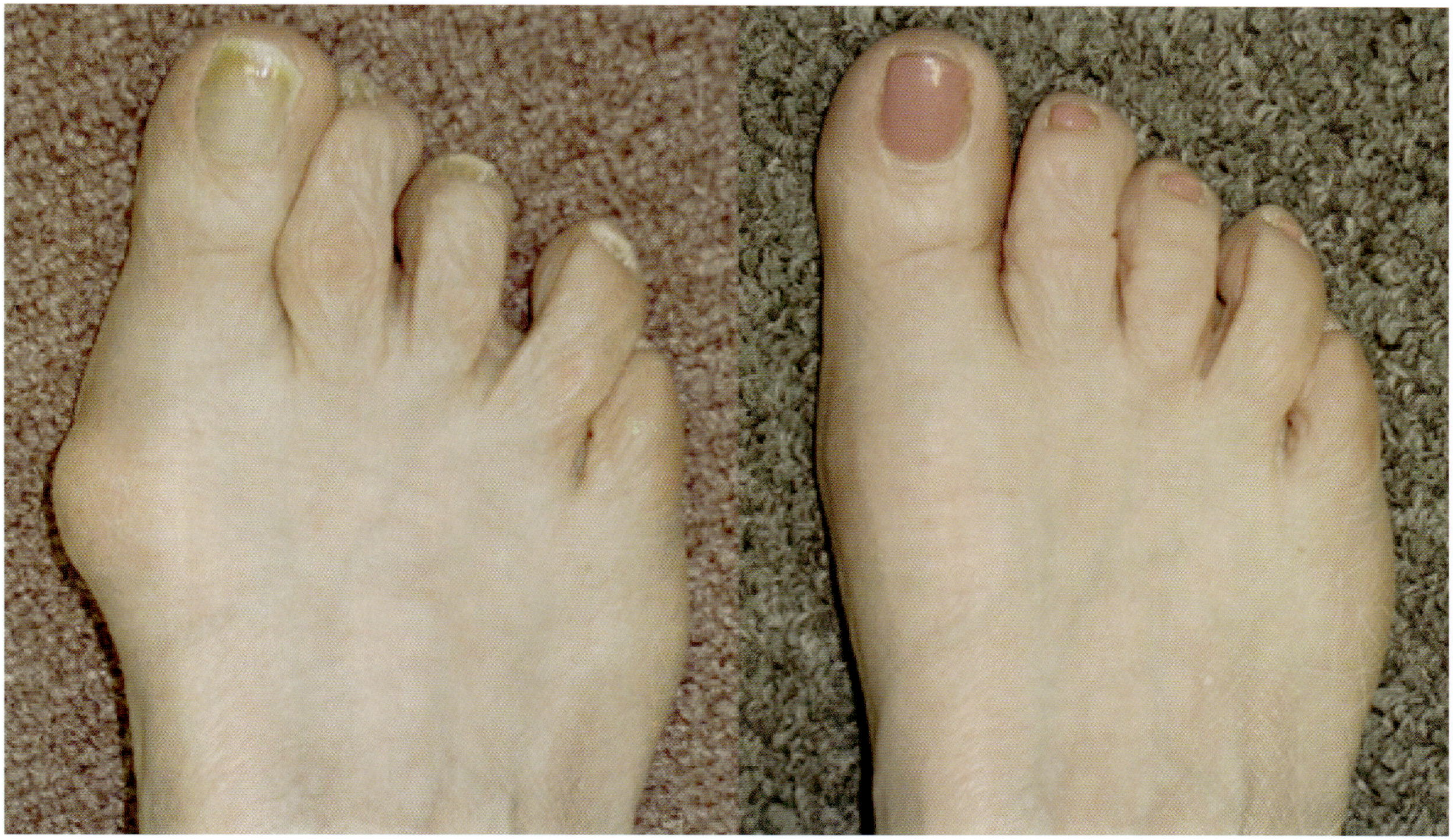

Courtesy of Dr. David Lee, DPM
www.arizonapodiatry.com

BUNION

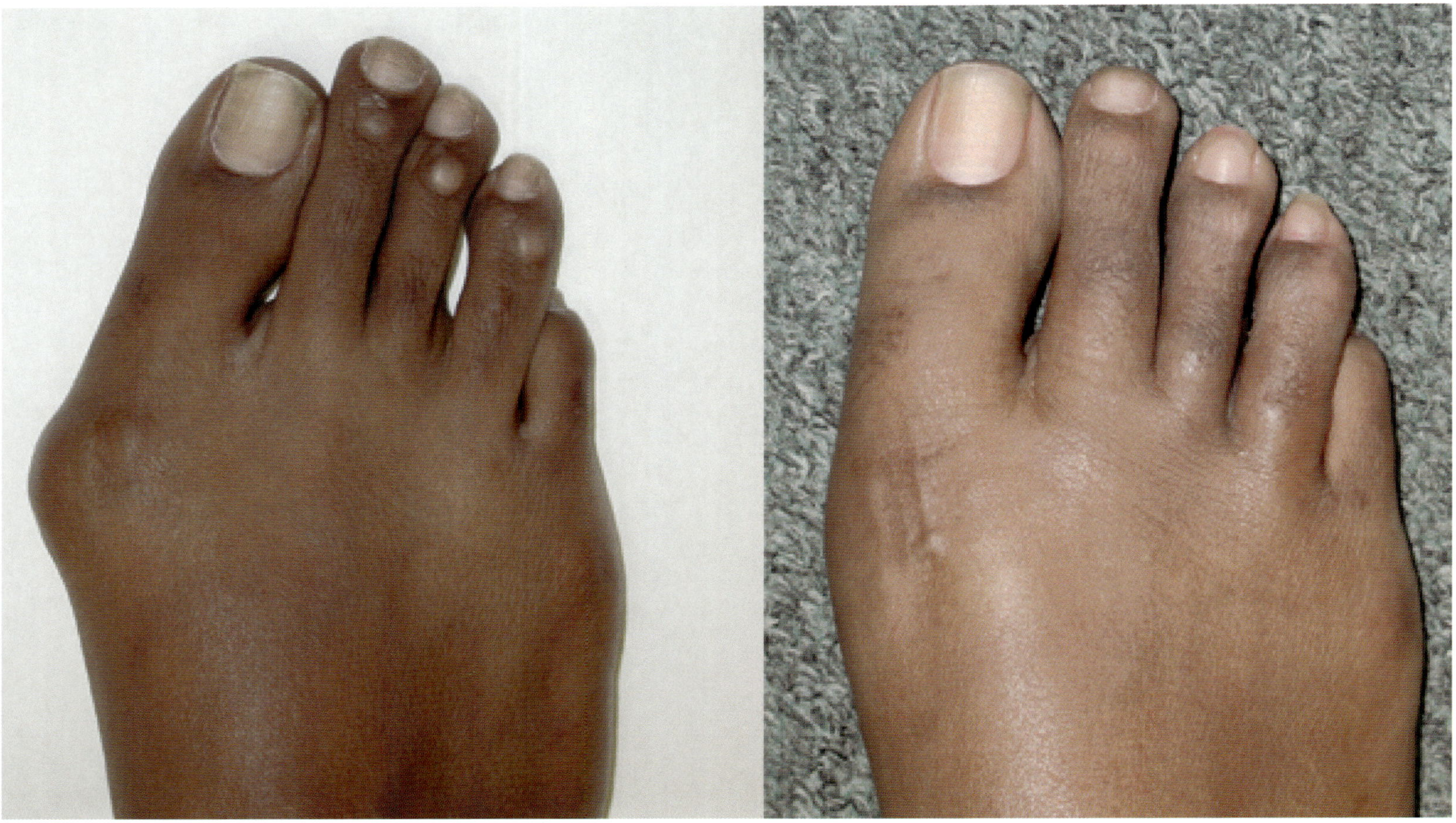

Courtesy of Dr. David Lee, DPM
www.arizonapodiatry.com

WEBBING SYNDROME

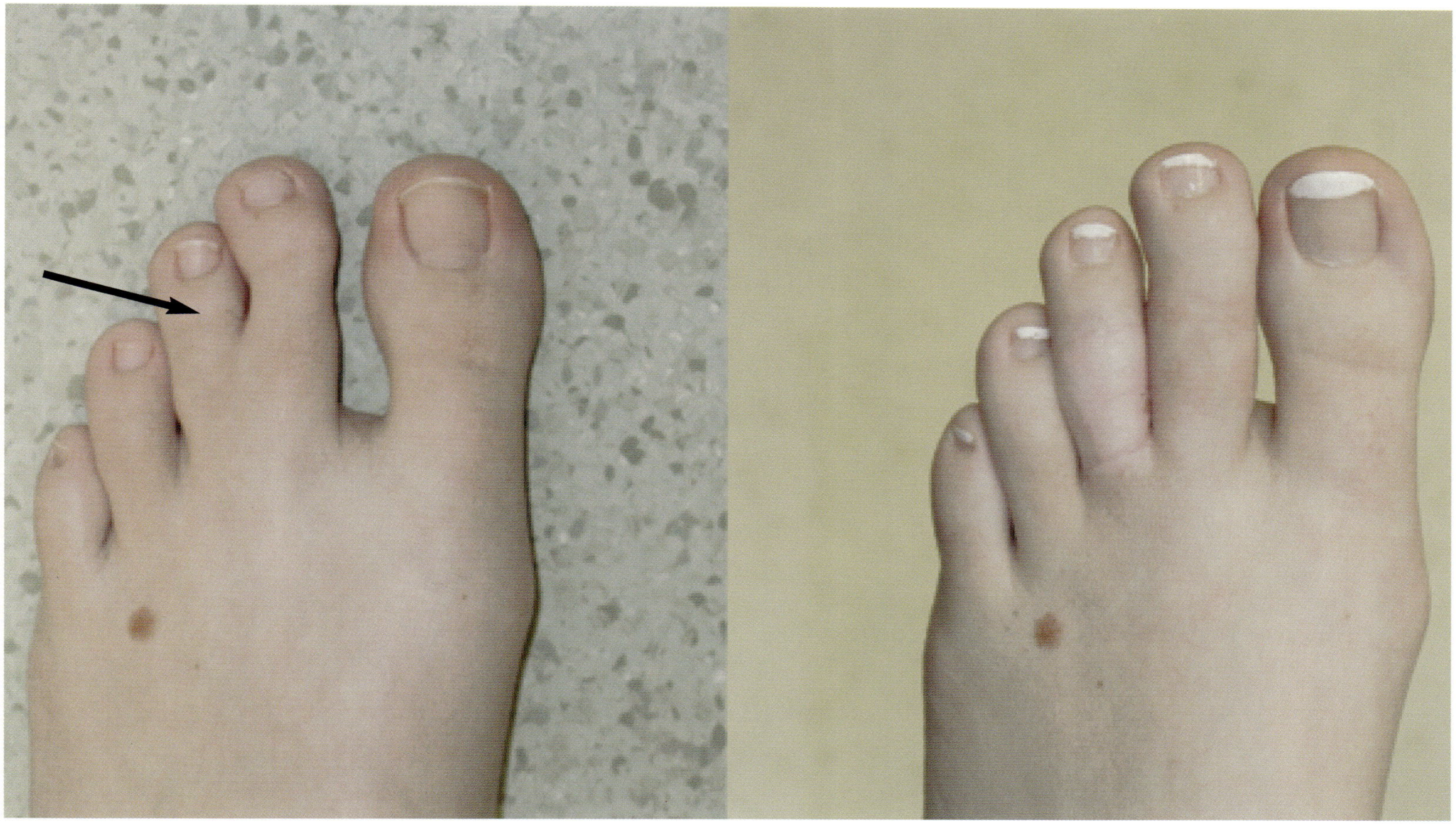

Courtesy of Dr. David Lee, DPM
www.arizonapodiatry.com

CURRENT STATISTICS REGARDING COSMETIC SURGERY
According to the American Society of Plastic Surgeons

ASPS Procedural Statistics represent procedures performed by ASPS Member Surgeons certified by The American Board of Plastic Surgery, Inc.® as well as other physicians certified by American Board of Medical Specialties-recognized boards. © ASPS, 2007

2006 Average Surgeon/Physician Fees

Cosmetic Procedures

Top Five Cosmetic Surgical Procedures:

	NATIONAL AVERAGE SURGEON/PHYSICIAN FEE	**TOTAL EXPENDITURE**
Breast augmentation (Augmentation Mammaplasty)	$3,600	$1,185,920,285
Nose reshaping (Rhinoplasty)	$3,841	$1,180,064,233
Liposuction	$2,750	$832,747,086
Eyelid surgery (Blepharoplasty)	$2,877	$670,978,018
Tummy tuck (Abdominoplasty)	$5,063	$740,343,243

Top Five Minimally-Invasive Cosmetic Procedures:

	NATIONAL AVERAGE SURGEON/PHYSICIAN FEE	**TOTAL EXPENDITURE**
Botox®**	$492	$2,011,283,275
Chemical peel	$686	$729,527,236
Laser hair removal	$466	$412,970,414
Microdermabrasion	$264	$215,959,054
Hyaluronic acid (Hylaform®, Hylaform Plus®, Restylane®)	$585	$455,217,308

COSMETIC SURGICAL PROCEDURES:

	NATIONAL AVERAGE SURGEON/PHYSICIAN FEE	TOTAL EXPENDITURE
Breast implant removals (Augmentation patients only)	$2,319	$63,669,776
Breast lift (Mastopexy)	$4,220	$437,952,317
Breast reduction in men (Gynecomastia)	$3,124	$62,108,293
Buttock implants	$4,409	$2,817,144
Buttock lift	$4,527	$16,796,076
Calf augmentation	$2,982	$1,499,811
Cheek implant (Malar augmentation)	$2,279	$20,060,863
Chin augmentation (Mentoplasty)	$1,910	$27,983,274
Dermabrasion	$951	$65,899,805
Ear surgery (Otoplasty)	$2,388	$71,967,156
Facelift (Rhytidectomy)	$4,856	$505,305,441
Forehead lift	$2,846	$149,483,588
Hair transplantation	$4,347	$121,137,729
Lip augmentation(other than injectable materials)	$1,603	$41,074,423
Lower body lift	$7,578	$8,229,506
Pectoral implants	$3,518	$1,438,998
Thigh lift	$4,376	$53,806,950
Thread lift	$2,443	$12,834,874
Upper arm lift	$3,513	$52,293,458
Vaginal rejuvenation	$2,229	$2,295,688

COSMETIC MINIMALLY-INVASIVE PROCEDURES:

	NATIONAL AVERAGE SURGEON/PHYSICIAN FEE	TOTAL EXPENDITURE
Cellulite treatment	$192	$6,453,888
Laser skin resurfacing	$2,160	$567,947,705
Laser treatment of leg veins	$400	$57,876,537
Sclerotherapy	$332	$201,446,347
Soft Tissue Fillers:		
(Radiesse™, formerly Radiance™)	$810	$63,899,055
Collagen	$390	$104,359,120
Fat	$1,380	$72,982,096
Polylactic acid (Sculptra™)	$1,042	$57,240,587

TOTAL 2006 EXPENDITURES $11,355,870,657

All figures are projected. Fees generally vary according to region of country and patient needs.
These fees are averages only. Fees do not include anesthesia, operating room facilities or other related expenses.

Email media@plasticsurgery.org and **Website** www.plasticsurgery.org

Arm Lift

Description: Procedure to restructure the upper arm by reducing skin and fatty deposits. Could be preformed in conjunction with liposuction.

Average Cost: 3,000.00 to 10,000.00

In/Out Patient: Outpatient

Anesthesia: General anesthesia or local with sedation.

Risks: Asymmetry, scar formation, infection, numbness, complications related to anesthesia.

Duration of Results: Permanent, if weight is stable. Aging could affect the results.

Breast lift

Description: Surgical procedure to raise and or reshape saggy breasts

Average cost: $4,000 to $10,000

In/out patient: Either

Anesthesia: General or local with IV sedation

Body lift

Description: A surgical procedure performed to reshape the lower torso and upper legs, the stomach, hips, back, thighs and buttocks. Sometimes more than one surgery is necessary for desired results.

Average cost: $15,000 – $35,000

In/out patient: Inpatient

Anesthesia: General

Breast enlargement

Description: Placement of silicone or saline filled implant to increase breast size, improve appearance of asymmetrical breast and to replace volume after weight loss or childbirth.

Average cost: $3,500 – $10,000

In/out patient: Out-patient.

Anesthesia: General or local with IV sedation.

Longevity of results: Very long lasting. Gravity, age, weight gain and/or loss may affect breast shape and size.

Breast reduction

Description: Removal of fat, fatty tissue and skin to decrease breast size, make them lighter and firmer.

Average cost: $4,000 to $15,000

In/out patient: An overnight stay at an accredited surgical facility may be recommended.

Anesthesia: General

Longevity of results: Permanent. Gravity, age, weight gain and/or loss may affect breast shape and size.

Liposuction

Description: Body sculpting through removal of fat from areas of the body. Variations of techniques include tumescent, ultrasound-assisted and power assisted lipoplasty.

Average cost: $1,500 – $5,000 per area

In/out patient: Out-patient or depending on the amount of surgery and health status of patient.

Anesthesia: Local, local with intravenous sedation or general.

Longevity of results: Results will remain if proper diet and exercise program is maintained.

Thigh lift

Description: Surgery to reshape the thighs by removing excess skin and fat.

Average cost: $6,000 – $20,000

In/out patient: Either

Anesthesia: General

Longevity of results: Permanent but aging, weight gain or loss may affect the desired results.

Tummy tucks

Description: Flattening of the abdomen by removal of excess skin and/or fat – can be done both non-invasively or invasively while tightening the muscles.

Average cost: $4,000 to $15,000

In/out patient: Extent of surgery can determine as well as the surgeons preference.

Anesthesia: General

Longevity of results: Permanent but weight loss, gain or pregnancy can affect desired results.

Buttock implants

Description: Solid silicone implants are placed under, over or inside the buttock muscles to add volume.

Average cost: $6,000 to $12,000

In/out patient: Outpatient

Anesthesia: General

Recovery time: Usually prone positioned for a required amount of days can return to work within 2 weeks. Return to normal activity 6 weeks.

Longevity of results: Permanent, weight gain or loss and aging can affect desired results.

Eyelid surgery

Description: Removal of fat and excess skin from the upper and/or eyelids.

Average cost: $1,500 to $3,000 for each upper & lower eyelids.

In/out patient: Out

Anesthesia: Local with sedation or general.

Longevity of results: Can last up to 10 years, may be affected by lifestyle, such as sun damage and heredity.

Brow lift/forehead lift

Description: Procedure to improve the appearance to the upper third of the face, including the forehead and brow region.

Average cost: $3,500 to $8,000

In/out patient: Out

Anesthesia: Local with sedation or general

Longevity of results: can be long lasting, aging can eventually affect the results.

Face-lift

Description: Repositioning and/or tightening facial muscles and tissue.

Average cost: $4,000 – $25,000

In/out patient: Either

Anesthesia: Local with sedation of general.

Longevity or results: Usually an 8-10 year improvement of overall appearance. Effects of aging, lifestyle and gravity continue to affect results.

Facial implants (chin, midfacial (cheek) & jaw)

Description: Chin, jaw or midfacial implants are designed to improve facial contours.

Average cost: \$2,000 – \$6,000 (each implant may have separate cost)

In/out patient: Out

Recovery time: Return to work within one week. Resume strenuous exercise 3 to 4 weeks.

Longevity of results: Permanent

Lip augmentation

Description: Surgical procedure to create fuller, plumper lips and reduce fine lines around mouth.

Average cost: \$2,000

In/out patient: Out

Anesthesia: Local

Longevity of results: Permanent

Neck lift

Description: Surgical procedure to tighten the sagging neck muscles, remove any excess or hanging skin and fat.

Average cost: $3,500 – $10,000

In/out patient: Out

Anesthesia: General or local with sedation.

Longevity of results: Long lasting. Aging, weight fluctuation and gravity can affect results over time.

Nose reshaping

Description: Surgery to reshape the nose, nostrils or tip by changing its size and/or proportions.

Average cost: $3,500 to $14,000

In/out patient: Out

Longevity of results: Permanent. Aging may affect results.

Hair restoration surgery

Description: Surgical procedure where hair is removed from a donor site and transplanted into thinning or balding area of the scalp.

Average cost: $3-$10 per individual graft / $2,500 to $10,000 per complete series of treatments.
In/out patient: Out

Anesthesia: Local or general – depending on technique chosen.

Longevity of results: Permanent

Teeth bonding

Description: The enamel of the tooth or teeth is etched to enhance the adhesion of a color match resin compound to correct a crooked, chipped, short or broken tooth. Light is used to harden and bond it to the tooth underneath.

Average cost: $500 - $2,000

Anesthesia: None

Longevity of results: Usually five to eight years.

Crowns

Description: Caps & crowns can be used in place of veneers to make a crooked smile look straighter, to repair broken or damaged teeth or to cover a bridge or implant. The surface of the tooth is reduced then covered with a cap in porcelain, porcelain bonded to metal or other durable material.

Average cost: $1,000 – $4,000 per crown.

Anesthesia: Local – sedation may be offered.

Longevity of results: 5 - 15 years.

Bleaching

Description: Teeth whitening by a professional can be significantly more effective than over the counter home remedies. A dentist can polish away superficial stains, applies a bleaching solution.

Average cost: In office – 500.00 to 1,500.00 – follow up at home 200.00 to 600.00

Longevity of results: Lifestyle and habits can reduce results of bleaching.

Invisalign

Description: Straightening the teeth almost invisibly with a series of 18 to 30 thin, clear removable plastic aligners worn for a period of months.

Average cost: $5,000 and up.

Anesthesia: None

Longevity of results: Comparable to traditional braces.

Public Faces - Reality

Cosmetic Surgery is very popular among all strata of society including people who are in the public eye.

At times the results are very satisfactory and sometimes the results are less than desirable.

Following is a collection of recognizable faces who have had a variety of cosmetic surgery.

You be the judge…

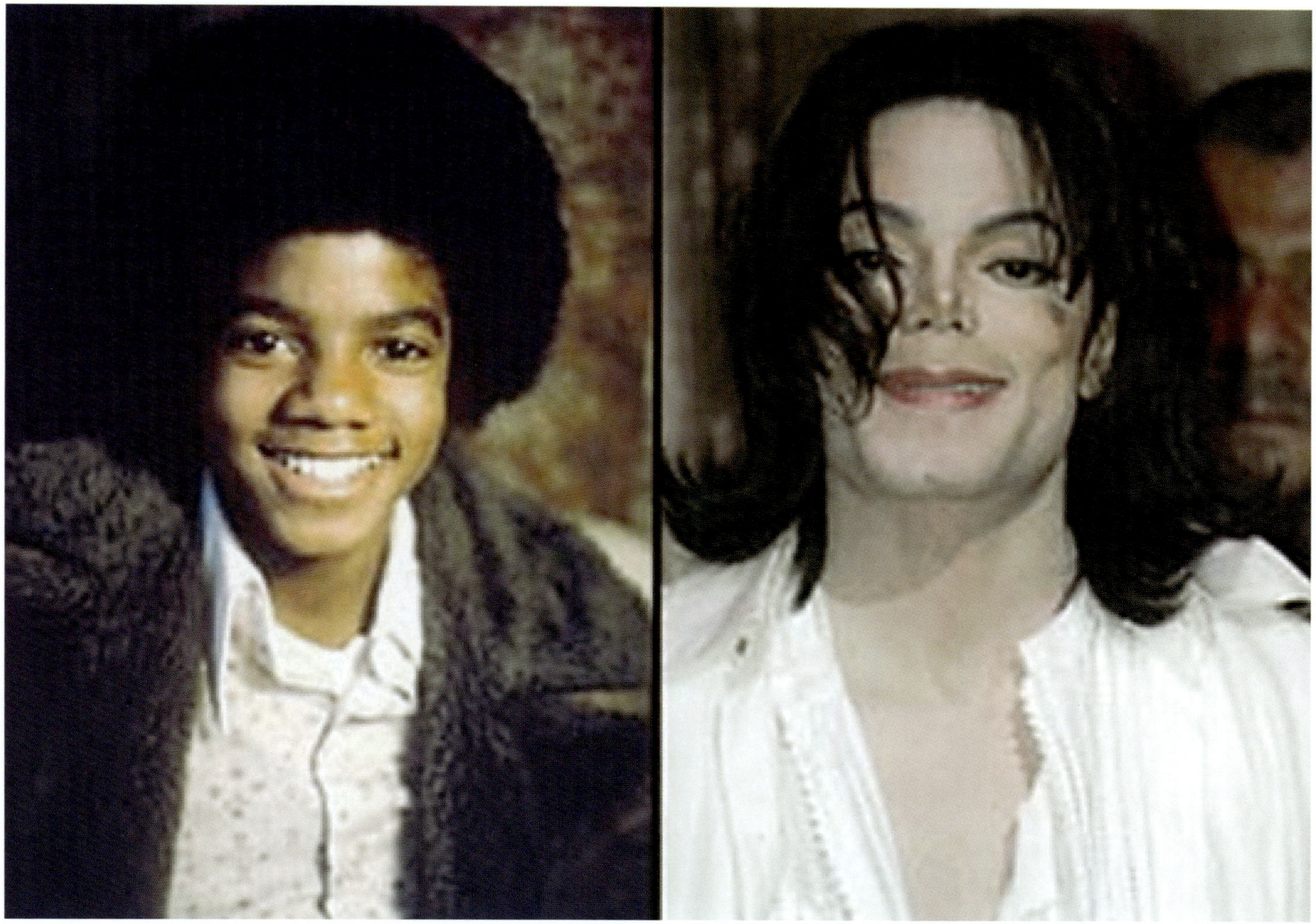

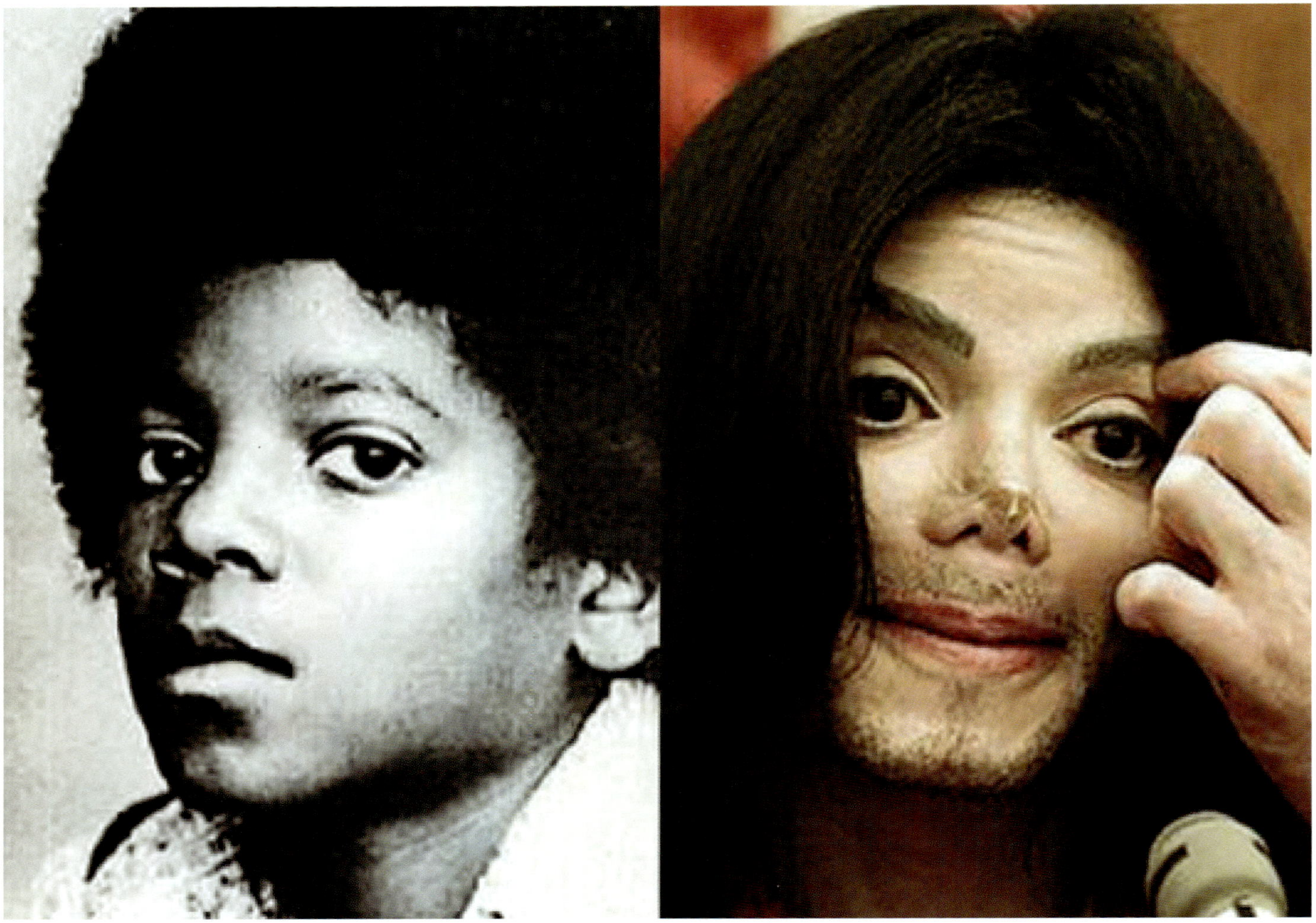

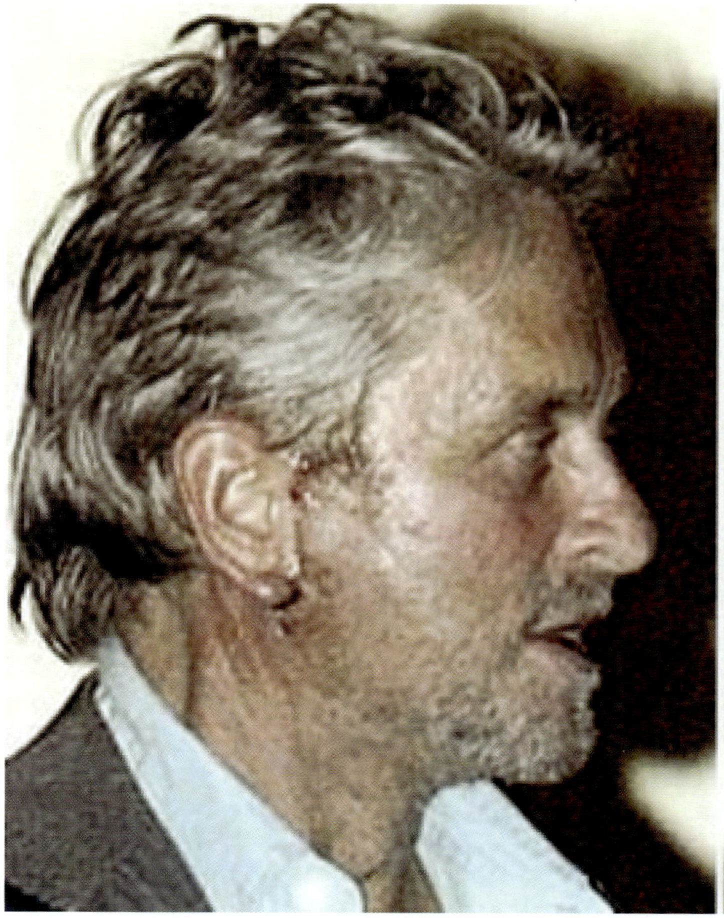

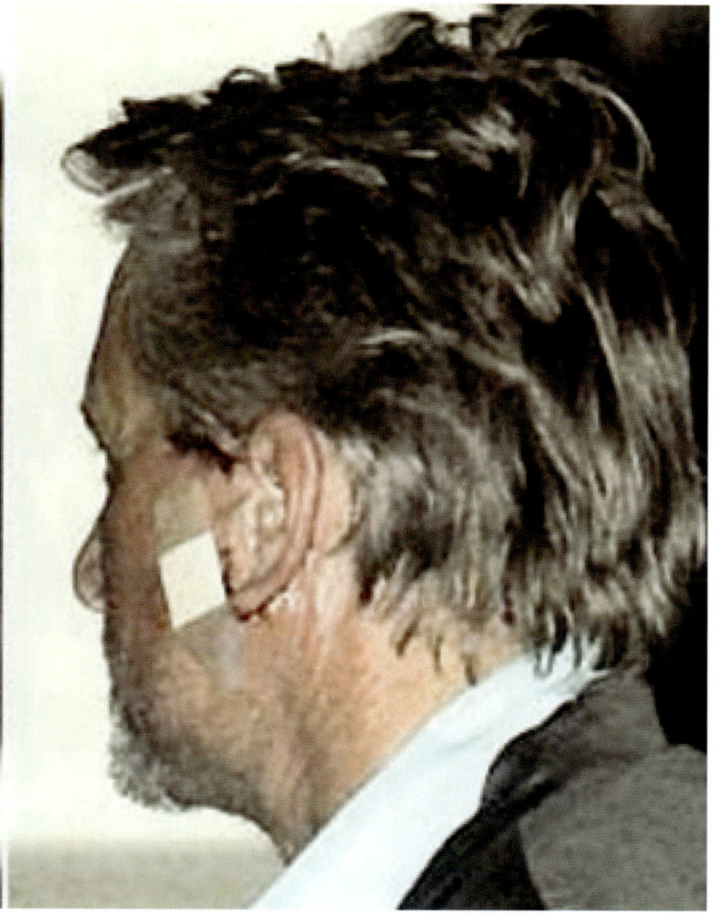

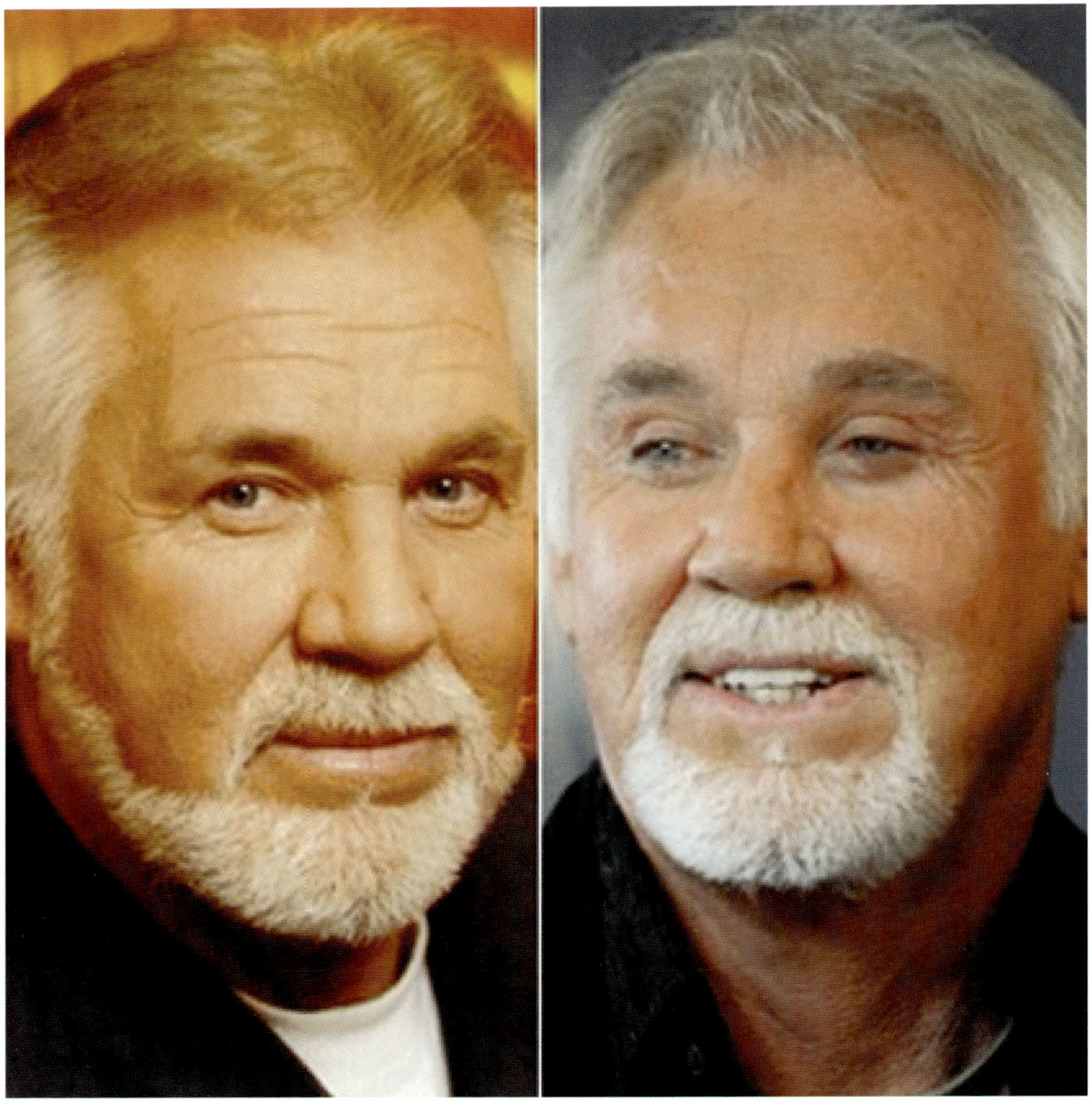

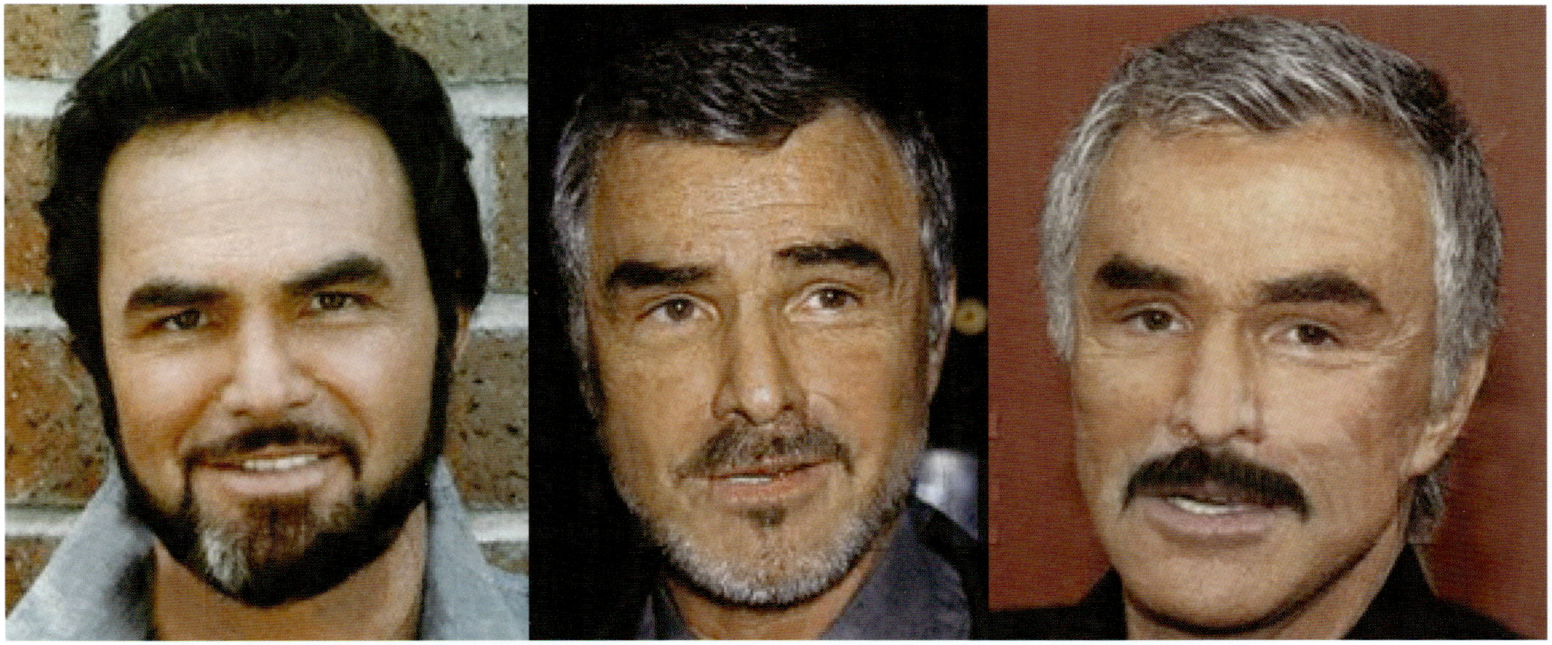

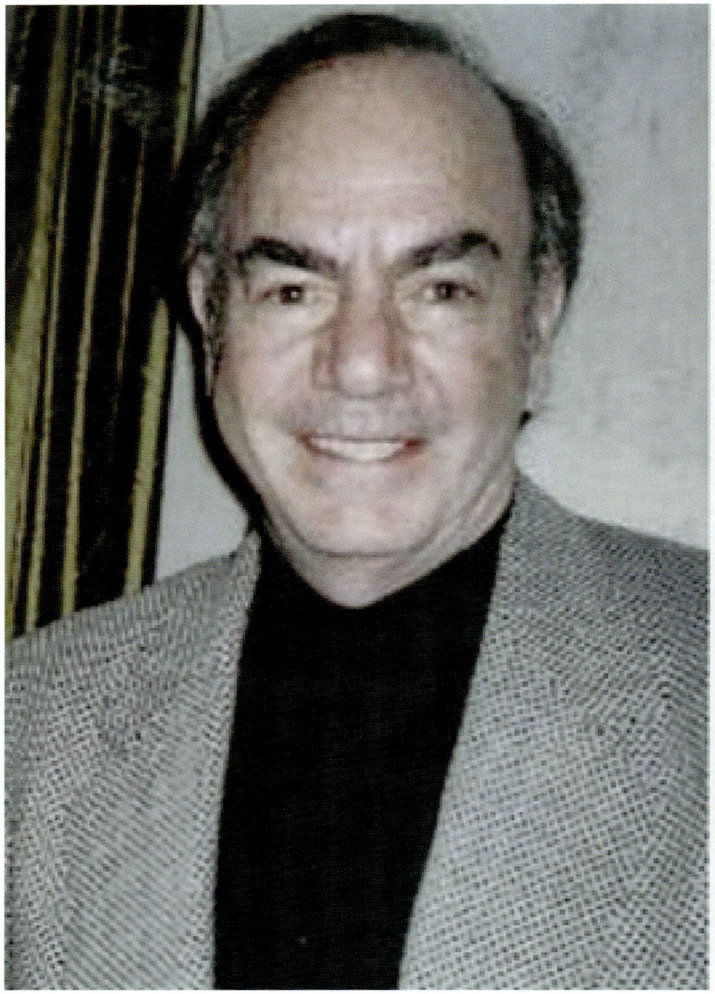

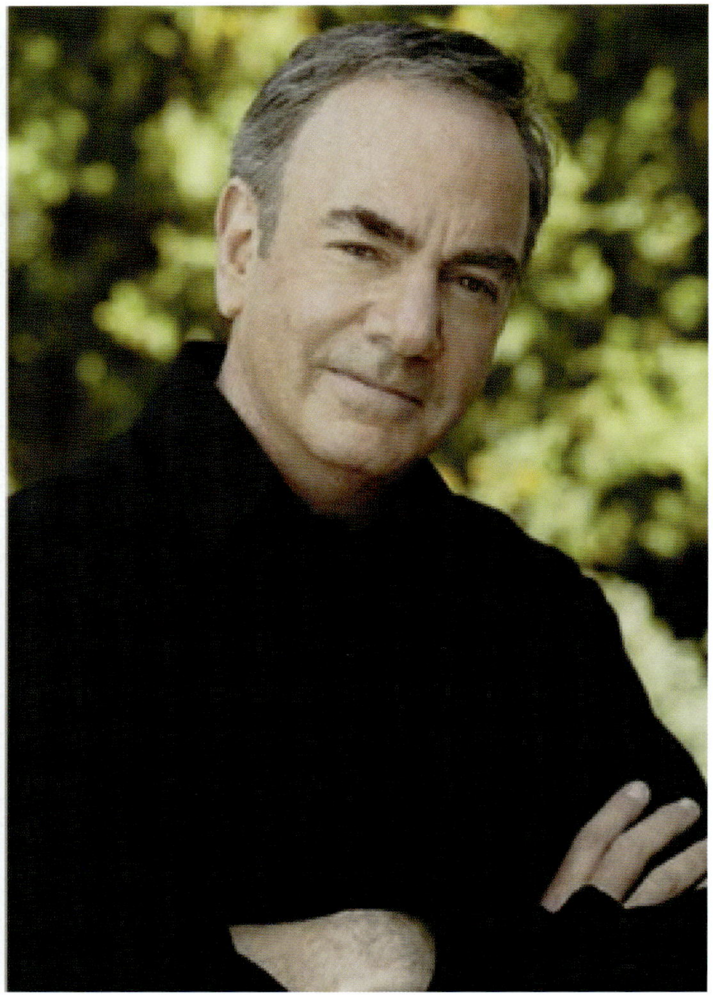

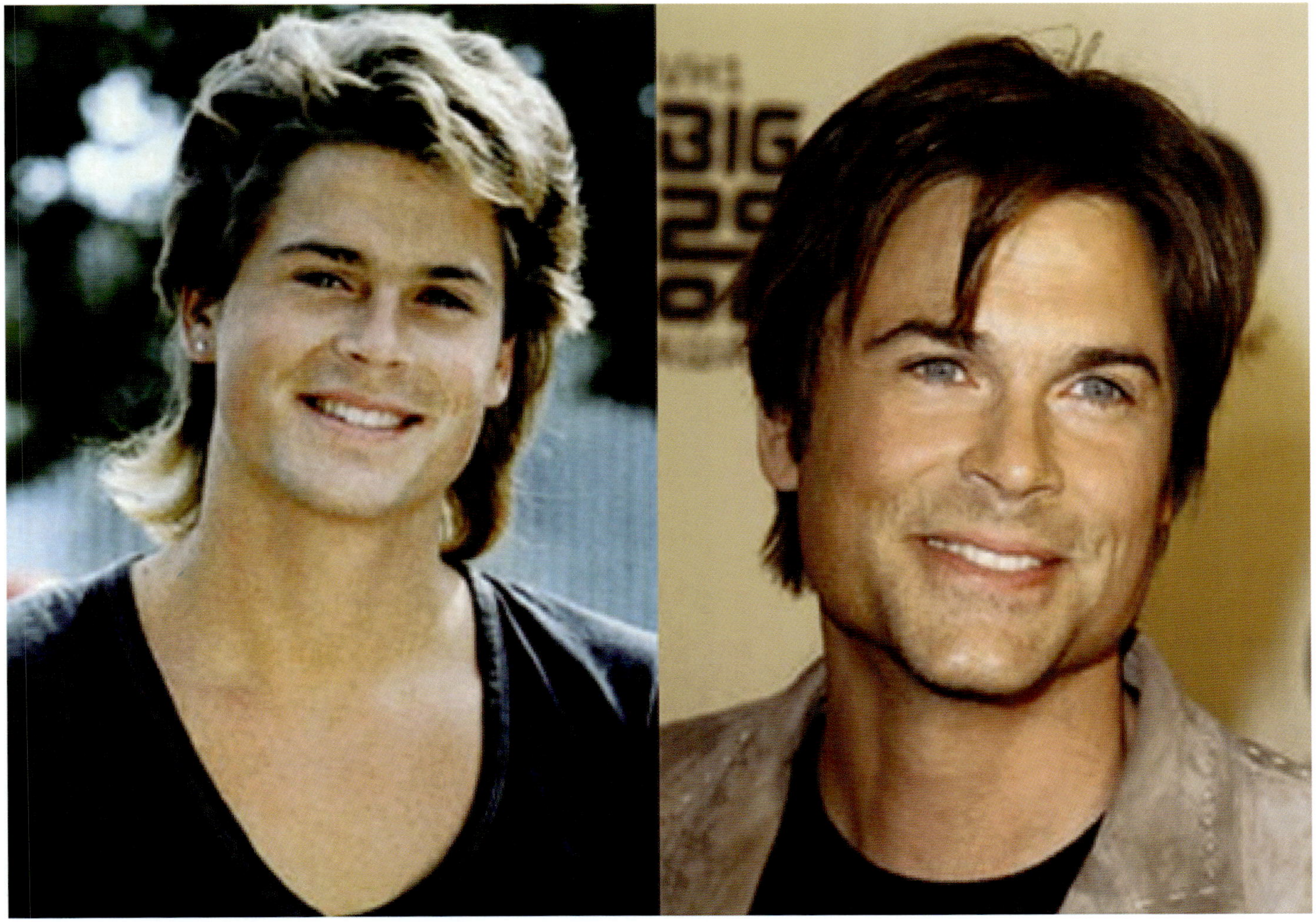

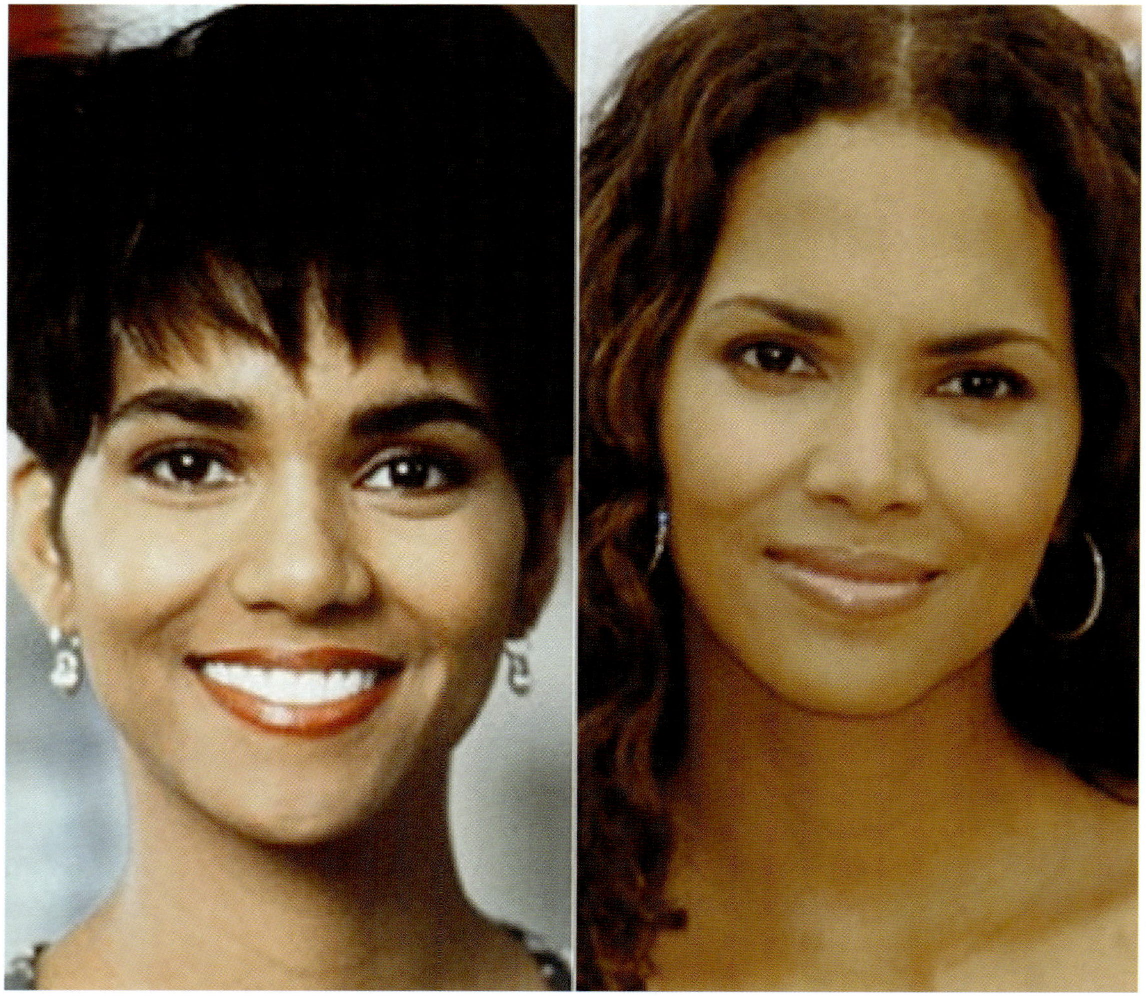

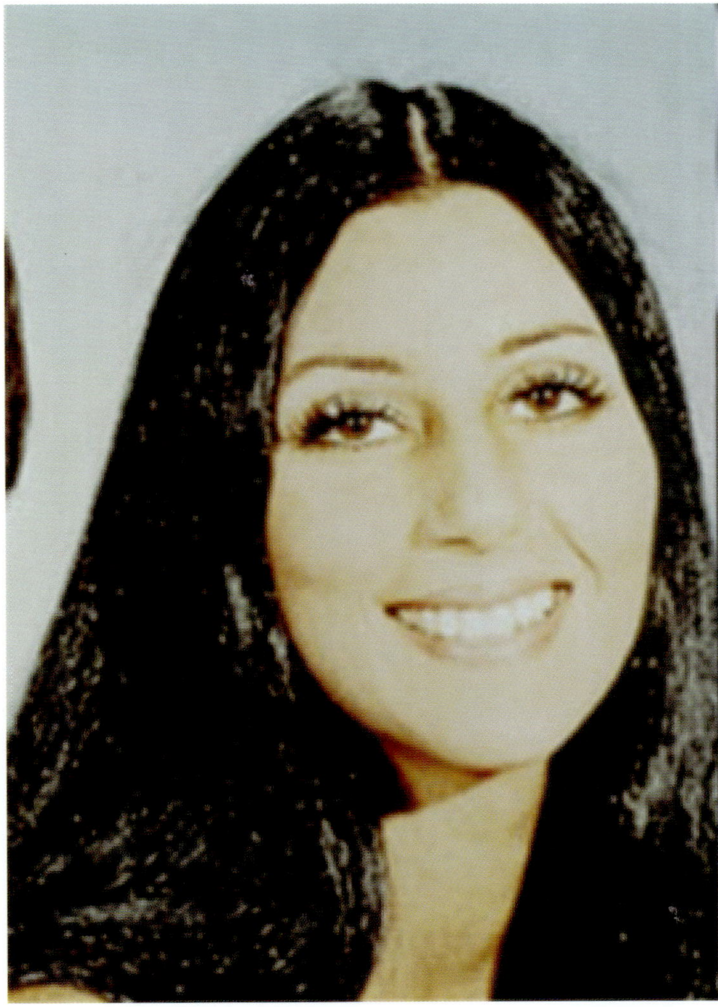
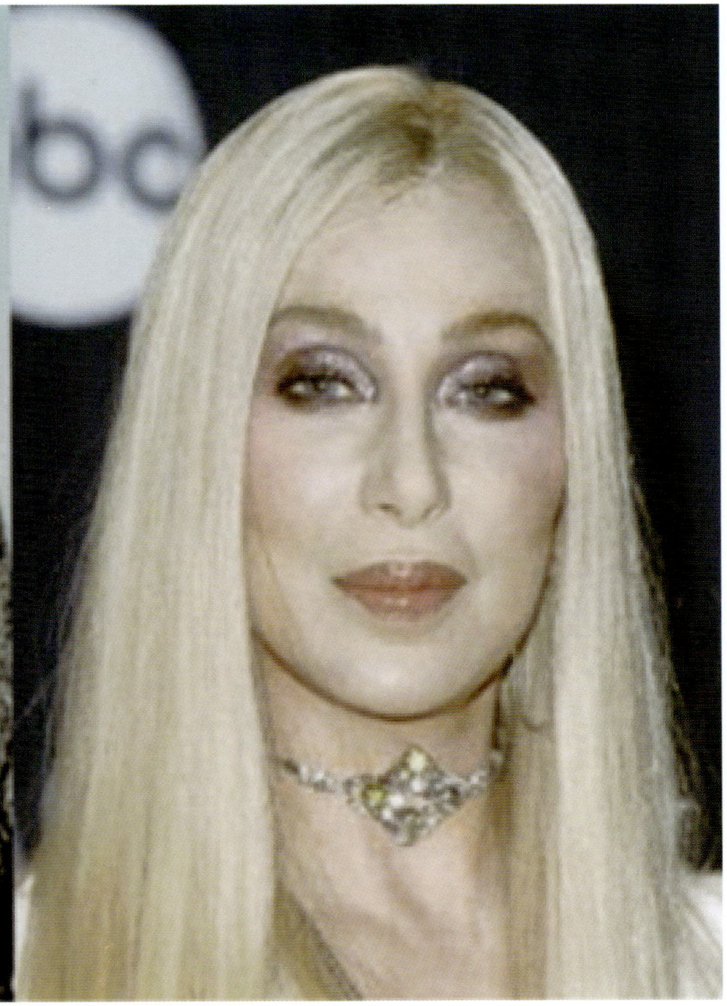

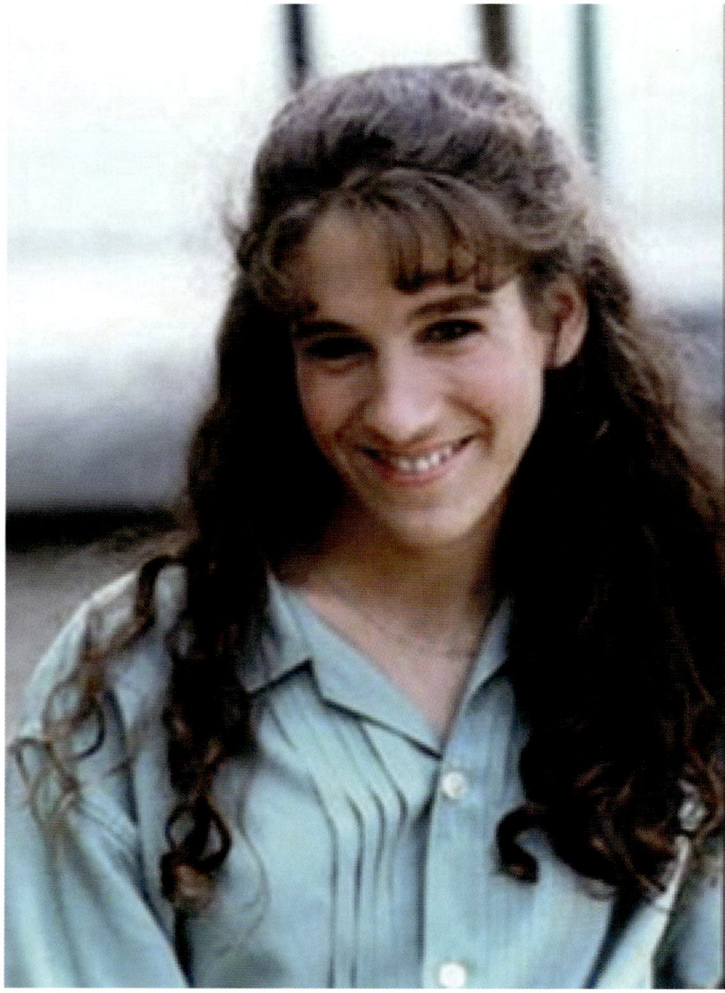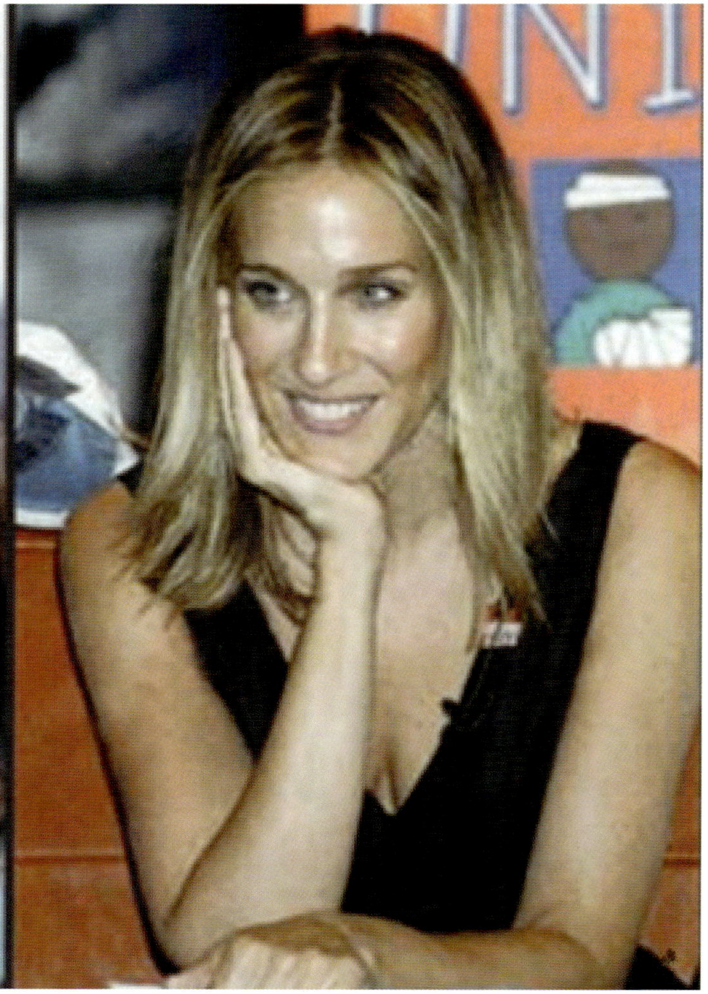

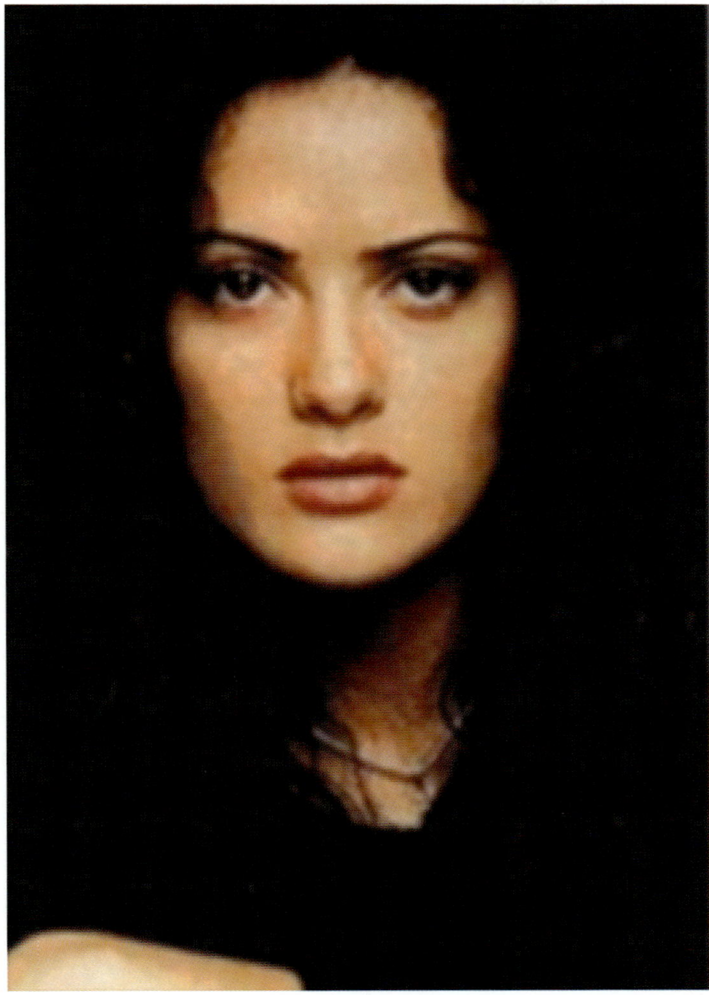

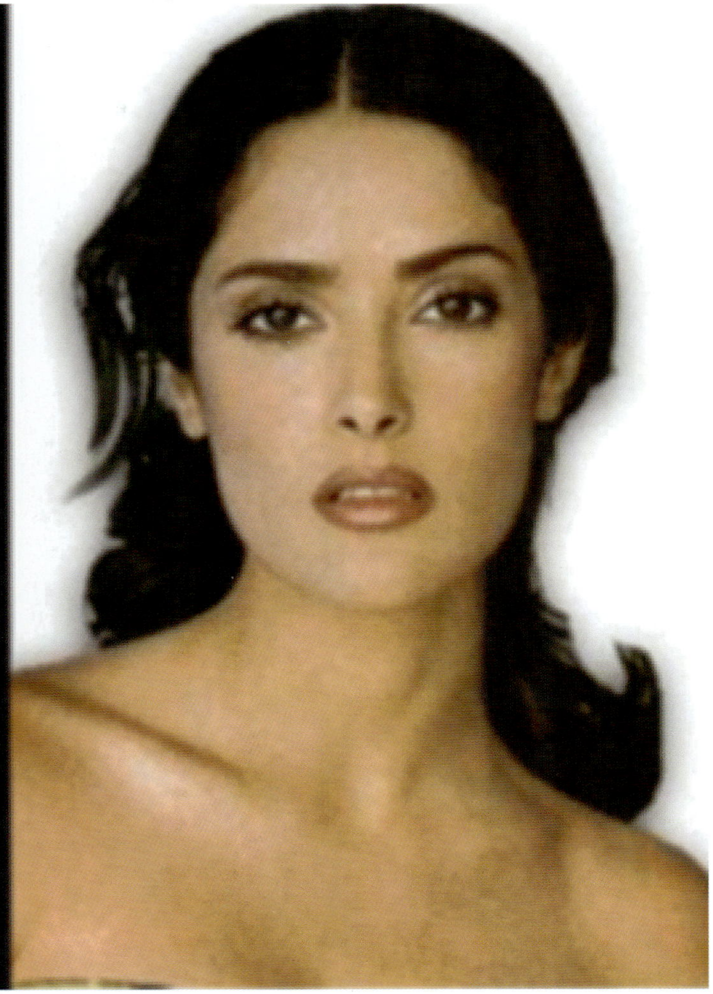

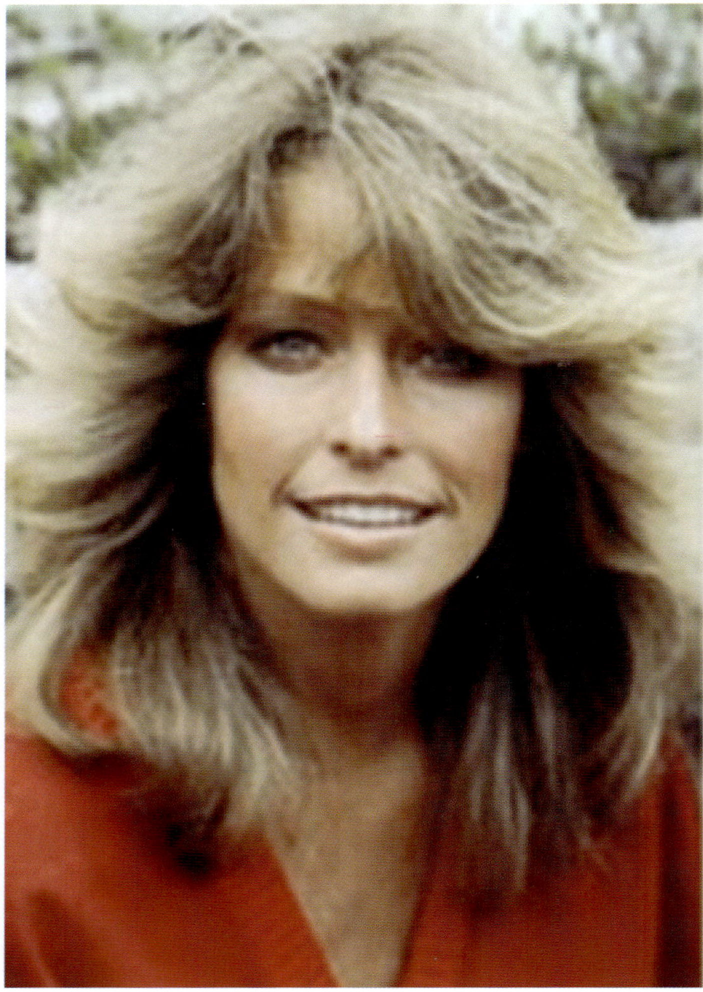 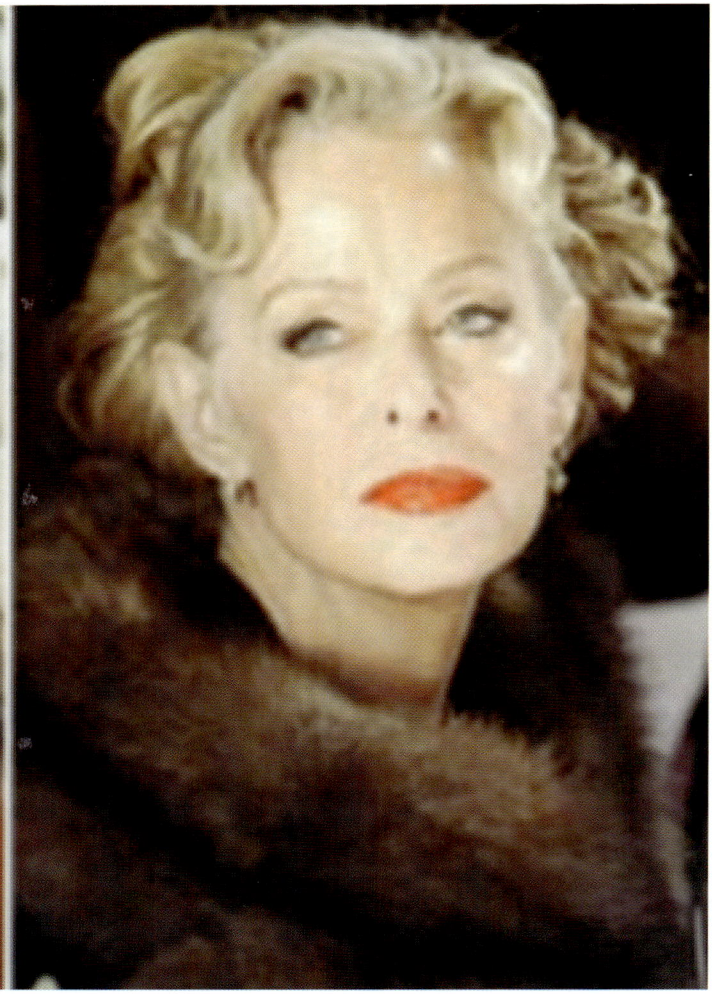

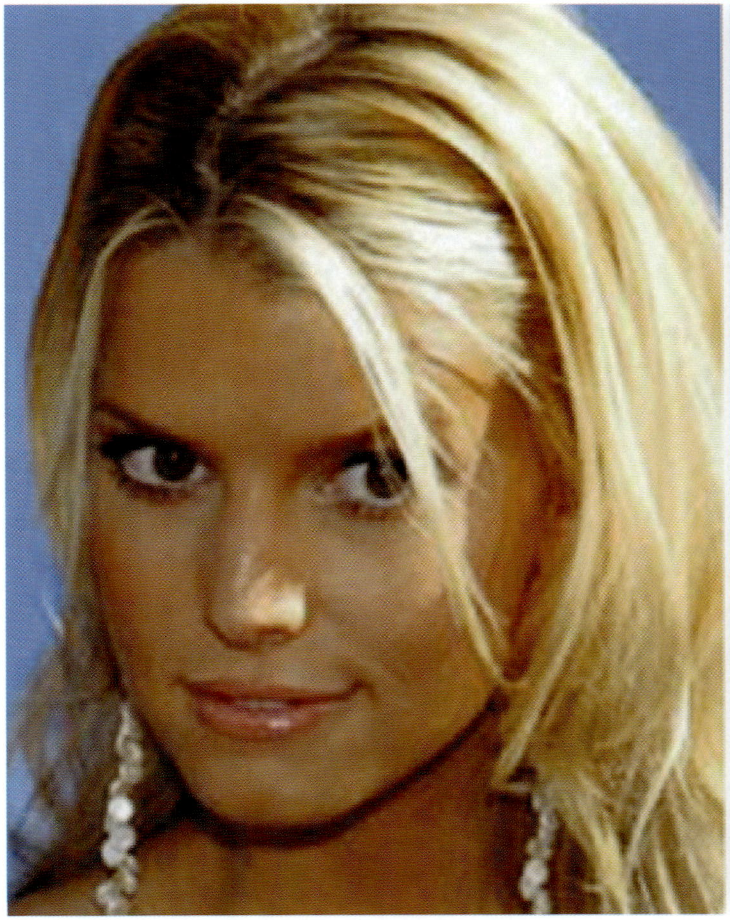

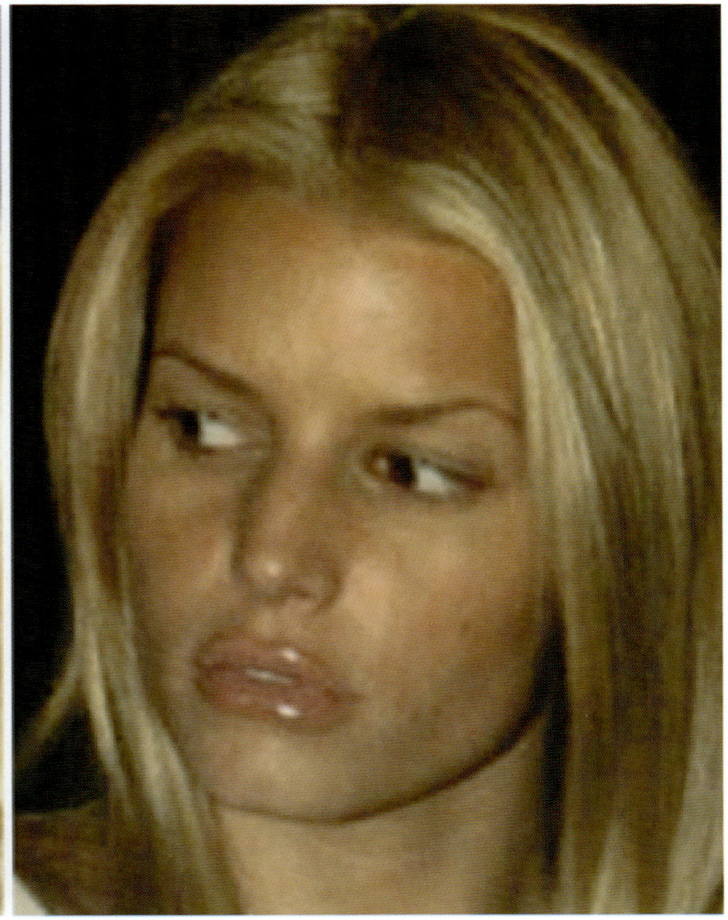

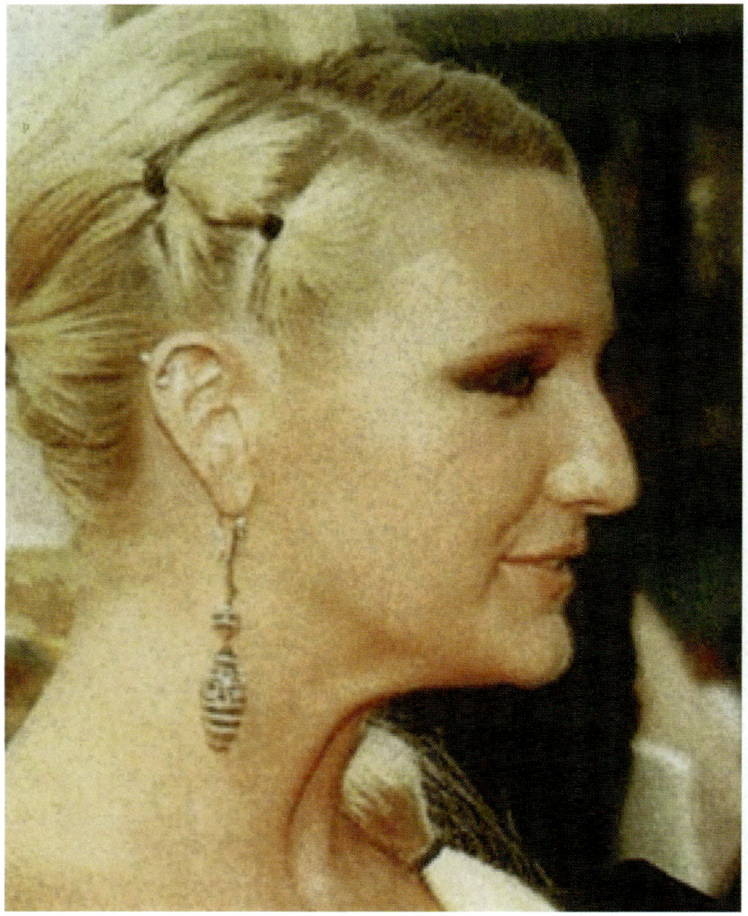

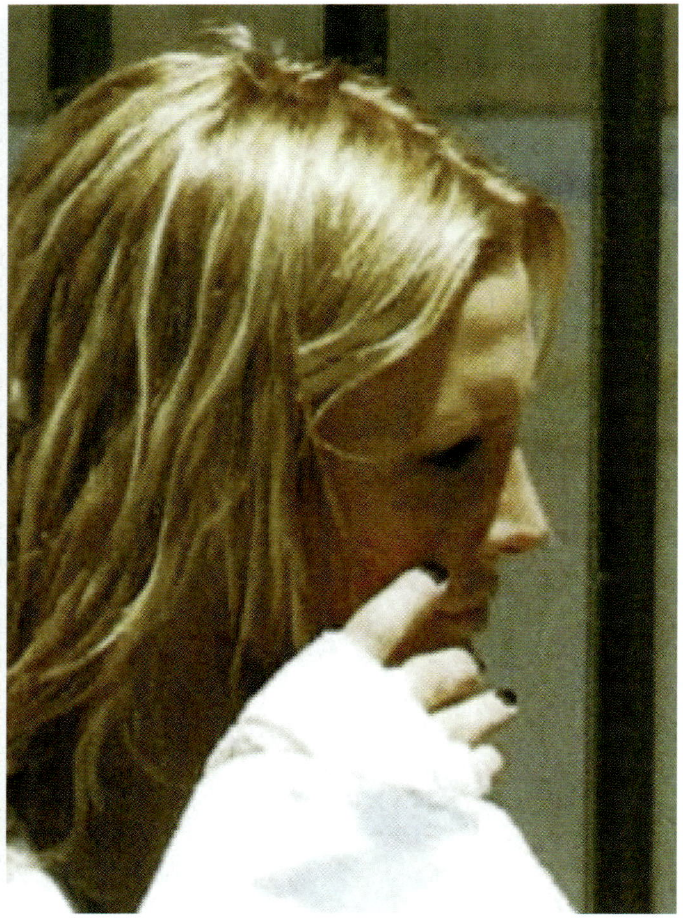

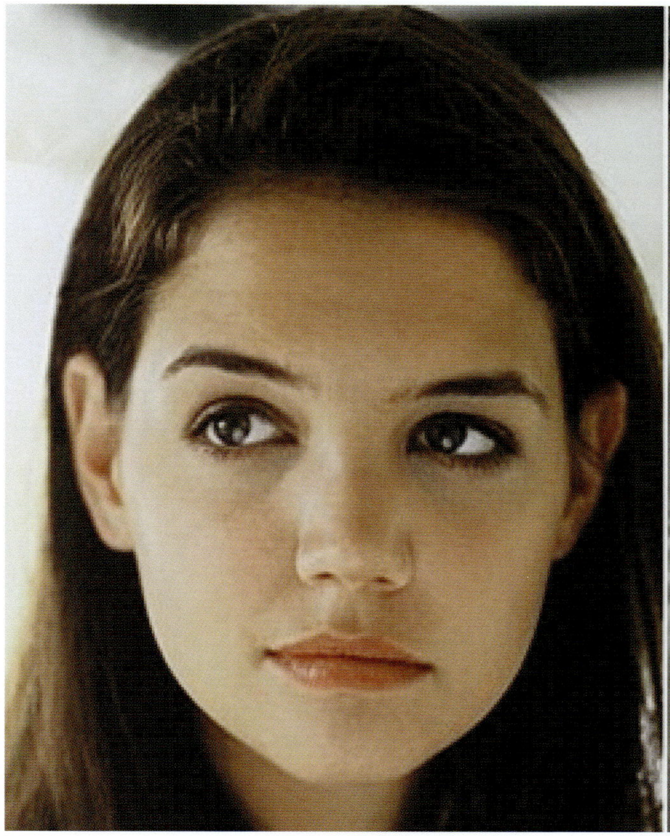
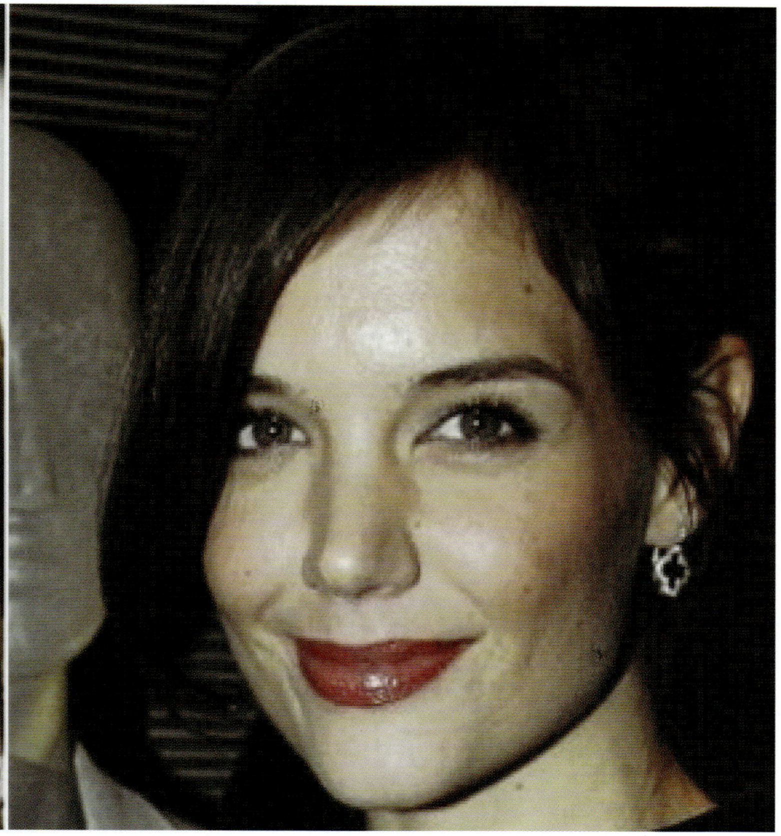

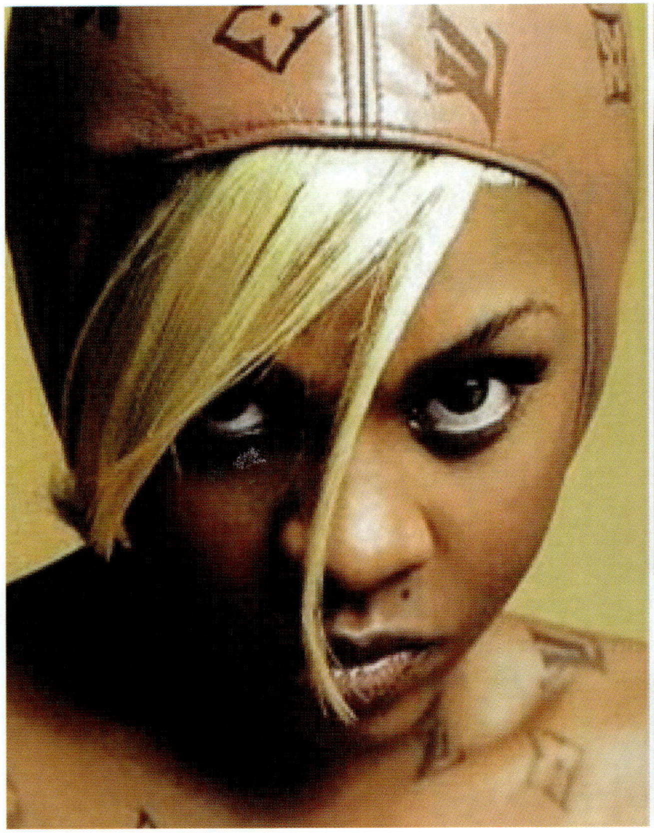

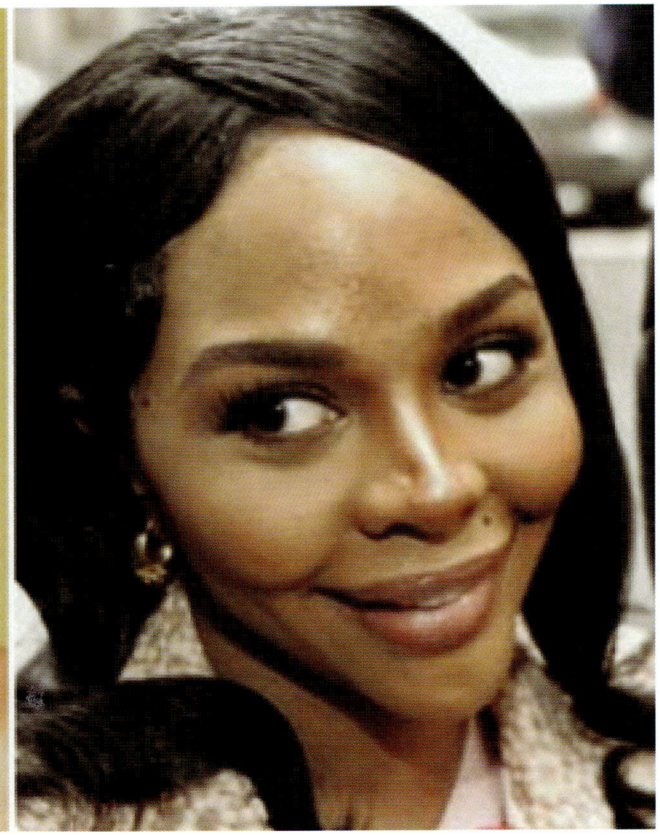

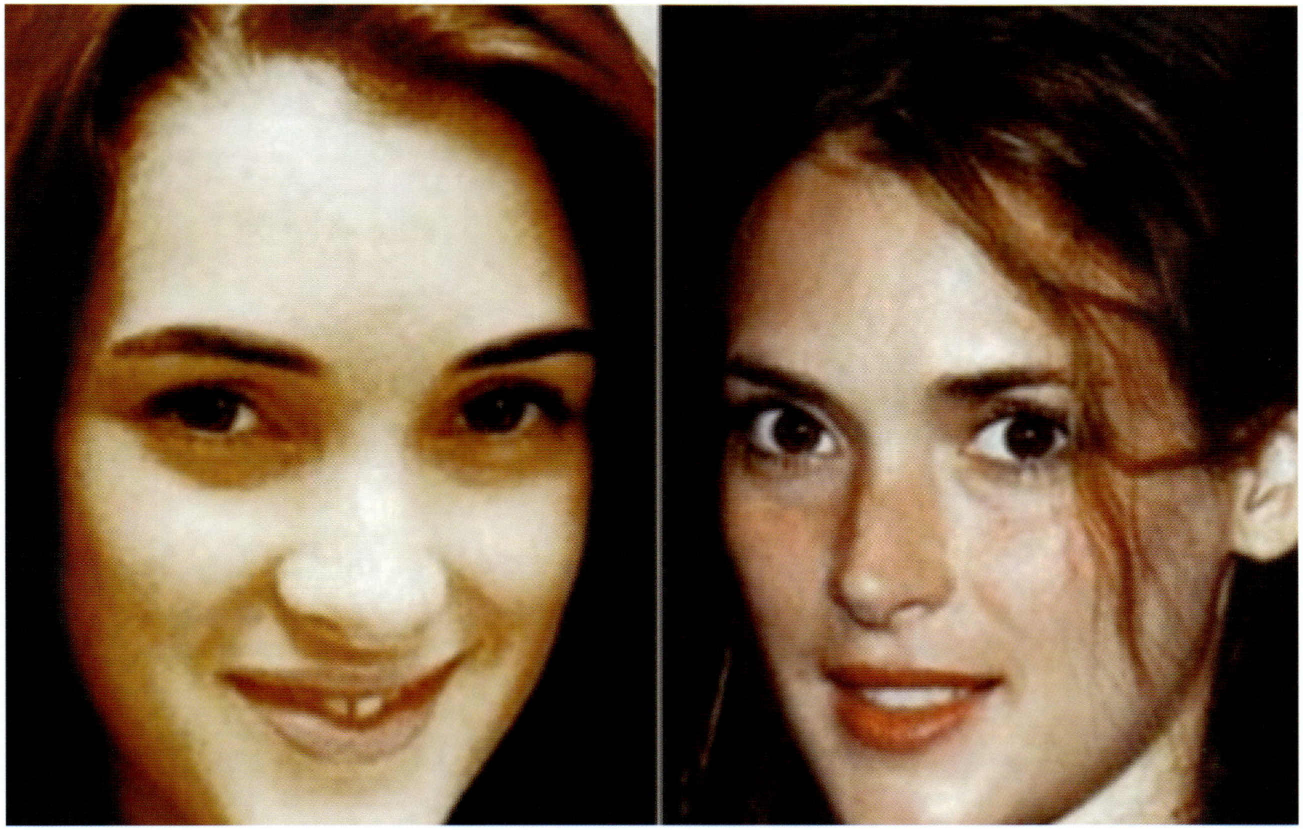

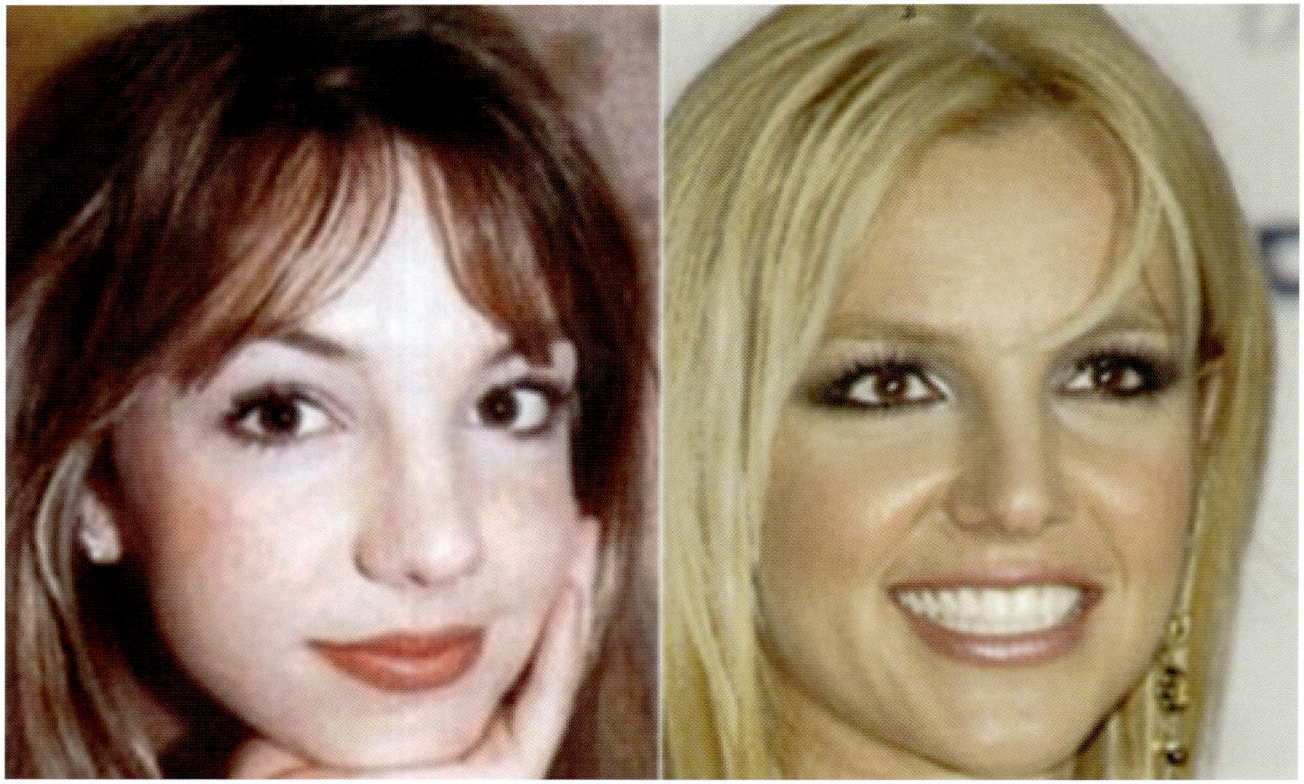

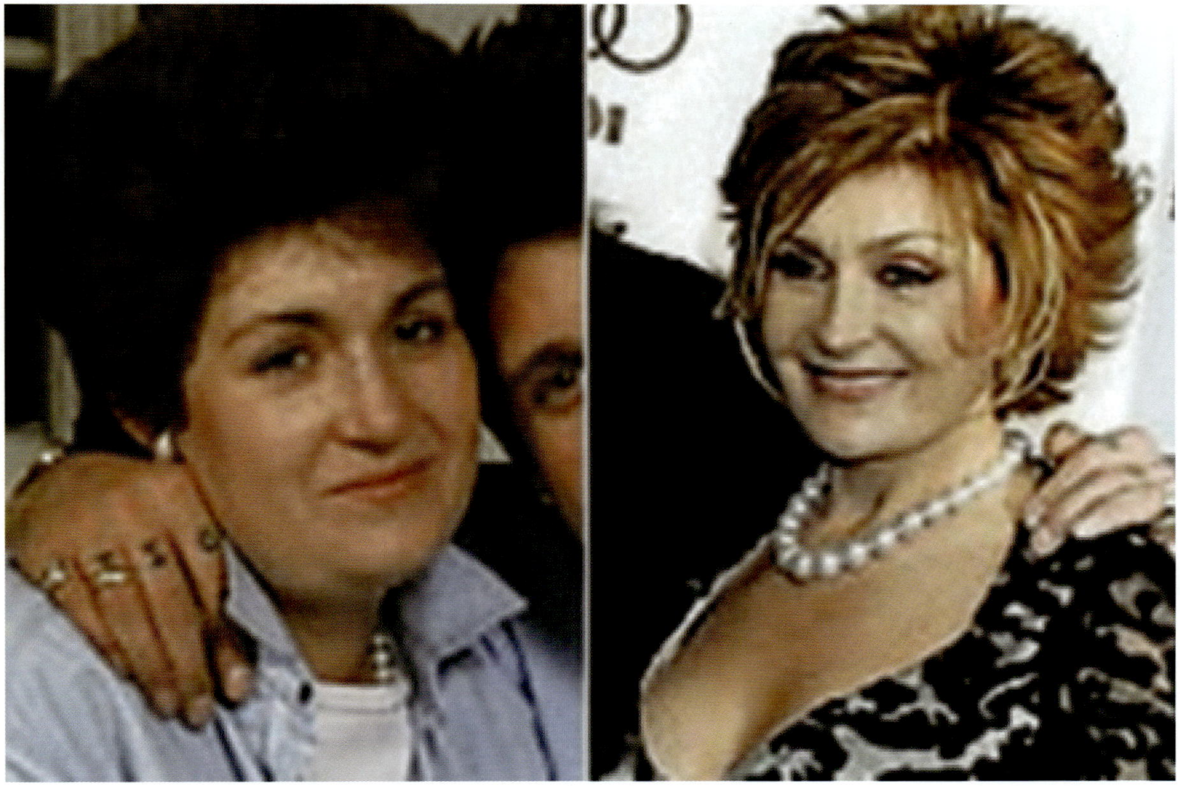

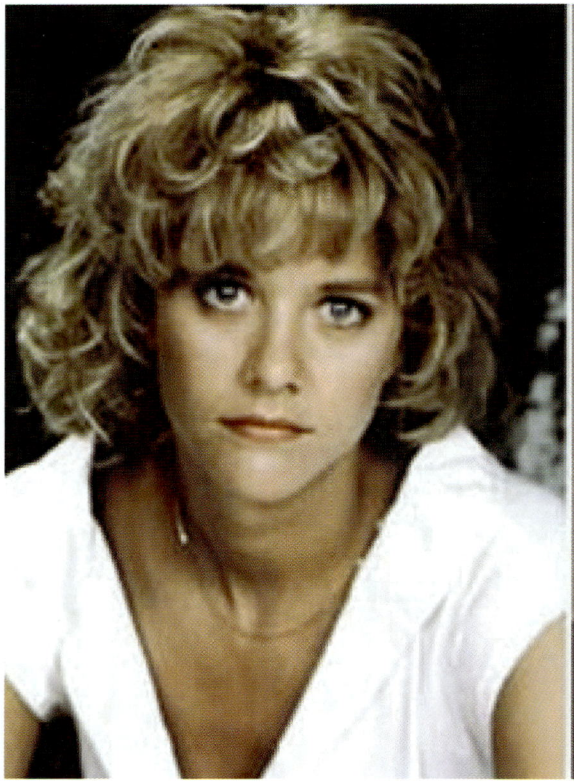
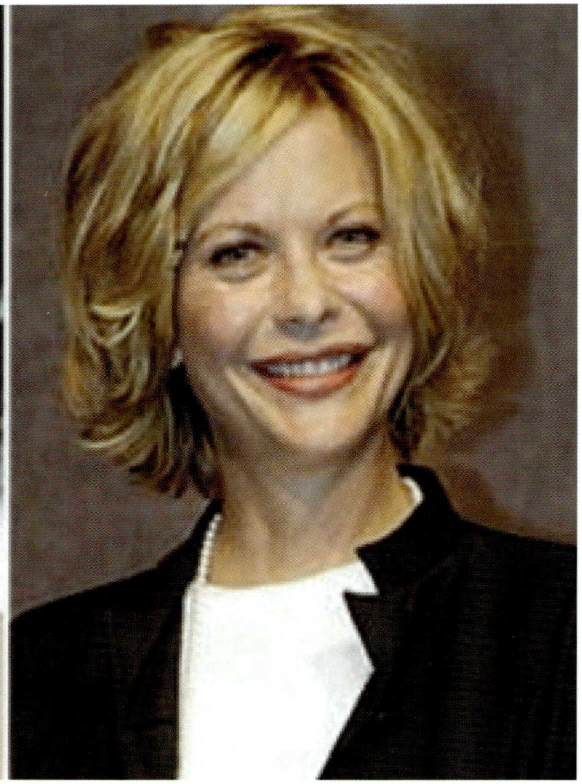

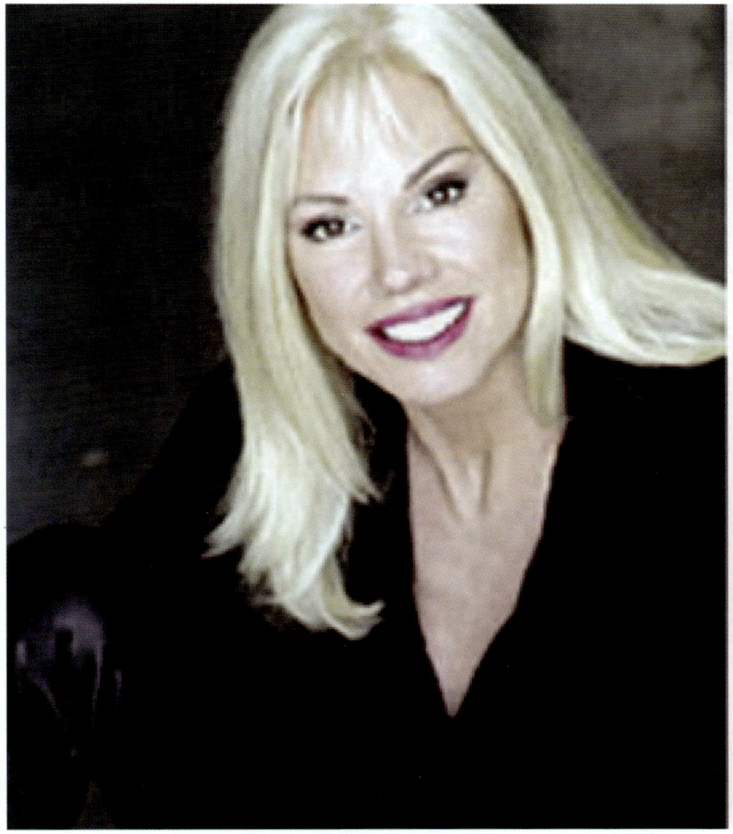

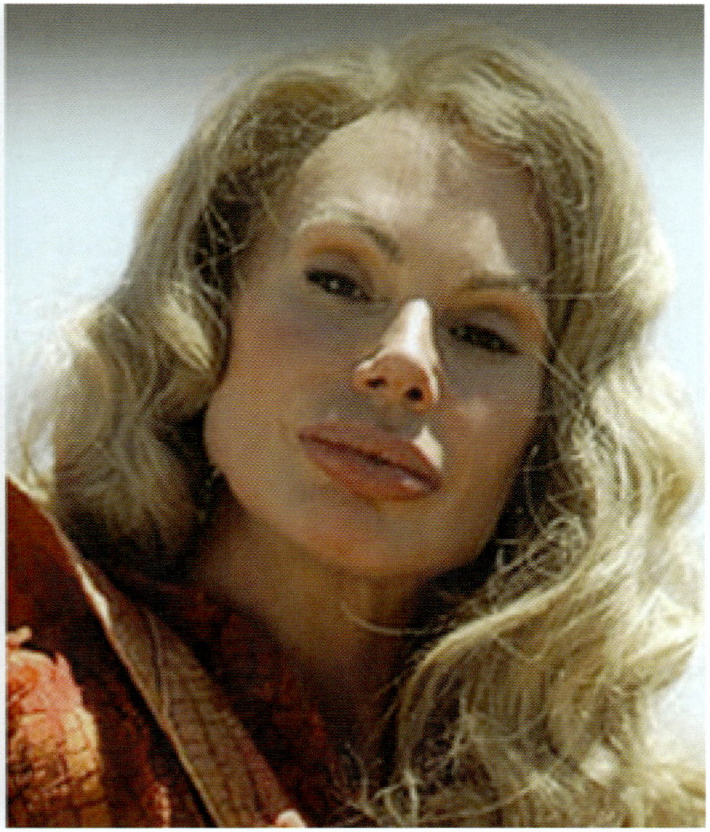

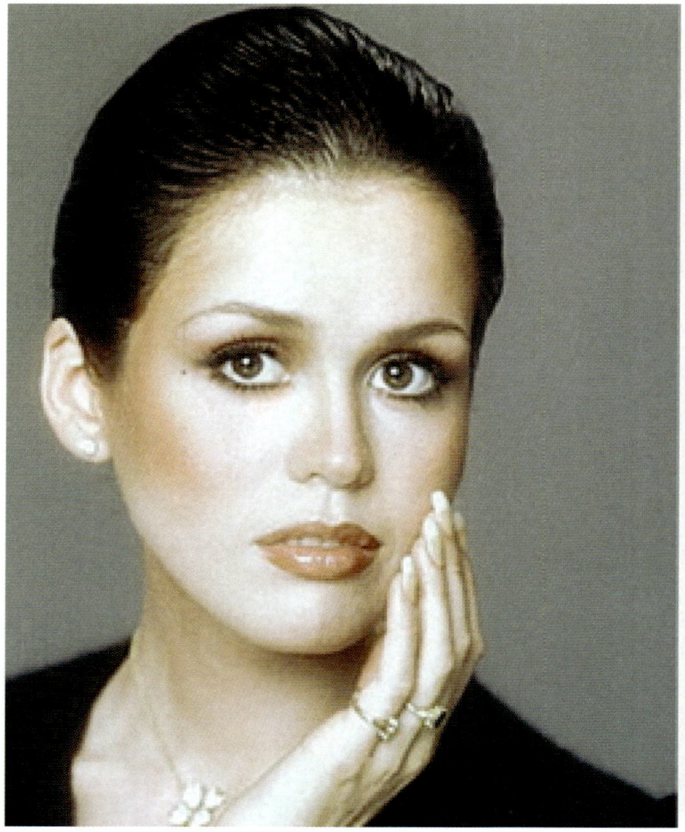

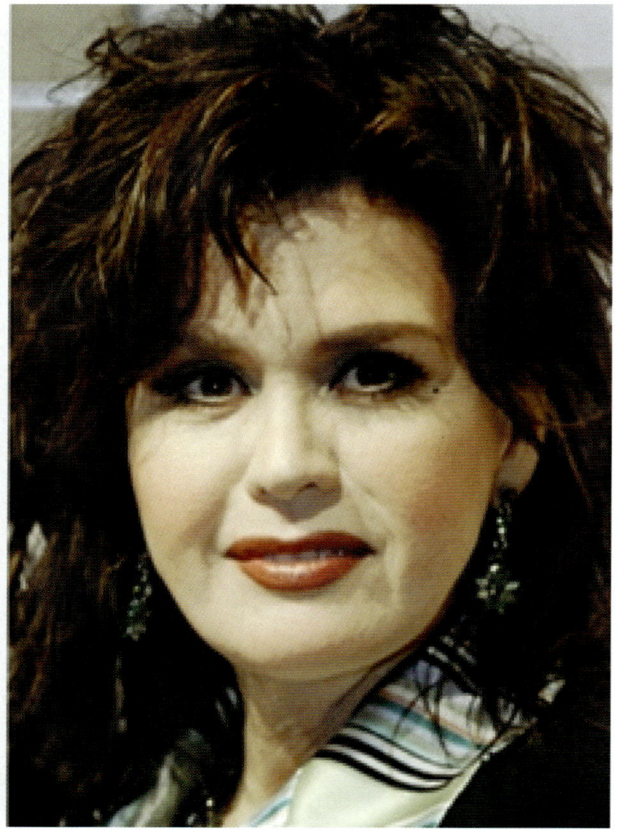

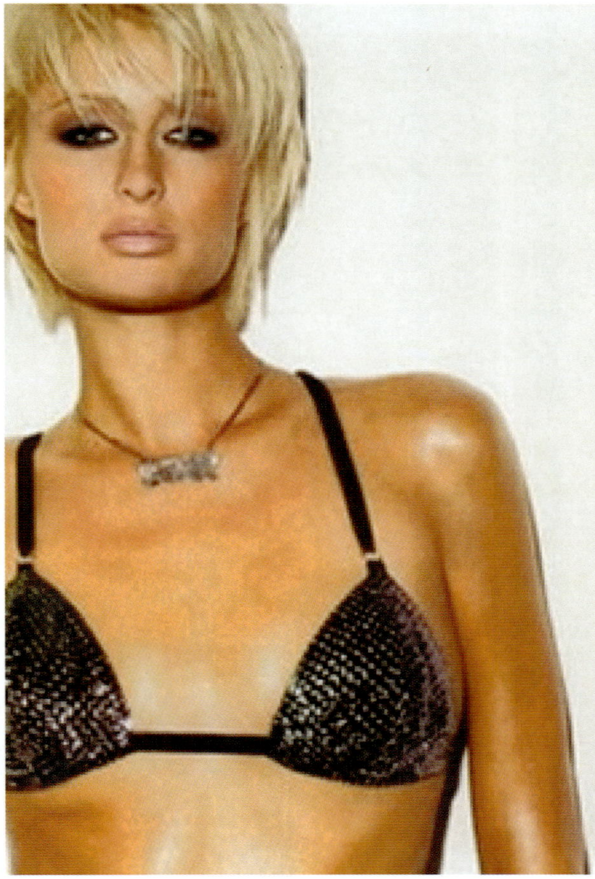

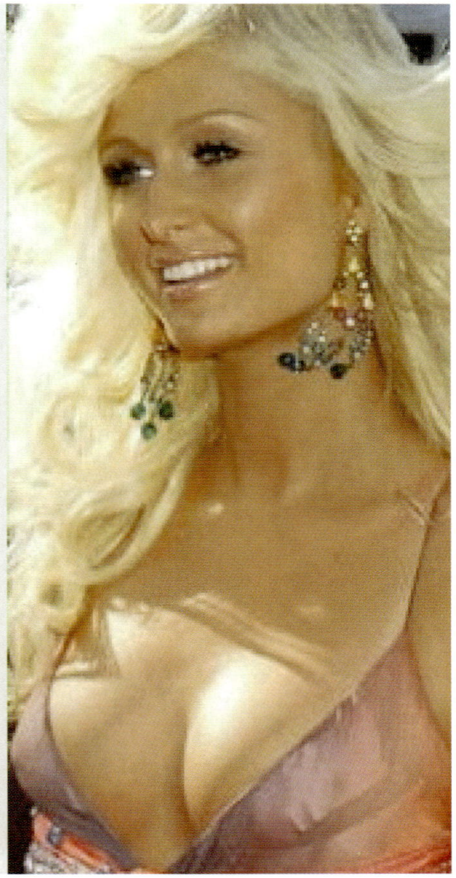

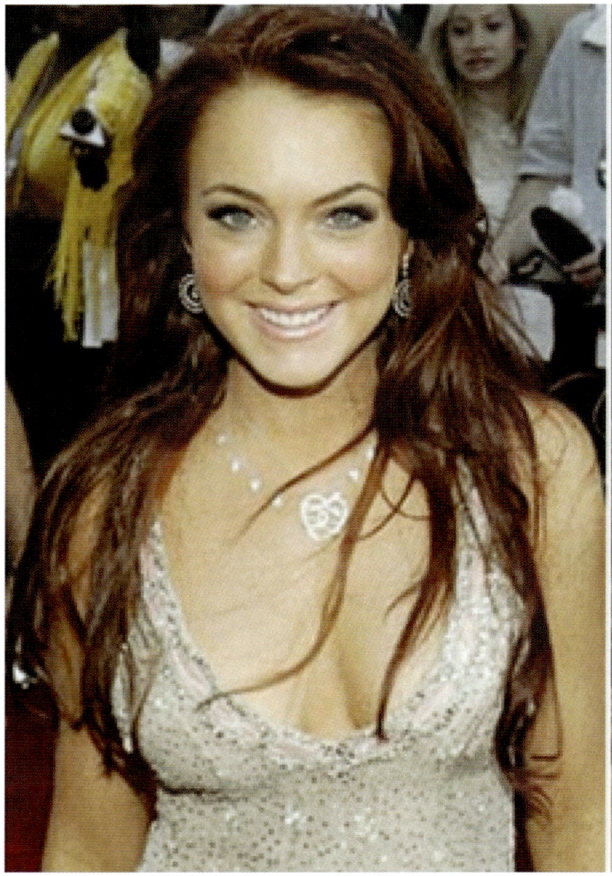

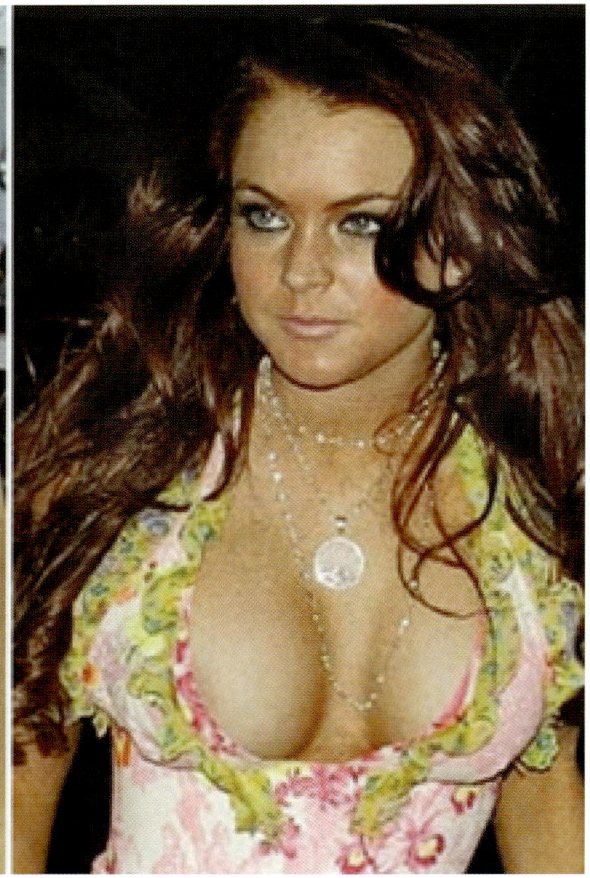

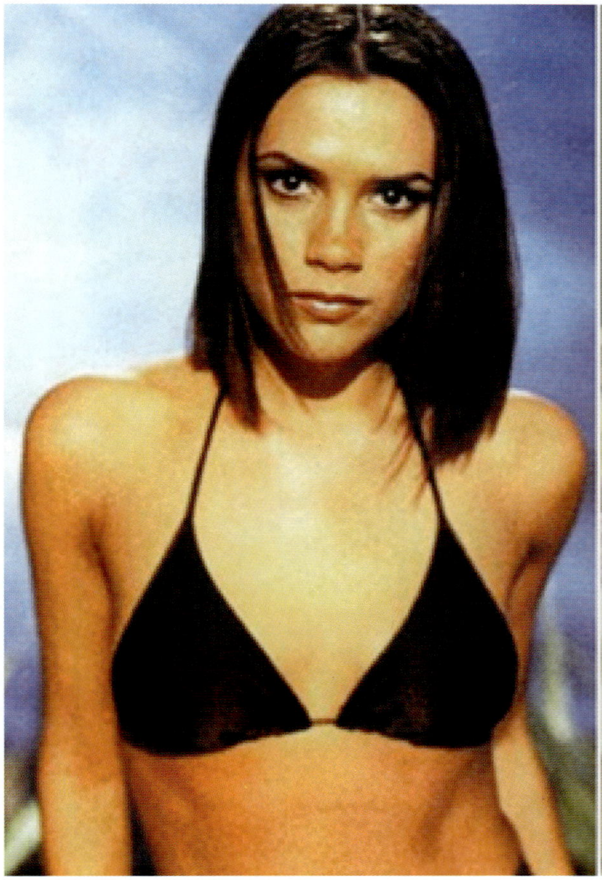

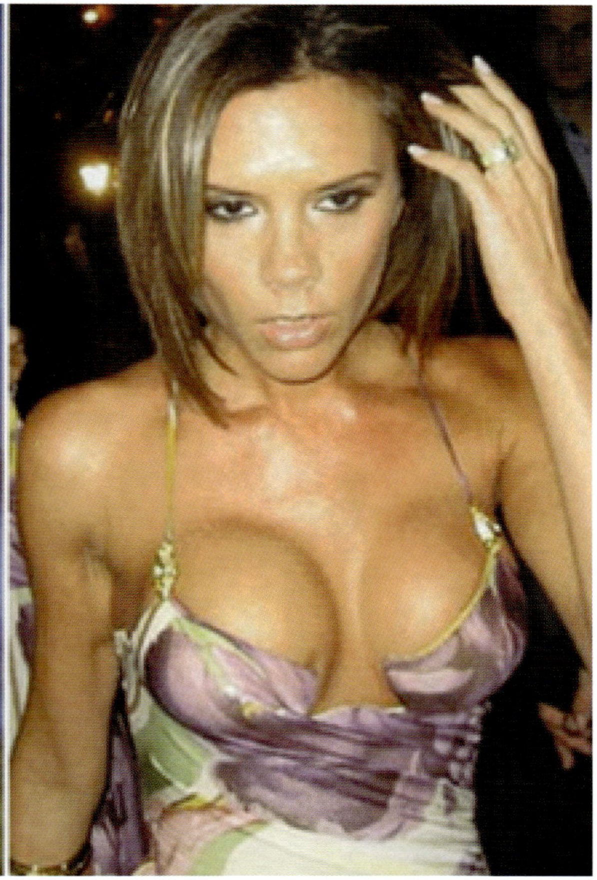

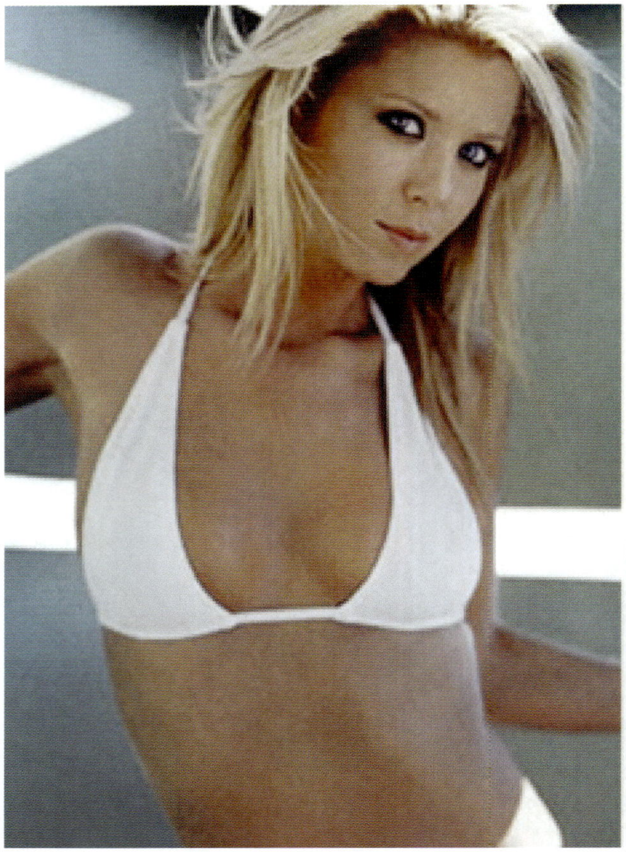

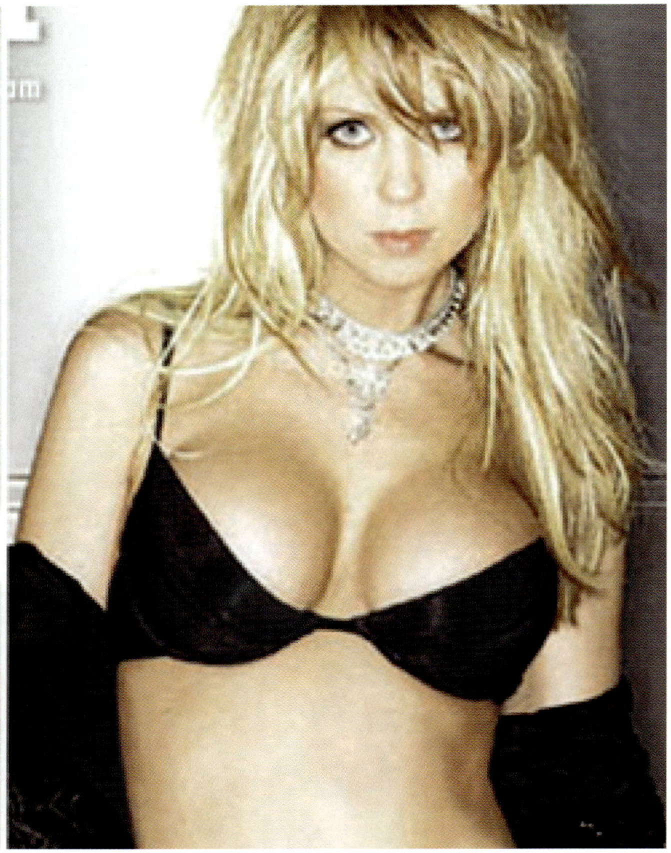

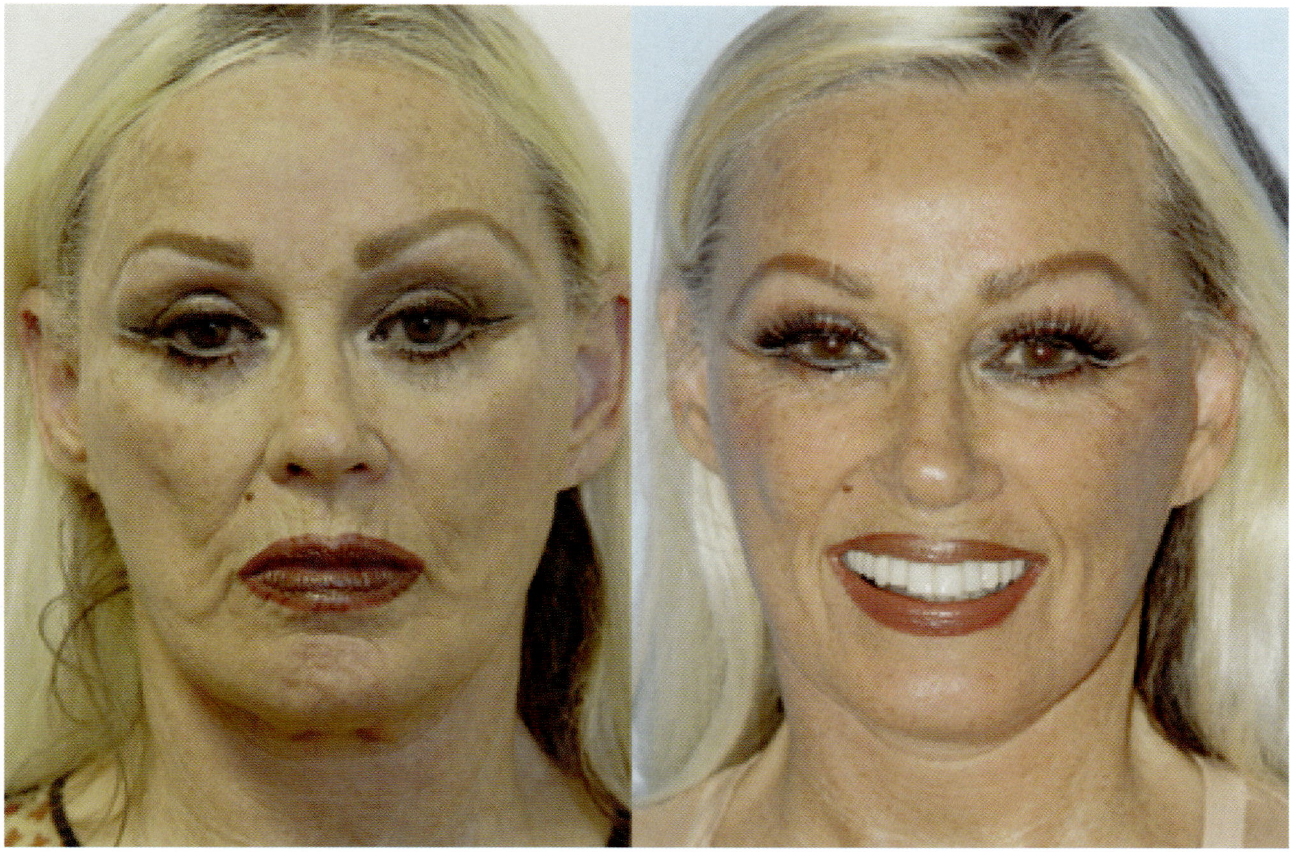

Mamie VanDoren:

In addition to Marilyn Monroe and Jane Mansfield, Mamie VanDoren is one of the original three Hollywood blonde bombshells. Here she is today still looking beautiful courtesy of Dr. H. George Brennan.

Public Faces - "What ifs?"

By: Cherie Lundquist-Grochow

Computer imaging can be used to simulate potential results for the prospective patient.
This is a very useful tool for patients considering cosmetic surgery.

It is also fascinating to contemplate results in public faces if they were to choose to have cosmetic surgery.

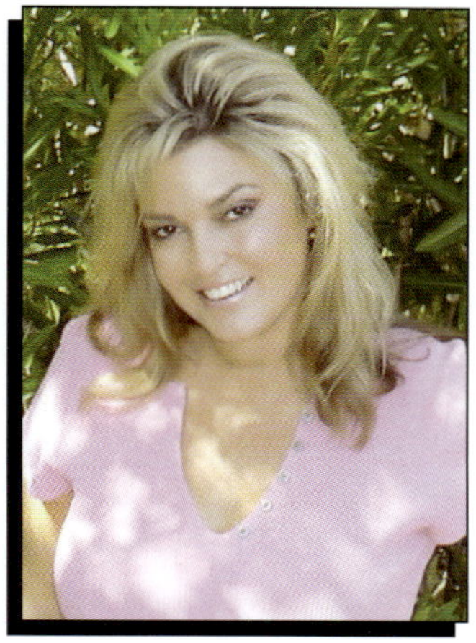

SIMULATION OF LOWER FACE REJUVENATION AND LOWER EYELID SURGERY

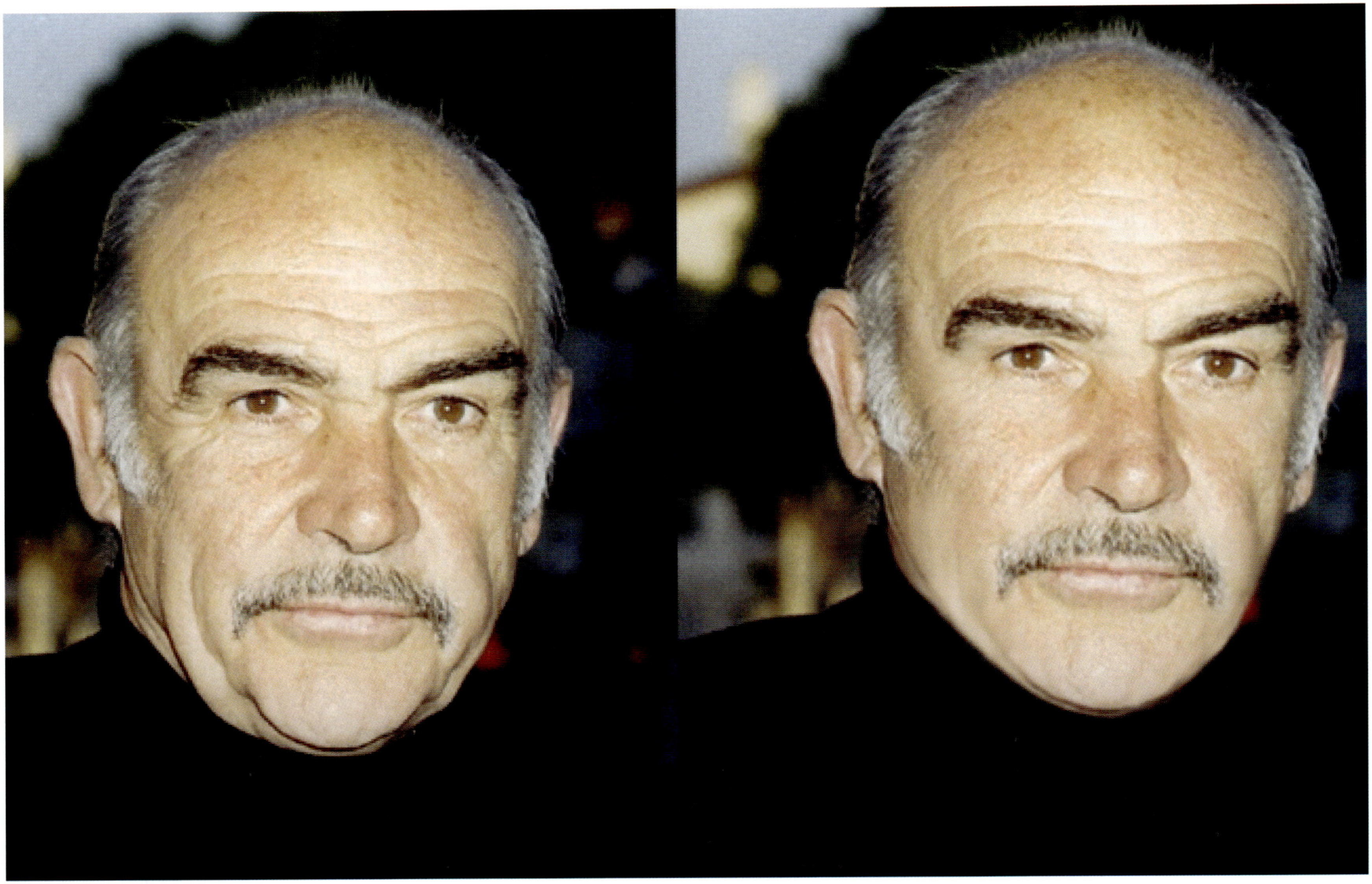

SIMULATION OF NASAL & EYELID SURGERY

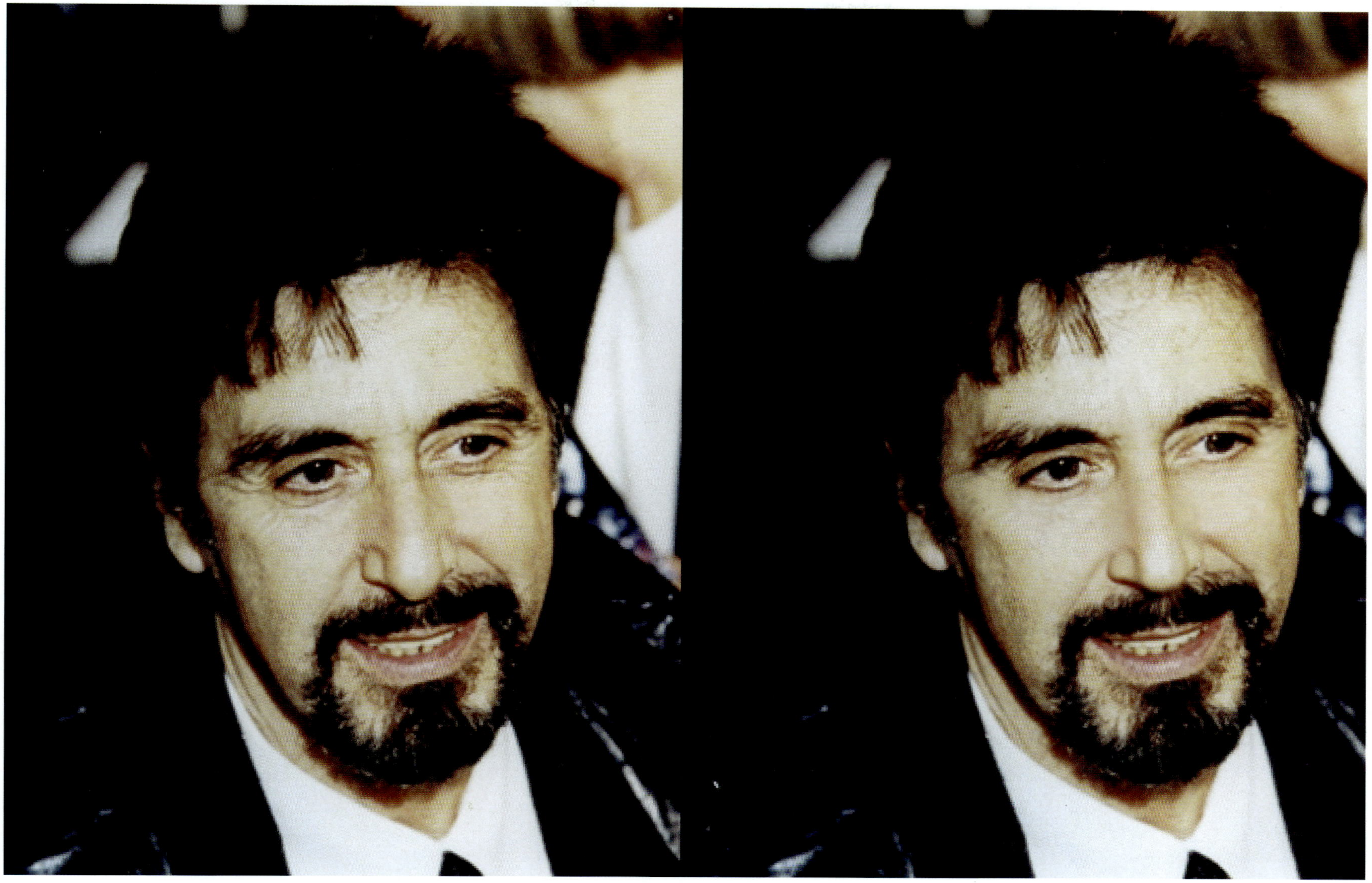

SIMULATION OF NASAL ALIGNMENT

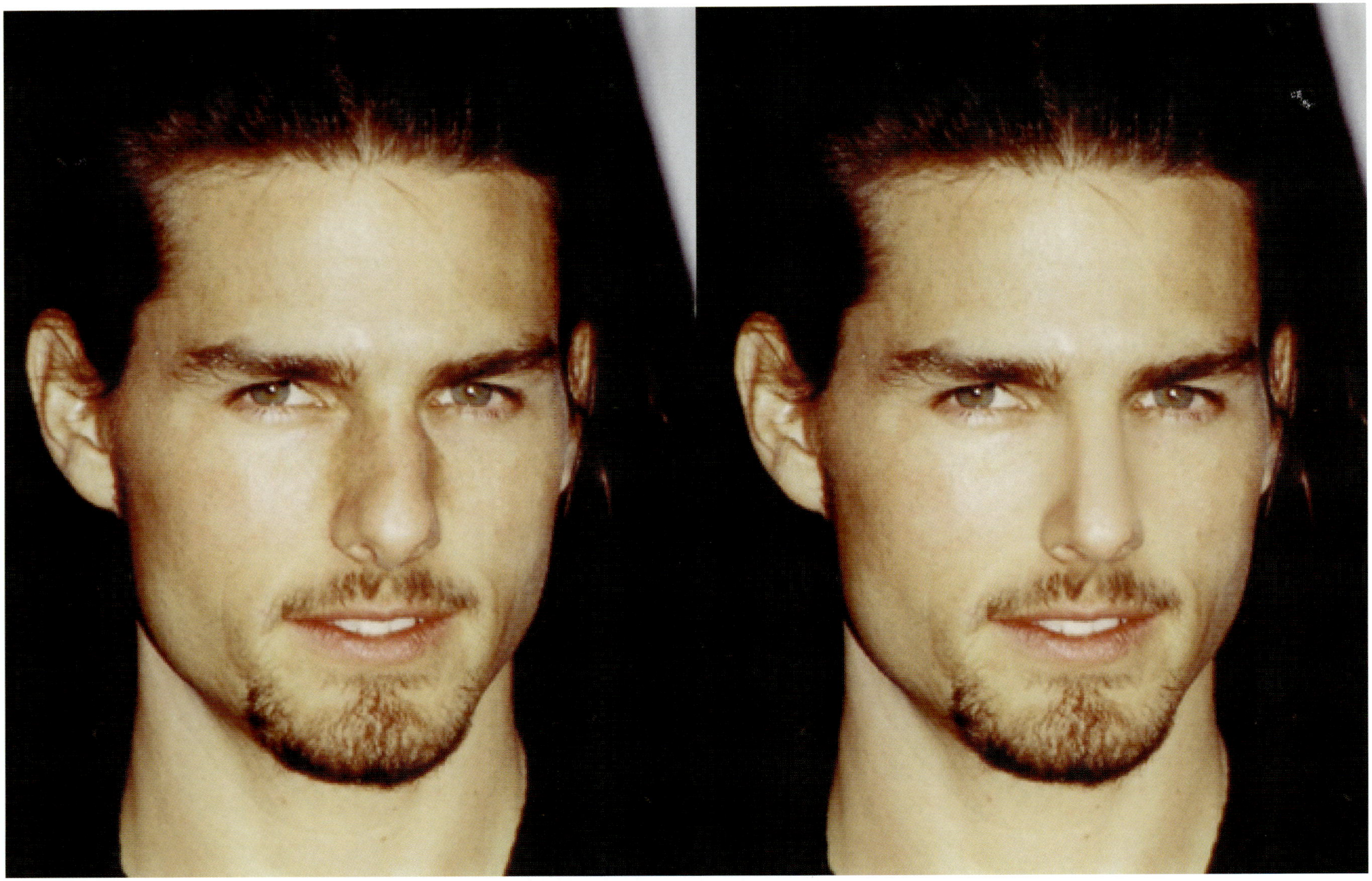

SIMULATION OF FACIAL REJUVENATION

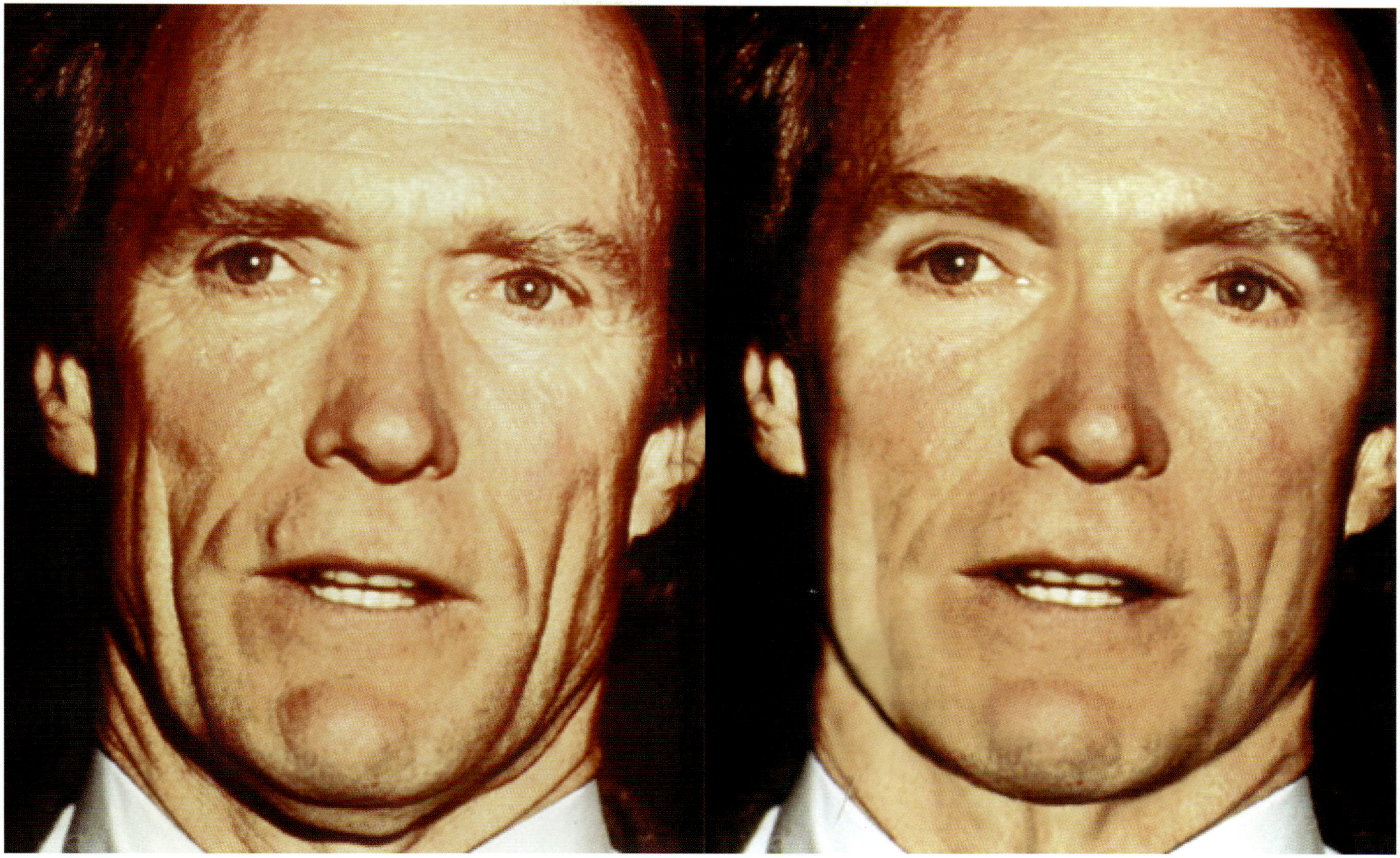

SIMULATION OF ELEVATING LOWER EYELIDS

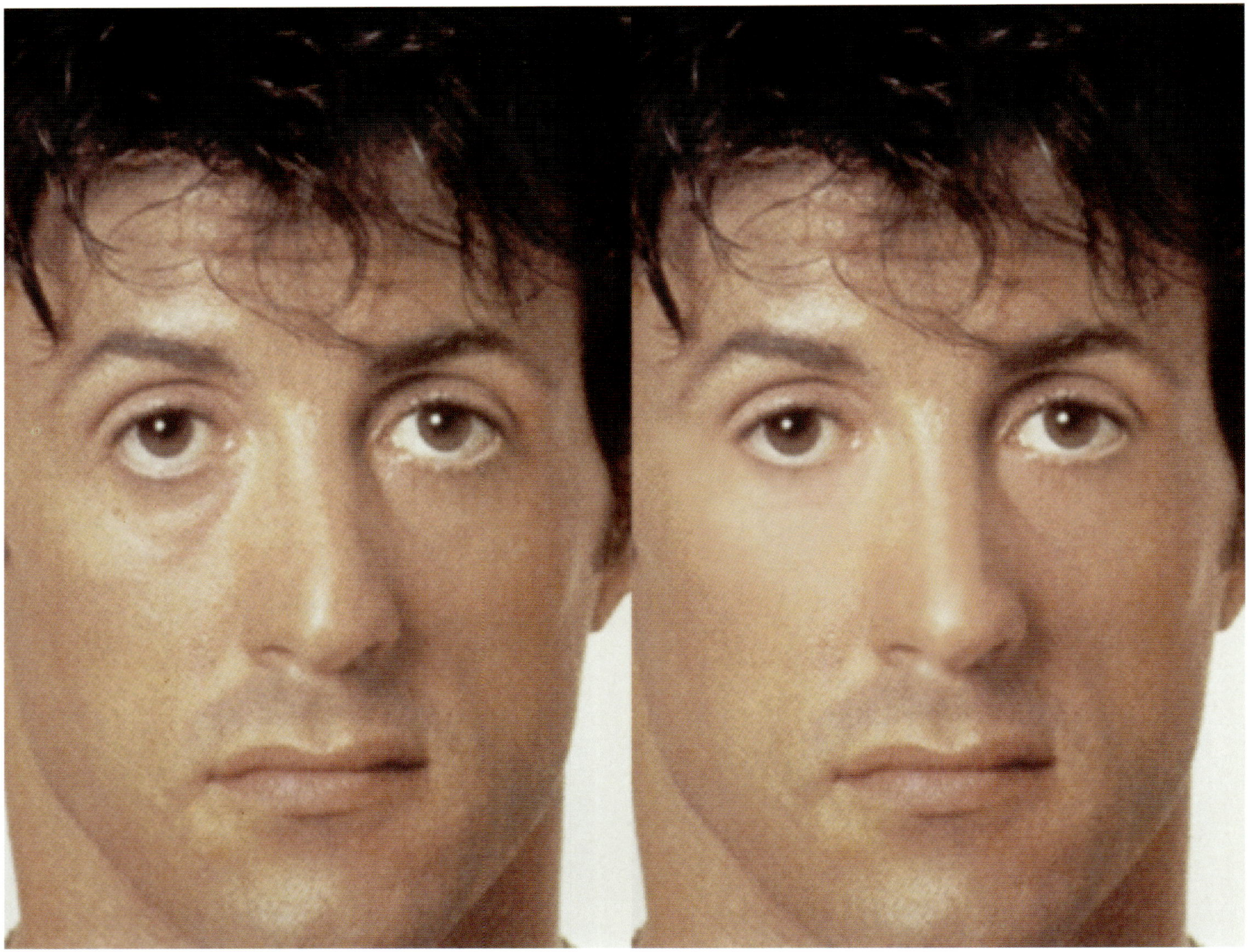

SIMULATION OF EYELIDS AND NASAL SURGERY

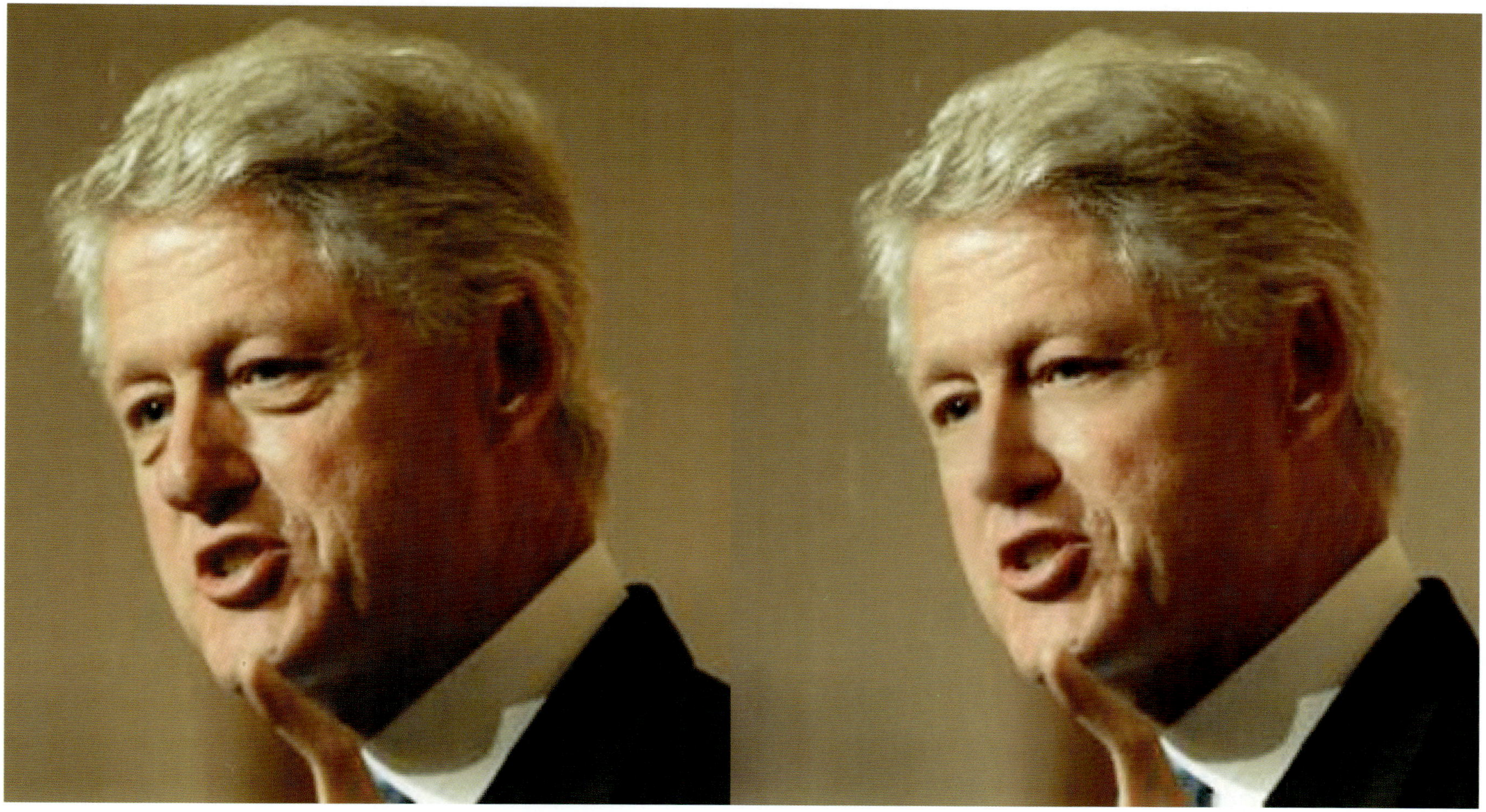

SIMULATION OF CHIN REDUCTION

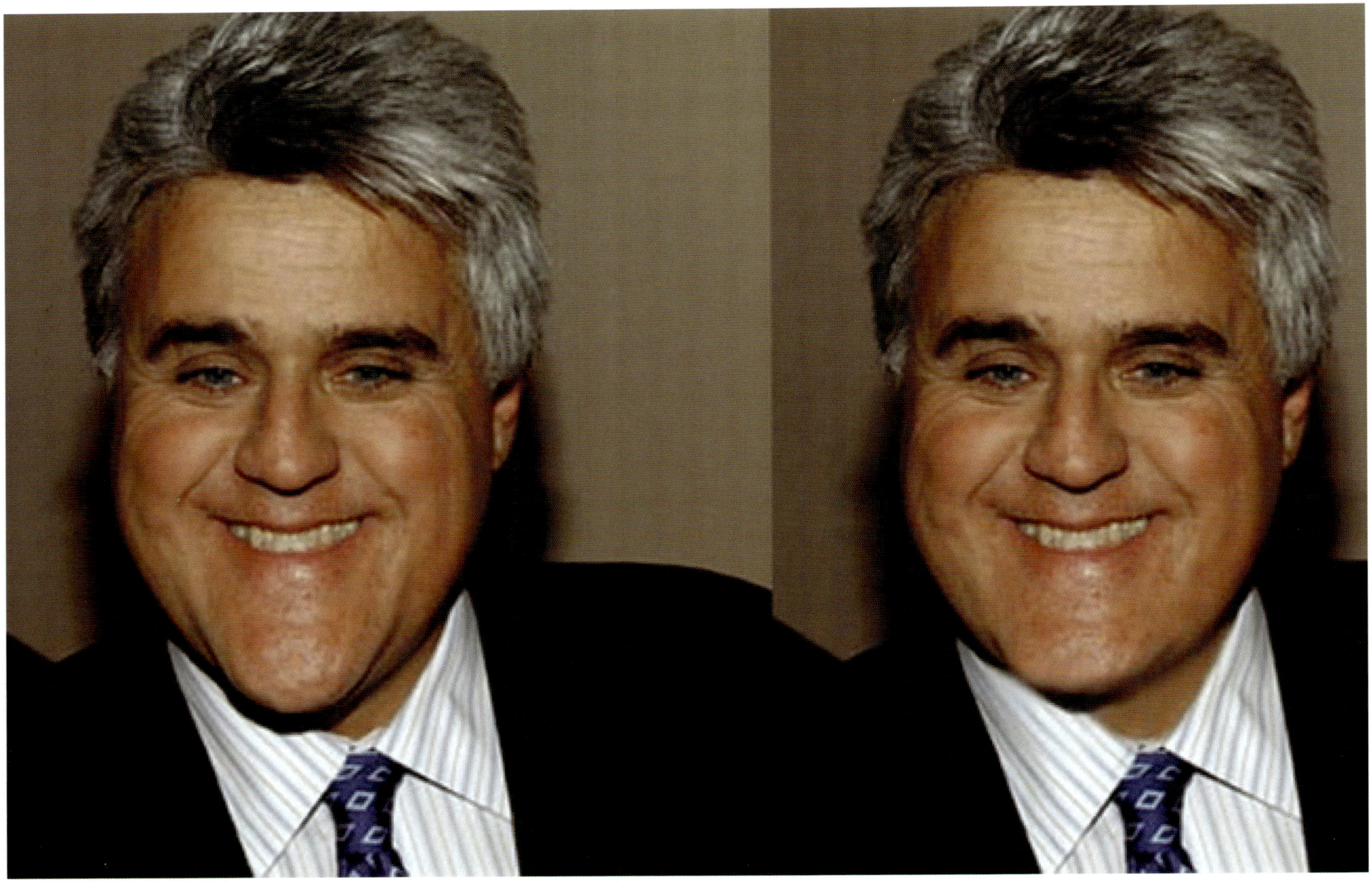

EAR REPOSITIONING

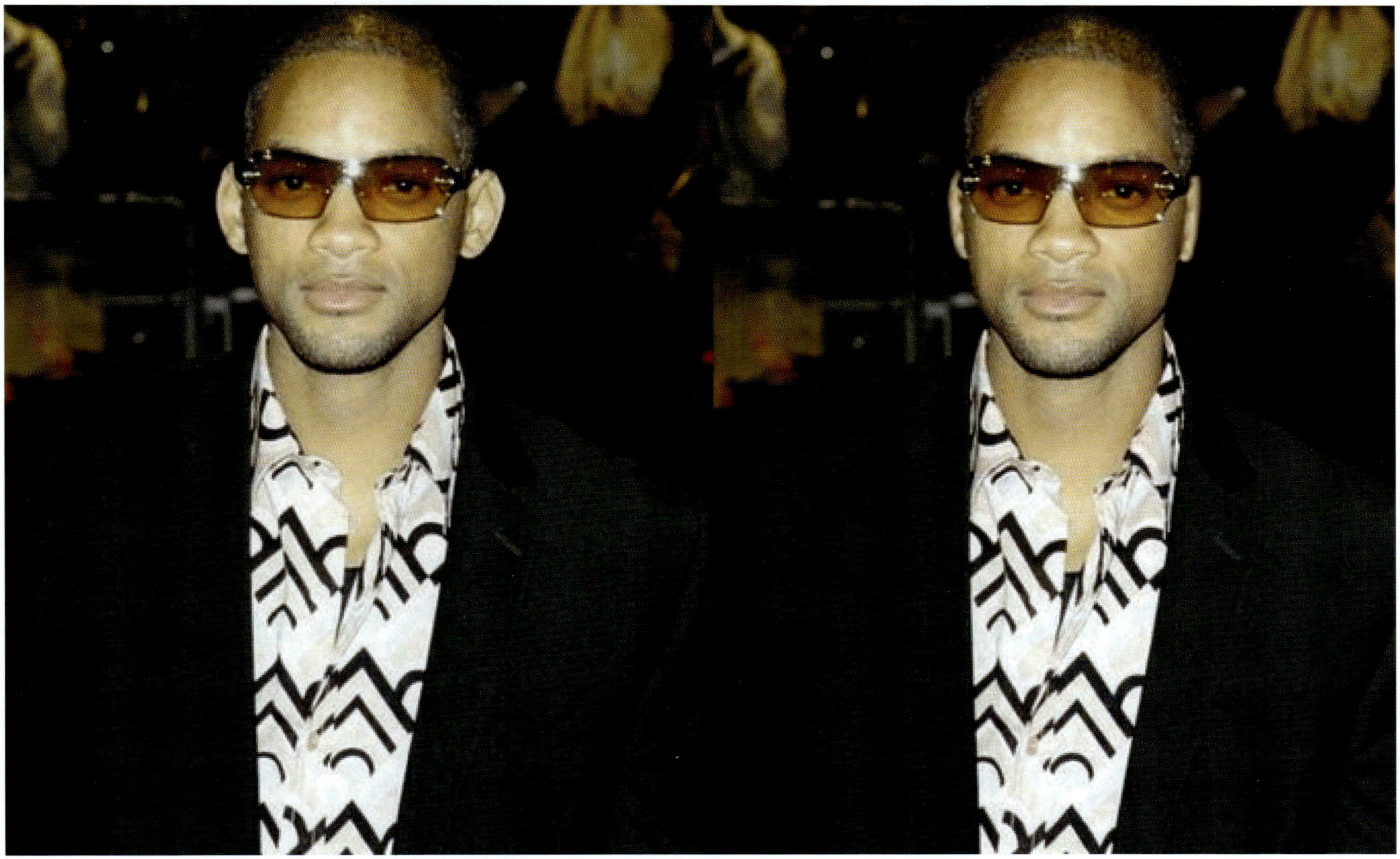

SIMULATION OF NASAL SURGERY

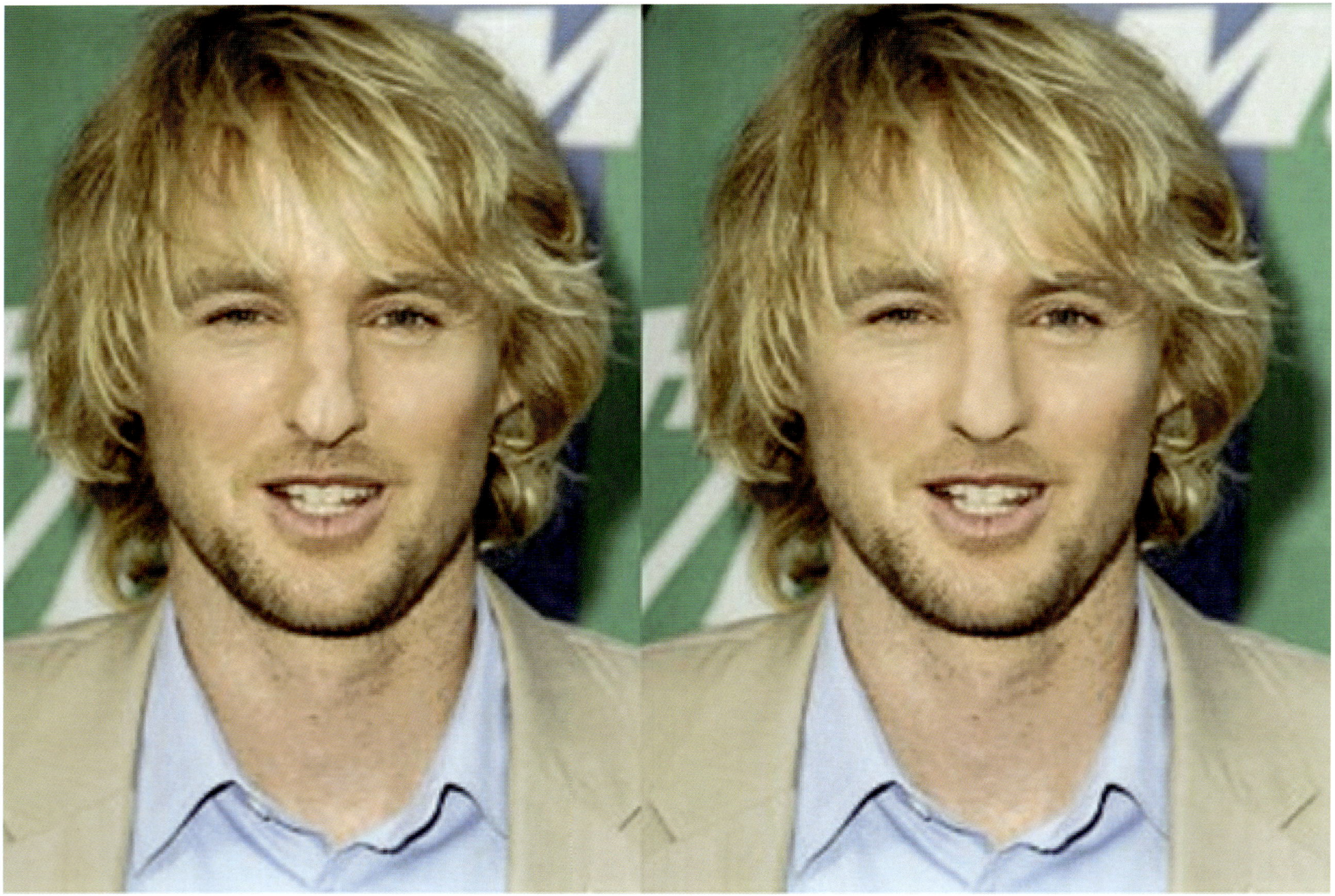

SIMULATION OF NASAL & LIP SURGERY

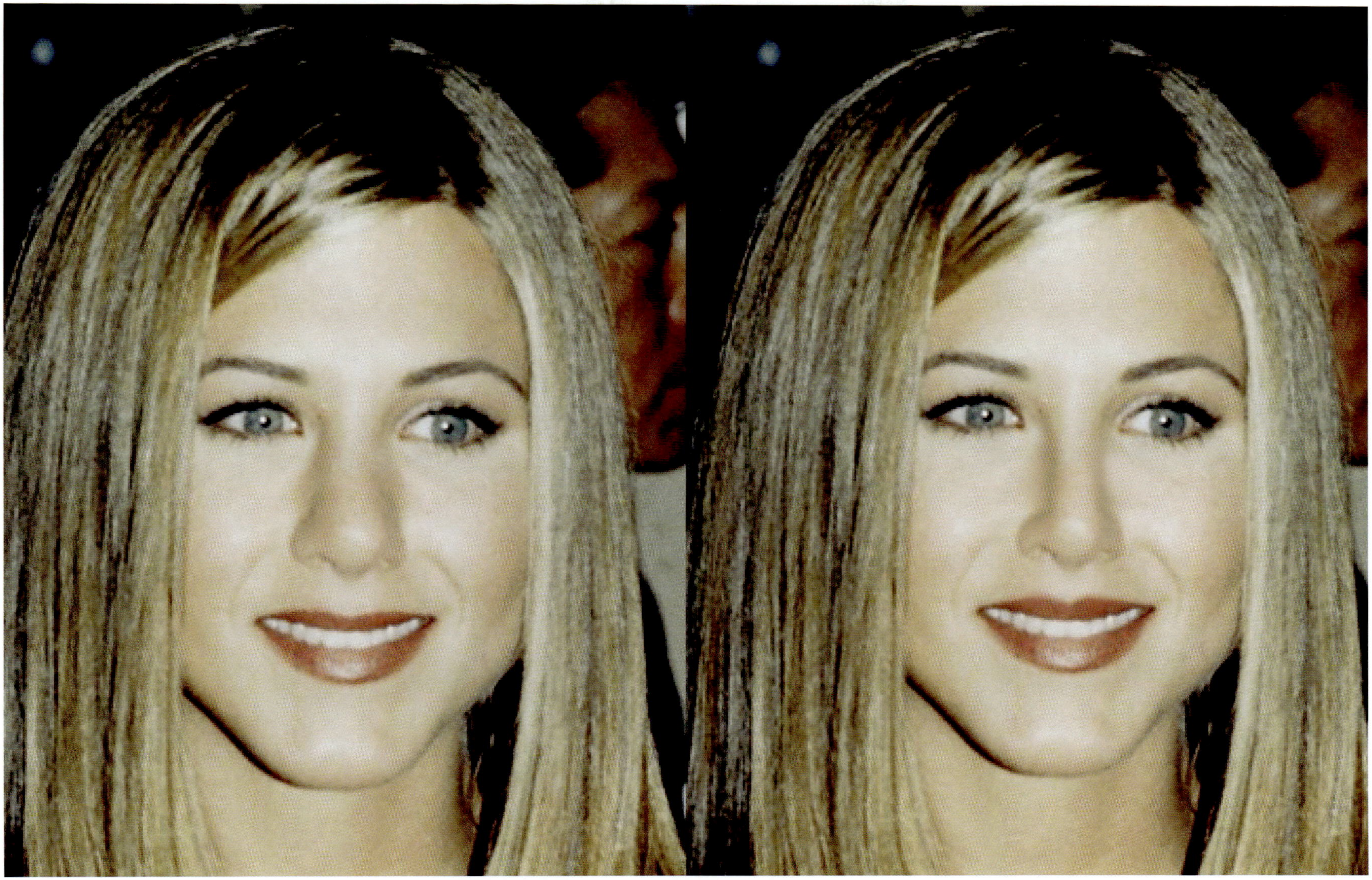

SIMULATION OF SHORTENING OF THE NOSE

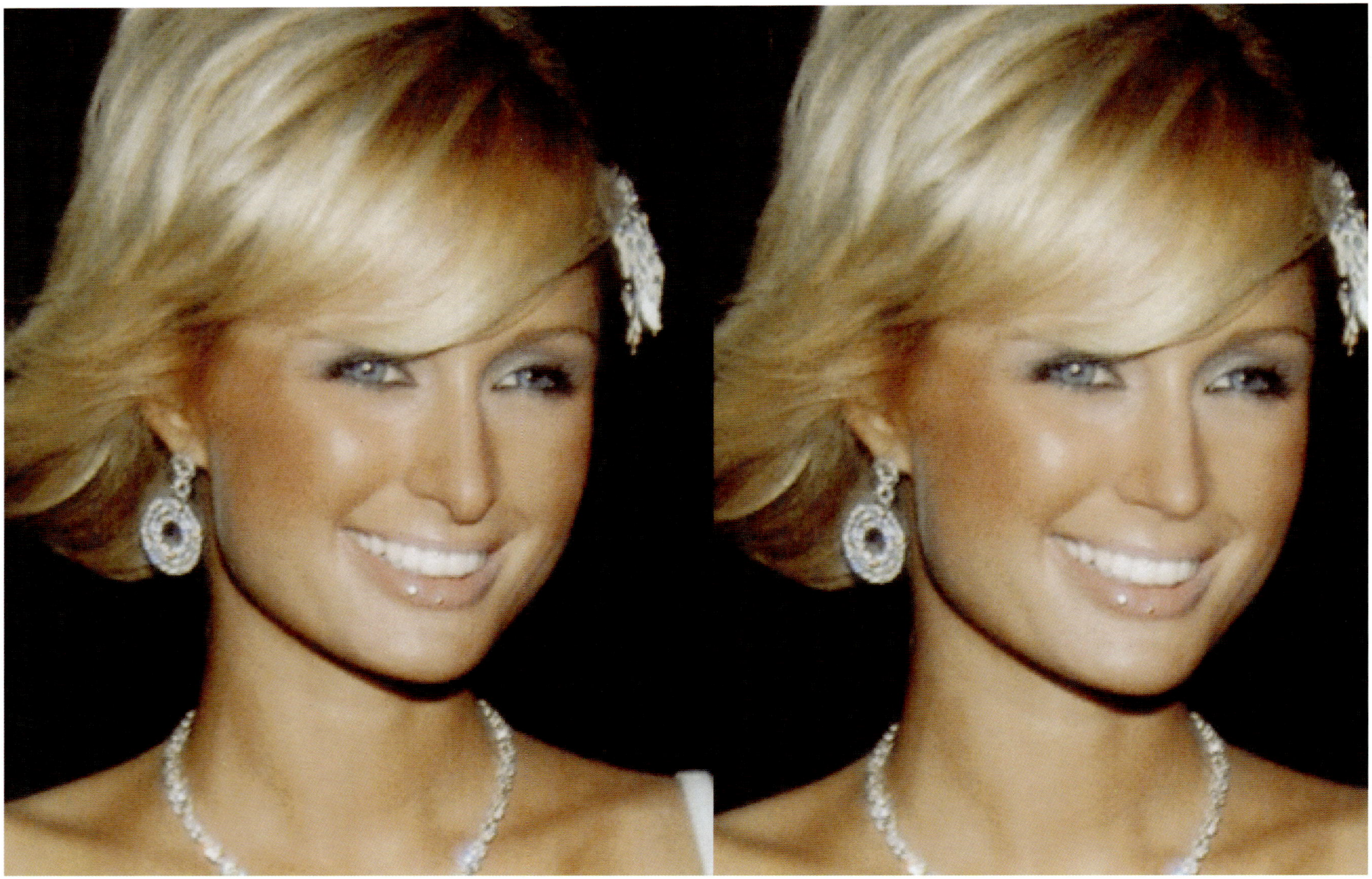

SIMULATION OF COSMETIC DENTISTRY

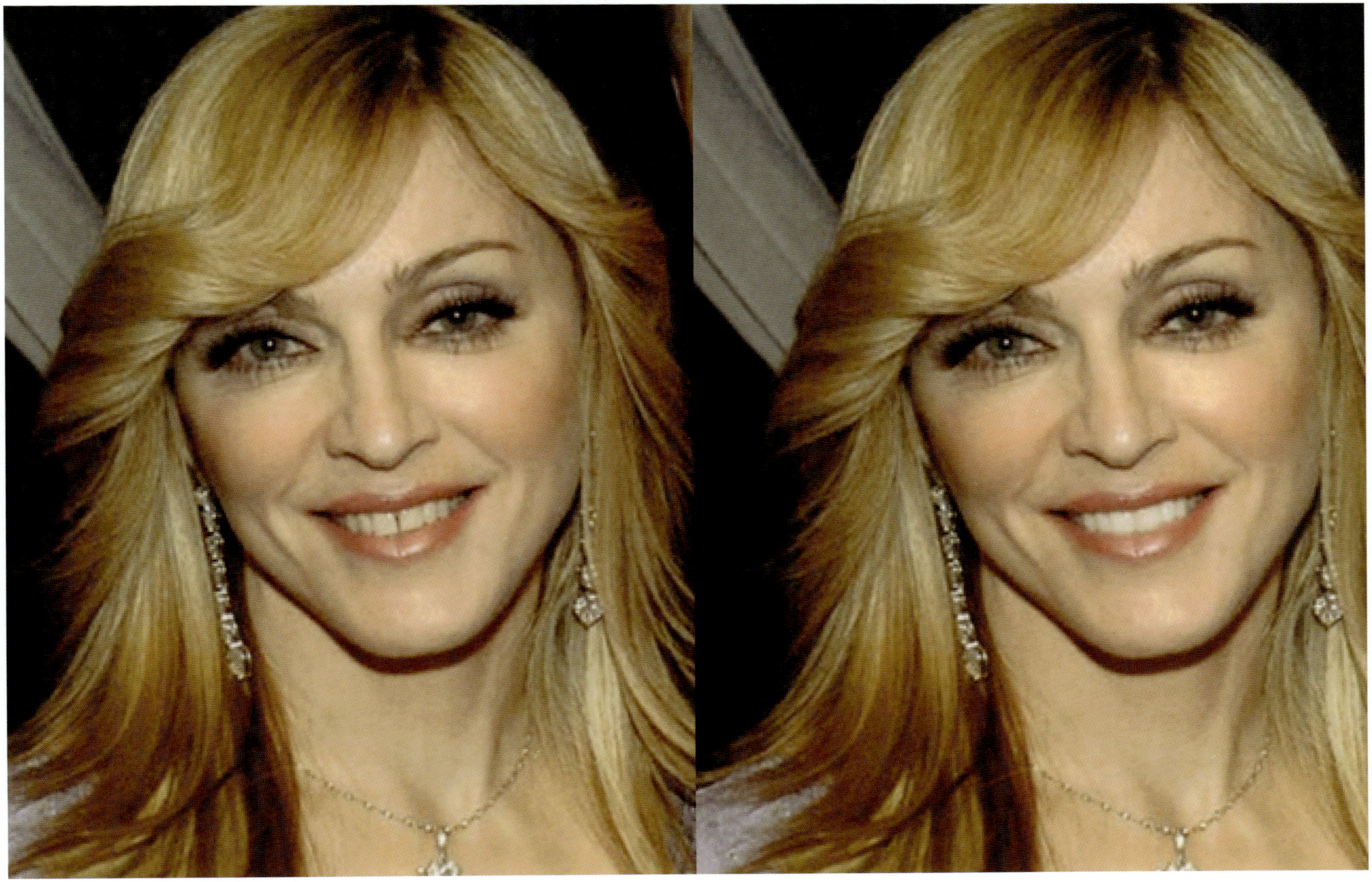

SIMULATION OF COSMETIC DENTISTRY (LENGTHENING THE TEETH)

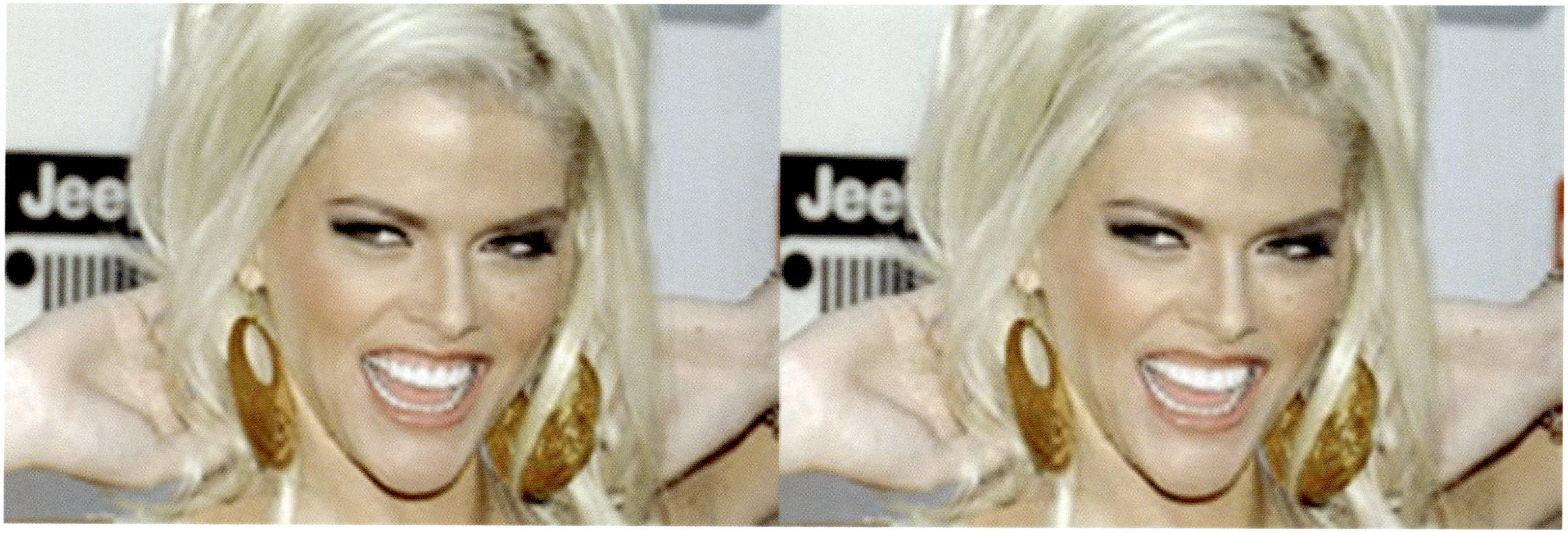

SIMULATION OF SHORTENING THE NOSE

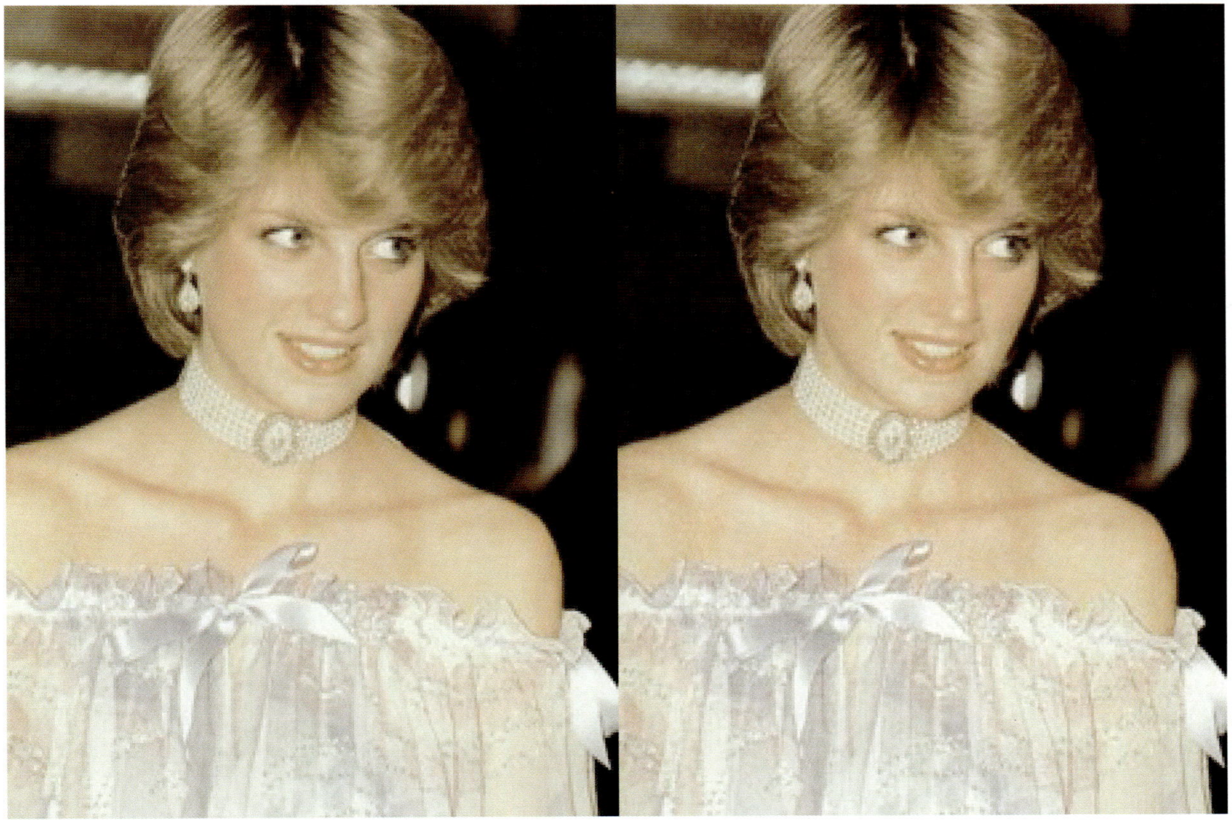

Maintaining Results

Maintaining Results

You've made a choice to create beauty now you have made a "partnership" with your surgeon to maintain your results.

This chapter will inform you on how to keep up your end of the partnership. Various lifestyles, environmental and self induced habits can work against you.

DIET

Thousands of diet plans contribute to a $40-billion-a-year weight-loss industry. However, while the weight-loss industry continues to grow, obesity has reached epidemic proportions.

Scientific-sounding "facts" and hocus-pocus "research" can dazzle and confuse the average consumer. Diet-plan marketers go to great lengths to explain how their diet can work for everyone, or claim that it is carbohydrate intake (or any other dieters "enemy-of-the-month) that is the culprit. However, the bottom line is that a caloric deficit (more calories burned than consumed) causes weight loss. The average American consumes 300 calories more today than he did 30 years ago. He also burns 260 less calories each day due to increased automation, technology and sedentary occupations.

While fad diets may initially offer rapid weight loss, the result is too often temporary, leaving the dieter defeated, angry and often with a few extra pounds just for good measure. The problem with fad diets is that they are just fads. The key to long-term weight loss is adopting a healthy lifestyle for life.

The list below is merely just a few of the most popular diet plans out there for someone to choose from:

Weight Watchers	www.weightwatchers.com	South Beach	www.southbeachdiet.com
Lindora	www.lindora.com	The Zone	www.zonedietathome.com
Jenny Craig	www.jennycraig.com	Slim Fast	www.slimfast.com
Nutri-System	www.nutrisystem.com	Atkins	www.atkins.com

SMOKING

"It may be hard, but the best thing you can do for a beautiful, glowing complexion is to stop smoking. Smoking both dehydrates and deprives your skin of oxygen, so you will see real benefits - skin will become smoother and more radiant." Sarah Monzani, make-up artist to Madonna.

Nicotine is highly addictive. It is both a stimulant and a sedative to the central nervous system. The ingestion of nicotine results in an almost immediate "kick" because it causes a discharge of epinephrine from the adrenal cortex. This stimulates the central nervous system, and other endocrine glands, which causes a sudden release of glucose. Stimulation is then followed by depression and fatigue, leading the abuser to seek more nicotine. Nicotine is absorbed readily from tobacco smoke in the lungs, and it does not matter whether the tobacco smoke is from cigarettes, cigars, or pipes.

Nicotine also is absorbed readily when tobacco is chewed. With regular use of tobacco, levels of nicotine accumulate in the body during the day and persist overnight. Thus, daily smokers or chewers are exposed to the effects of nicotine for 24 hours each day. Nicotine taken in by cigarette or cigar smoking takes only seconds to reach the brain but has a direct effect on the body for up to 30 minutes.

Women who smoke generally have earlier menopause. If women smoke cigarettes and also take oral contraceptives, they are more prone to cardiovascular and cerebrovascular diseases than are other smokers; this is especially true for women older than 30.

In addition to nicotine, cigarette smoke is primarily composed of a dozen gases (mainly carbon monoxide) and tar. The tar in a cigarette, which varies from about 15 mg for a regular cigarette to 7 mg in a low-tar cigarette, exposes the user to a high expectancy rate of lung cancer, emphysema, and bronchial disorders.

The carbon monoxide in the smoke increases the chance of cardiovascular diseases. The Environmental Protection Agency has concluded that secondhand smoke causes lung cancer in adults and greatly increases the risk of respiratory illnesses in children and sudden infant death.

MORE INFORMATION ON THE HAZARDS OF SMOKING CAN BE OBTAINED AT NIDA.COM

ALCOHOL

Parties, celebrations, fancy dinners, or watching the basketball play-offs are all good reasons to indulge in your favorite cocktail. After all, alcohol is synonymous with festivities. But, while having a drink or two is never a terrible thing, the amount usually consumed on these occasions is what can be damaging. Sure, there are a few health benefits of drinking red wine, but most people will find themselves nursing a lot of martinis, Manhattans and everything in between on party night! Binge drinking is never good for you, and we're not just talking in terms of hangovers. We're talking about effects binge drinking has on your skin, beauty sleep and waistline…

Drinking should always be practiced in moderation, but that's rarely the case when it comes to the big celebrations. If you haven't decided on whether to drink moderately or go all out at your next social gathering or celebration, there are a few things to think about.

The "Ugly" Side of Binge Drinking

Skin Damage
You've probably heard of how the sun can damage your skin with its intense UV rays, but did you ever learn about the damage that alcohol can do to your skin?

Not only does drinking too much dehydrate and strip your skin of its natural oils, leaving it dry, cracked and peeling, but it also causes flushing of the cheeks that can lead to permanent damage. More specifically, alcohol causes tiny facial blood vessels called capillaries to dilate and carry more blood to the surface. This pressure can cause the capillaries to burst, leaving permanent damage on your face.

Your face can also suffer a dull, gray pallor which can last for days after your drinking binge. And, as if your face hasn't had enough at this point, binge drinking can also cause bloodshot eyes. Beautiful faces need a healthy glow, not damaged skin and eyes.

Poor Quality of Sleep

After a long night of drinking, you probably want to get a good night's rest to rejuvenate yourself for the morning, right? Well it might not do you much good. Going to bed after you've been drinking may seem like a smart idea, but the chances of you getting a good night's rest are slim to none. Although the initial effect of alcohol is to make you drowsy, after a few hours, a neurotransmitter known as norepinephrine is released. This chemical release gives you a jolt of energy that will wake you out of your slumber and disrupt your happy sleep.

Remember that eight hours of interrupted sleep is not the same as the benefits of eight hours of uninterrupted sleep.

Weight Gain

One of the most obvious consequences of binge drinking is rapid weight gain. Alcohol and weight gain are like peanut butter and jelly – you just can't have one with out the other!

After-all, for every gram of alcohol you drink, there are seven calories hidden there. So for every ounce of alcohol you drink, you'll be consuming between 100-200 empty calories. And that doesn't include the soda, juice or other flavorings in your drink that pack on even more empty calories.

If you drink "just a little" (let's say about three drinks), that's at least 600 calories, or if you drink heavily (about 5-6 drinks), that's over 1,000 calories!

On the bright side, a four-ounce glass of red wine has only 100 calories, and is full of beneficial antioxidants. Our advice? Do like the Italians and learn to love red wine. You'll save hundreds of calories just by switching over.

Severity of Effect

Alcohol affects women more severely than it affects men, but many women are still tempted to try and keep up with their male counterparts. Women simply have smaller frames, more body fat and less ability to process alcohol out of their systems.

These three factors add up when women consume more drinks than they can handle. Not only does the alcohol stay in their system longer, but the effects of binge drinking are increased and the side effects are not pretty – throwing up, fever and lack of conscious control.

Know your limits, and if you're not sure what your limits are, stick to one type of alcohol (i.e. vodka only instead of mixing vodka, gin and tequila). Make sure you drink slowly, and for every drink you do have, drink a full glass of water to keep you hydrated. Also, never drink on an empty stomach, which will magnify the binge drinking effects of alcohol on your body.

Parties are good! They're a time to celebrate and hang out with people you love and enjoy. But the results of binge drinking on your skin, beauty sleep and waistline can be downright ugly after a fun night out.

Drink in moderation and be smart about which types of alcohol you allow yourself to have. The smarter you drink, the more beautiful you'll be - inside and out. Courtesy of *http://www.lifescript.com/*

Health and Other Dangers of Alcohol and Drug Use

Alcohol

Alcohol travels to every cell in the body, every tissue, and every organ. Over time, using too much alcohol can damage your heart, raise your blood pressure, and cause cancer, liver disease, and brain damage; it can give you ulcers, weaken your muscles, and can even lead to death.

Problems with alcohol usually develop over time. Some people become sick quickly; others drink for years without knowing that their body is being damaged. Many people suffer withdrawal symptoms when they try to stop: headaches, anxiety, or the shakes. At work, the withdrawal can make it hard for you to concentrate, and you may become short-tempered.

As the addiction gets worse, so do the withdrawal symptoms – you become more and more anxious and have stronger cravings. In the late stages of the disease, some people in withdrawal see and hear things that aren't really there. Continuing to use alcohol once an addiction has developed can result in liver and brain damage that my not be reversible. It can tear your family apart. Also, a pregnant woman who drinks alcohol may have a baby born with fetal alcohol effects (FAE) or fetal alcohol syndrome (FAS), which are characterized by mental and physical problems.

Amphetamines (Speed) and Cocaine

As the addiction to these drugs gets worse, you become obsessed with getting the drug. You cannot stay focused on tasks. You lose your appetite. Your behavior becomes extreme; you are always either really excited or really depressed.

It's not that hard to overdose on speed or cocaine because once you start using, you want more and more of the drug to keep the high going. So that's what you do: get high again and again, usually until the money runs out. When the drug starts to wear off, you feel depressed and tired, so you keep using the drug. Before you know it, you're hooked.

Marijuana
Regular use of marijuana causes a loss of interest and motivation. You become lazy and don't care about making life better. You begin to feel depressed. It can also damage your lungs. It affects the brain and may cause you to become fearful as well as forgetful. Focusing on tasks is difficult. You become more interested in getting high than in spending time with friends; you may lose "straight" friends. You lose the energy and drive to be involved in fun activities that don't include using pot.

PCP, LSD, Designer Drugs
These drugs bring to mind hallucinations - seeing and hearing things that are not really there. When this happens to you at work, you could do foolish or dangerous things. These drugs make you think you are stronger and more powerful than you really are. Accidents are more likely to happen due to poor judgment, and concentrating becomes really hard. Sometimes people who are high on these drugs become anxious and violent, and this can lead to fights and other negative behaviors on the job.

Prescription Drugs
Sometimes drugs prescribed by a doctor for anxiety or pain can lead to abuse or addiction. Many people become hooked on these drugs without realizing it. Using prescription drugs that change your mood can affect your job performance and could contribute to accidents or costly mistakes at work. It is important that you talk to your doctor to be sure you understand the effects of any drug you might take. If you want to know about the risks, ask your doctor to explain them to you or ask any pharmacist. It's better to be careful than to risk becoming addicted.

Heroin and Other Opiates

An opiate is a drug that makes you sleepy and lessens pain at the same time. There are legal uses for some opiates: A doctor might give an opiate to ease pain, stop diarrhea, or calm a cough. Heroin is an opiate; its effects on the body are similar to the other opiates given by doctors. However, heroin often contains a lot of impurities that add to its harmful effects.

Sometimes opiates are taken as pills; other times they are injected. Whether a person starts using opiates given by a doctor or uses them to get high, long-term use can result in these problems: abuse or addiction; tolerance (when it takes more of the drug to get the same effect); and dependence (when pain occurs if the drug use is stopped). Being hooked on any type of opiate can disrupt your life, family, and job.

Top model, Kate Moss, demonstrates the early devastating effects of drug use on her God given beauty.

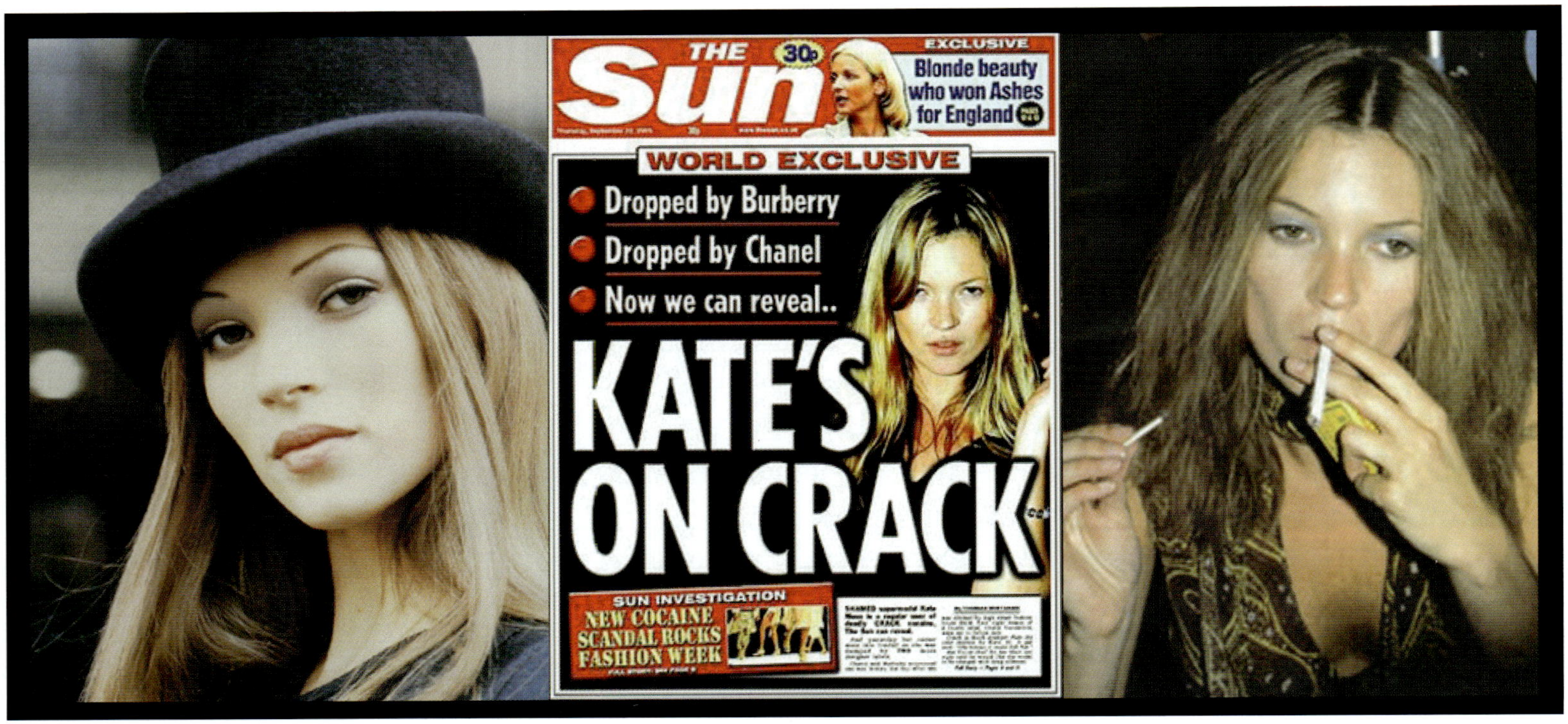
THE Sun
30p
EXCLUSIVE
Blonde beauty who won Ashes for England
WORLD EXCLUSIVE
Dropped by Burberry
Dropped by Chanel
Now we can reveal..
KATE'S ON CRACK
SUN INVESTIGATION
NEW COCAINE SCANDAL ROCKS FASHION WEEK

MENTAL HEALTH

There is more to beauty than meets the stranger's eye, according to results from three studies examining the influence of non-physical traits on people's perception of physical attractiveness.

The results, which show that people perceive physical appeal differently when they look at those they know versus strangers, are published in the recently released March issue of Evolution and Human Behavior.

In many studies evaluating physical attractiveness, people are often shown an array of strangers' photos, computer-generated images or line drawings and asked to identify which ones, based on differences in physical features, are most attractive. Results from these studies suggest that physically attractive traits include high degrees of bilateral facial symmetries, such as eyes that are identical in shape and size, and waist-to-hip ratios of 0.7 for women and 0.9 for men.

"You can find study after study that focuses on which waist-to-hip ratios or particular facial features people find physically attractive, and these studies have captured popular attention," says Kevin Kniffin, an honorary fellow in the anthropology department at the University of Wisconsin-Madison and an adjunct assistant professor at Binghamton University.

Kniffin co-authored the Evolution and Human Behavior paper with David Sloan Wilson, an evolutionary biologist at Binghamton University.

While these past studies do show which features people find physically appealing after just a glance, they overlook the non-physical traits that may influence a person's perception of another's beauty over time. In other words, people may see physical attractiveness differently when they know that person's other qualities, usually invisible to strangers, says Kniffin.

Maintaining Results

According to evolutionary theory, many animals, including humans, are attracted to those who are likely to increase their own fitness -- the likelihood of surviving and reproducing.

In the case of humans, "the fitness value of potential social partners depends at least as much on non-physical traits -- whether they are cooperative, dependable, brave, hardworking, intelligent and so on -- as physical factors, such as smooth skin and symmetrical features," says Wilson. "It follows that non-physical factors should be included in the subconscious assessment of beauty."

To systematically consider the influence of non-physical traits on how people who are familiar with each other perceive physical appeal, Kniffin and Wilson conducted three studies of beauty involving people who know each other and people who don't. For all studies, the participants were asked to rate physical attractiveness and non-physical traits such as liking, respect and talent. Strangers rated only physical attractiveness. In the first study, the participants rated people photographed in high school yearbooks, including one that belonged to each participant. In the second, members of a college sports team, as well as strangers, rated each team member. Finally, students in a summer archaeological excavation course rated each other on the first day of class and six weeks later at the end of the course.

"In each case, non-physical traits known only to familiars, such as how much the person was liked, respected and contributed to shared goals, had a large effect on the perception of physical attractiveness that was invisible to the strangers," says Wilson.

Maintaining Results

Each study provided an illustrative example of this finding. For instance, one middle-aged subject who had not seen the familiar person photographed in the yearbook for decades responded with absolute disgust when she recalled the person's character and described that person as ugly. In the sports team study, team members considered the slacker to be ugly and one of the leaders to be physically attractive, while strangers, blind to the members' relative contributions, rated them as equally attractive on the basis of photographs.

And, after six weeks of working together on an archaeological dig, students' perception of physical attractiveness changed based on interactions during the course.

Courtesy of *http://mentalhealth.about.com/*

Sunlight has a profound effect on the skin causing premature skin aging, skin cancer, and a host of skin changes. Exposure to ultraviolet light, UVA or UVB, from sunlight accounts for 90% of the symptoms of premature skin aging. Many skin changes that were commonly believed to be due to aging, such as easy bruising, are actually a result of prolonged exposure to UV radiation.

What is UV Radiation?

The sun gives off ultraviolet radiation that we divide into categories based on the wavelength.

- UVB - 290 to 320 nm
- UVA - 320 to 400 nm

UVB Radiation

UVB affects the outer layer of skin, the epidermis, and is the primary agent responsible for sunburns. It is the most intense between the hours of 10:00 am and 2:00 pm when the sunlight is brightest. It is also more intense in the summer months accounting for 70% of a person's yearly UVB dose. UVB does not penetrate glass.

UVA Radiation

UVA was once thought to have a minor effect on skin damage, but now studies are showing that UVA is a major contributor to skin damage. UVA penetrates deeper into the skin and works more efficiently. The intensity of UVA radiation is more constant than UVB without the variations during the day and throughout the year. UVA is also not filtered by glass.

Damaging Effects of UVA and UVB

Both UVA and UVB radiation can cause skin damage including wrinkles, lowered immunity against infection, aging skin disorders, and cancer. However, we still do not fully understand the process. Some of the possible mechanisms for UV skin damage are collagen breakdown, the formation of free radicals, interfering with DNA repair, and inhibiting the immune system.

Collagen Breakdown

In the dermis, UV radiation causes collagen to break down at a higher rate than with just chronologic aging. Sunlight damages collagen fibers and causes the accumulation of abnormal elastin. When this sun-induced elastin accumulates, enzymes called metalloproteinases are produced in large quantities. Normally, metalloproteinases remodel sun-injured skin by manufacturing and reforming collagen. However, this process does not always work well and some of the metalloproteinases actually break down collagen. This results in the formation of disorganized collagen fibers known as solar scars. When the skin repeats this imperfect rebuilding process over and over wrinkles develop.

Free Radicals

UV radiation is one of the major creators of free radicals. Free radicals are unstable oxygen molecules that have only one electron instead of two. Because electrons are found in pairs, the molecule must scavenge other molecules for another electron. When the second molecule looses its electron to the first molecule, it must then find another electron repeating the process. This process can damage cell function and alter genetic material. Free radical damage causes wrinkles by activating the metalloproteinases that break down collagen. They cause cancer by changing the genetic material, RNA and DNA, of the cell.

DNA Repair
UV radiation can affect enzymes that help repair damaged DNA. Studies are being conducted looking into the role a specific enzyme called T4 endonuclease 5 (T4N5) has in repairing DNA.

Immune System Effects
The body has a defense system to attack developing cancer cells. These immune system factors include white blood cells called T lymphocytes and specialized skin cells in the dermis called Langerhans cells. When the skin is exposed to sunlight, certain chemicals are released that suppress these immune factors.

Cell Death
The last line of defense of the immune system is a process called apoptosis. Apoptosis is a process of cell-suicide that kills severely damaged cells so they cannot become cancerous. This cell-suicide is seen when you peel after a sunburn. There are certain factors, including UV exposure, that prevent this cell death allowing cells to continue to divide and possibly become cancerous.

Cosmetic Surgery & Organized Medicine

Accreditation Agencies, Scientific Organizations and Certifying Boards for Cosmetic Surgery in Organized Medicine

By: Candace Chatham

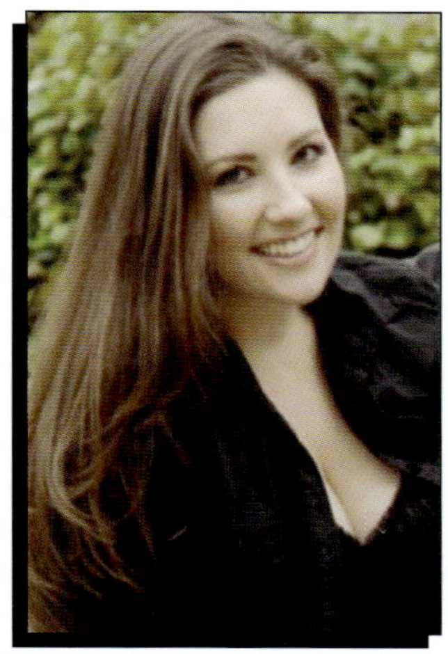

Accreditation Agencies For Out-Patient Surgical Facilities

The Accreditation Association for Ambulatory Health Care
The Accreditation Association for Ambulatory Health Care, also known as AAAHC or the Accreditation Association, is a private, non-profit organization formed in 1979. It is the preeminent leader in developing standards to advance and promote patient safety, quality and value for ambulatory health care through peer-based accreditation processes, education and research. Accreditation is ultimately awarded to organizations that are found to be in compliance with the Accreditation Association standards.
http://www.aaahc.org

American Association for Accreditation of Ambulatory Surgery Facilities
It is the mission of the American Association for Accreditation of Ambulatory Surgery Facilities, Inc. (AAAASF) to develop and implement standards of excellence to ensure the highest quality of patient care through an accreditation program that serves both the medical community and the public interest by establishing a means for measuring medical competence and providing an external source for evaluating patient safety in the ambulatory surgery setting.
http://www.aaaasf.org

Our Mission: To continuously improve the safety and quality of care provided to the public through the provision of health care accreditation and related services that support performance improvement in health care organizations.

The Joint Commission," formerly 'Joint Commission on Accreditation of Healthcare Organizations'.

The mission of The Joint Commission is to continuously improve the safety and quality of care provided to the public through the provision of health care accreditation and related services that support performance improvement in health care organizations."

This mission statement continues to reflect the fundamental purposes set forth by the American College of Surgeons when it created its Hospital Standardization Program in 1917. That program would transition into the Joint Commission on Accreditation of Hospitals in 1951 when it acquired a group of additional major professional organization sponsors.
http://www.jointcommission.org/

Scientific Organizations

American Academy of Cosmetic Dentistry (AACD)
The American Academy of Cosmetic Dentistry is dedicated to advancing excellence in the art and science of cosmetic dentistry and encouraging the highest standards of ethical conduct and responsible patient care. The AACD fulfills its mission by: offering superior educational opportunities; promoting and supporting a respected Accreditation credential; serving as a user-friendly and inviting forum for the creative exchange of knowledge and ideas; and providing accurate and useful information to the public and the profession.
www.aacd.com

American Academy of Cosmetic Surgery (AACS)
The American Board of Cosmetic Surgery is the only certifying board exam devoted to examining a surgeon's skill in cosmetic surgery of the face and body. It is an independent sub-specialty board that examines and certifies physicians in general, facial and dermatological cosmetic surgery.
www.cosmeticsurgery.org

American Academy of Facial Plastic and Reconstructive Surgery (AAFPRS)
The AAFPRS was founded in 1964 as an autonomous professional society representing the specialty of facial plastic surgery. The mission of the AAFPRS is:

- To promote the highest quality facial plastic surgery through education, dissemination of professional information, and the establishment of professional standards.
- To achieve understanding and recognition of the specialty of facial plastic surgery by the medical profession, hospitals, and other medical care entities, legislative and regulatory bodies, and the public at large.
- To define facial plastic surgery as a specialty that requires intensive training and competence embodies high ethical standards, artistic ideals, commitment to humanitarian service, and a desire to enhance the quality of human life.
- To serve as the public's information source on facial plastic surgery.

- To assist members in the practice of facial plastic and reconstructive, guiding them in the delivery of high quality, cost-effective medicine and surgery.
  www.aafprs.org

American Society of Aesthetic Plastic Surgery (ASAPS)
The mission of the American Society of Plastic Surgeons is to support its members in their efforts to provide the highest quality patient care and maintain professional and ethical standards through education, research, and advocacy of socioeconomic and other professional activities.
www.plasticsurgery.org

American Society of Cosmetic Breast Surgery (ASCBS)
What we are about is that we bring together a group of experienced surgeons who perform and have performed tens of thousands of cosmetic breast operations over many years. We learn from each other and we invite all surgeons who do breast surgery to come and join us in our educational efforts to improve the care and cosmetic results of surgery on women all over the world.
http://www.ascbs.org

American Society of Dermatologic Surgery (ASDS)
The American Society for Dermatologic Surgery is an organization whose primary purpose is to promote optimal quality care for patients as well as support and develop investigative knowledge in the field of dermatologic surgery. The Society carries out this mission in order to further the interests and needs of the specialty, with the underlying purpose of contributing to the delivery of quality care in the ambulatory setting.
www.asds-net.org

American Society of Ophthalmic Plastic and Reconstructive Surgery (ASOPRS)
The mission of the ASOPRS Foundation is to foster ASOPRS' educational, research and humanitarian projects, both nationally and internationally.
www.asoprs.org

American Society of Plastic Surgeons (ASPS)
The mission of ASPS is to advance quality care to plastic surgery patients by encouraging high standards of training, ethics, physician practice and research in plastic surgery. The society advocates for patient safety, such as requiring its members to operate in accredited surgical facilities that have passed rigorous external review of equipment and staffing. The society works in concert with the **Plastic Surgery Educational Foundation (PSEF)**, founded in 1948, which supports research and educational programs for plastic surgeons.
www.plasticsurgery.org

Certifying Boards

American Board of Cosmetic Surgery (ABCS)
The mission of the American Board of Cosmetic Surgery (ABCS) is to serve the public by promoting the safe and ethical practice of the specialty of cosmetic surgery. Diplomates of the ABCS shall demonstrate the highest standards of training, knowledge, and expertise, as determined by a process of peer review and standardized examination and certification.
www.americanboardcosmeticsurgery.org

American Board of Dermatology (ABD)
The American Board of Dermatology is a voluntary, non-profit, private, autonomous organization formed for the primary purpose of protecting the public interest by establishing and maintaining high standards of training, education and qualifications of physicians rendering care in dermatology. The objective of all of its activities is to provide assurance that a diplomate of the Board possesses the knowledge and skills essential for the provision of superior, specialized care to patients with cutaneous diseases.
www.abderm.org

American Board of Facial Plastic and Reconstructive Surgery (ABFPRS)
The specific objectives of the Board are:

- To establish standards of qualification for facial plastic and reconstructive surgeons.
- To determine which candidates fulfill these standards of qualification.
- To conduct examinations of such candidates and issue certificates upon satisfactory completion of requirements.
- To improve and broaden the opportunities for graduate education and training of facial plastic and reconstructive surgeons.

www.abfprs.org

American Board of Ophthalmology (ABO)
The mission of the American Board of Ophthalmology is to serve the public by improving the quality of ophthalmic practice through a certification and maintenance of certification process that fosters excellence and encourages continual learning.
www.aborp.org

American Board of Oral Maxillofacial Surgery (ABOMS)
The Mission of the American Board of Oral and Maxillofacial Surgery is to help set the standards for the confluence of education, training, and experience for the specialty of Oral and Maxillofacial Surgery to assure the public of an acceptable level of attainment by those who are Board Certified. To this end, the Board's mission includes examination and certification of candidates, and recertification of Diplomates.
www.aboms.org

American Board of Otolaryngology (ABOto)
The mission of the American Board of Otolaryngology (ABOto) is to assure that, at the time of certification and recertification, diplomates certified by the ABOto have met the ABOto's professional standards of training and knowledge in otolaryngology - head and neck surgery.
www.aboto.org

American Board of Hair Restoration Surgery (ABHRS)
The Mission of the ABHRS is to act for the benefit of the public to establish specialty standards and to examine surgeons' skill, knowledge and aesthetic judgment in the field of hair restoration surgery.
http://www.abhrs.com

American Board of Plastic Surgery Inc.
The mission of The American Board of Plastic Surgery, Inc.® is to promote safe, ethical, efficacious plastic surgery to the public by maintaining high standards for the education, examination, certification and recertification of plastic surgeons as specialists and subspecialists.
www.abplsurg.org